SOCIAL AND COMMUNICATION DEVELOPMENT IN AUTISM SPECTRUM DISORDERS

Social and Communication Development in Autism Spectrum Disorders

Early Identification, Diagnosis, and Intervention

Edited by

TONY CHARMAN
WENDY STONE

THE GUILFORD PRESS
New York London

Library of Congress Cataloging-in-Publication Data

Social and communication development in autism spectrum disorders : early identification,
diagnosis, and intervention / edited by Tony Charman, Wendy Stone.
      p. cm.
   Includes bibliographical references and index.
   ISBN 10: 1-59385-284-3   ISBN-13: 978-1-59385-284-9 (hard cover : alk. paper)
   1. Autistic children.   2. Autistic children—Language.   3. Developmentally disabled
children—Language.   4. Language disorders in children—Treatment.   5. Social skills
in children.   6. Communicative disorders in children.   I. Charman, Tony.
II. Stone, Wendy.

RJ506.A9.S628   2006
618.92′85882—dc22
                                                        2005034925

*To Jane. And for all the children and families
who have taught me so much about autism
over the years—long may I carry on learning.*
                                        —T. C.

*To my husband, Mark, who has been my rock
and my buoy through this journey. And with deep
admiration for and gratitude to the many
children and families who have been
my inspiration and my guides.*
                                        —W. S.

About the Editors

Tony Charman, PhD, is Reader in Neurodevelopmental Disorders in the Behavioural and Brain Sciences Unit at the Institute of Child Health, University College London. He is also an honorary clinical psychologist at Great Ormond Street Hospital for Children National Health Service Trust, where he works in a diagnostic service for children with complex neuro-developmental conditions. Dr. Charman's main research interest is the investigation of early social-cognitive development in children with autism and the clinical application of this work via screening, diagnostic, outcome, early intervention, and epidemiological studies. His work has been funded by the Medical Research Council, the Wellcome Trust, and the Department of Health, as well as by a number of U.K. and U.S. charities. He will be Editor-in-Chief of the *Journal of Child Psychology and Psychiatry* from 2007 to 2010, is currently Associate Editor of the *Journal of Autism and Developmental Disorders,* and is on the Editorial Boards of *Autism: The International Journal of Research and Practice,* the *British Journal of Developmental Psychology,* and the *Journal of Intellectual Disability Research.* Dr. Charman is a scientific member of the Advisory Group to the All Party Parliamentary Group on Autism as well as a member of the "College of Experts" for the Medical Research Council (Mental Health and Neuroscience Board), and in 2003 served on the National Institutes of Health/National Institute of Mental Health Interagency Autism Coordinating Committee Science Panel.

Wendy Stone, PhD, is Professor of Pediatrics and Psychology and Human Development at Vanderbilt University, director of the Treatment and Research Institute for Autism Spectrum Disorders (TRIAD) at the Vanderbilt

Kennedy Center, and director of the Marino Autism Research Institute–Vanderbilt. Dr. Stone's primary research interests are in early identification and early intervention for children with autism spectrum disorders. Much of her work has focused on identifying and characterizing the early-emerging behavioral features of autism, and she has received federal funding for this research since 1993. She has studied several aspects of early social-communicative development, including play, motor imitation, and prelinguistic communication, examining their contributions to later behavioral and diagnostic outcomes. Her research with young children led to the development of the Screening Tool for Autism in Two-Year-Olds (STAT), which is now being adapted for use at younger ages. Current research projects include the identification of social-communicative markers in children under 24 months, the prediction of responsiveness to early intervention, and the early social development of later-born siblings of children with autism. Dr. Stone serves on the editorial boards of the *Journal of Autism and Developmental Disorders* and *Infants and Young Children,* as well as on several National Institutes of Health work groups and the Baby Siblings Research Consortium.

Contributors

Nadra Aouka, PhD, Centre National de Recherche Scientifique (CNRS), Université Pierre et Marie Curie, Paris, France

Simon Baron-Cohen, PhD, Departments of Experimental Psychology and Psychiatry, Cambridge University, Cambridge, United Kingdom

Tony Charman, PhD, Behavioural and Brain Sciences Unit, Institute of Child Health, University College London, London, United Kingdom

Patricia Howlin, PhD, Department of Psychology, St. George's, University of London, London, United Kingdom

Jennifer J. Hurley, PhD, Department of Psychology and Human Development, Vanderbilt University, Nashville, Tennessee

Catherine Lord, PhD, Autism and Communication Disorders Center, University of Michigan, Ann Arbor, Michigan

Andrea S. McDuffie, PhD, Department of Psychology and Human Development, Vanderbilt University, Nashville, Tennessee

Peter Mundy, PhD, Department of Psychology and the Marino Autism Research Institute, University of Miami, Coral Gables, Florida

Jacqueline Nadel, PhD, Centre National de Recherche Scientifique (CNRS), Université Pierre et Marie Curie, Paris, France

Jennifer Richler, MA, Autism and Communication Disorders Center, University of Michigan, Ann Arbor, Michigan

Sally J. Rogers, PhD, The M.I.N.D. Institute, Department of Psychiatry and Behavioral Sciences, University of California, Davis, Medical Center, Sacramento, California

Adriana L. Schuler, PhD, Department of Special Education, San Francisco State University, San Francisco, California

Wendy Stone, PhD, Vanderbilt Kennedy Center and Department of Pediatrics, Vanderbilt University, Nashville, Tennessee

Danielle Thorp, PhD, Louis de la Parte Florida Mental Health Institute, University of South Florida, Tampa, Florida

Tedra A. Walden, PhD, Department of Psychology and Human Development, Vanderbilt University, Nashville, Tennessee

Amy M. Wetherby, PhD, Department of Communication Disorders, Florida State University, Tallahassee, Florida

Pamela J. Wolfberg, PhD, Department of Special Education, San Francisco State University, San Francisco, California

Paul J. Yoder, PhD, Department of Special Education, Vanderbilt University, Nashville, Tennessee

Lonnie Zwaigenbaum, MD, Department of Pediatrics, McMaster University, Hamilton, Ontario, Canada

Preface

More than 25 years of research have refined our recognition and understanding of the impairments in early social-communicative behavior that are characteristic of toddlers and preschool children with autism spectrum disorders (ASD) (Mundy, Sigman, Ungerer, & Sherman, 1986; Ricks & Wing, 1975; Wetherby & Prutting, 1984). Delay and atypical development in the acquisition of joint attention, social orienting, imitation, and play are among the most robust and earliest recognized symptoms of ASD (Charman, 2000; Rogers, 2001; Stone, 1997; Stone, Hoffman, Lewis, & Ousley, 1994). The advances of the past two and a half decades have been supported by—and at times led—new research into the course and underlying processes of these behaviors in typically developing infants. Indeed, much of the impetus and inspiration for research into social-communication development in autism was not only the recognition that social impairments were core to the disorder (Rutter, 1970; Wing & Gould, 1979) but also the lessons being learned from the psycholinguistic revolution in developmental psychology in the 1970s (Bates, Benigni, Bretherton, Camaioni & Volterra, 1979; Bruner, 1975).

Innovative empirical methodologies and theoretical expositions of social and communication development have continued to evolve, informing our understanding of both typical and atypical development in ASD (e.g., Klin, Jones, Schultz, & Volkmar, 2003; Kuhl, Coffey-Corina, Padden, & Dawson, 2005; Tomasello, Carpenter, Call, Behne, & Moll, 2005). Of the many critical contributions to the study of ASD, two stand out. First is the recognition that nonverbal communication interchanges are the building blocks through which typical infants develop language understanding (and subsequently language use). Second is the delineation of the recursive nature of early social and language development. Not only does a child's level of social engagement affect his or her language-learning environment, but limitations in the ability to avail oneself of language opportunities also contribute to further impairment in social understanding (see Wetherby, 1986; Mundy & Thorp, Chapter 11, this volume; and Walden & Hurley, Chapter 10, this volume, for theoretical expositions of such accounts).

Improved understanding of early social-communicative impairments in children with ASD has informed a range of developments in the clinical field. These innovations include the development of instruments that measure early social-communicative behavior as an aid to diagnosis (see Lord & Richler, Chapter 2, this volume and Wetherby, Chapter 1, this volume), screening instruments to prospectively identify children with ASD (Charman & Baron-Cohen, Chapter 3, this volume; Zwaigenbaum & Stone, Chapter 4, this volume), and intervention approaches that specifically target these behaviors and thus the "core deficits" that characterize toddlers and preschool children with ASD (Howlin, Chapter 9, this volume; Koegel, 2000; Lord, 2000; Nadel & Aouka, Chapter 8, this volume; Rogers, 2000, Chapter 6, this volume; Wolfberg & Schuler, Chapter 7, this volume; and Yoder & McDuffie, Chapter 5, this volume). However, it is only more recently that social-communication intervention approaches have been evaluated systematically with toddler and preschool children with ASD, and initial studies show some promise in improving verbal and nonverbal communicative abilities (Aldred, Green, & Adams, 2004; Drew et al., 2002; Whalen & Schreibman, 2003).

This volume brings together leading experts from the autism field and from the study of typical development to provide a state-of-the-art summary of these advances and to set out clinical and research agendas for the coming decade. The focus of the book is on the application of empirical knowledge to assessment and treatment settings. We intend the volume to be a resource for clinicians and clinical researchers involved in assessment and diagnosis, intervention, and preventative approaches, so each chapter draws out the lessons for clinical practice on the basis of the extant empirical literature. We are fortunate that all the contributors are also well versed in the theoretical literature that underpins the application of social-communication-based approaches to understanding and intervening with children with ASD. Thus the volume also serves as an up-to-date forum for researchers within the broader field of developmental psychopathology interested in the social and communication impairments seen in young children with ASD.

REFERENCES

Aldred, C., Green, J., & Adams, C. (2004). A new social communication intervention for children with autism: Pilot randomized controlled treatment study suggesting effectiveness. *Journal of Child Psychology and Psychiatry, 45*, 1420–1430.

Bates, E., Benigni, L., Bretherton, I., Camaioni, L., & Volterra, V. (1979). *The emergence of symbols: Cognition and communication in infancy.* New York: Academic Press.

Bruner, J. S. (1975). From communication to language. *Cognition, 3*, 255–287.

Charman, T. (2000). Theory of mind and the early diagnosis of autism. In S. Baron-Cohen, H. Tager-Flusberg, & D. Cohen (Eds.), *Understanding other minds: Perspectives from autism and developmental cognitive neuroscience* (2nd ed., pp. 422–441). Oxford, UK: Oxford University Press.

Drew, A., Baird, G., Baron-Cohen, S., Cox, A., Slonims, V., Wheelwright, S., et al. (2002). A pilot randomized control trial of a parent training intervention for pre-school children with autism: Preliminary findings and methodological challenges. *European Child and Adolescent Psychiatry, 11*, 266–272.

Klin, A., Jones, W., Schultz, R., & Volkmar, F. (2003). The enactive mind, or from actions to cognition: Lessons from autism. *Transactions of the Royal Society of London: Series B. Biological Sciences, 358*, 345–360.

Koegel, L. K. (2000). Interventions to facilitate communication in autism. *Journal of Autism and Developmental Disorders, 30*, 383–391.

Kuhl, P. K., Coffey-Corina, S., Padden, D., & Dawson, G. (2005). Links between social and linguistic processing of speech in preschool children with autism: Behavioral and electrophysiological measures. *Developmental Science, 8*, F1–F12.

Lord, C. (2000). Commentary: Achievements and future directions for intervention research in communication and autism spectrum disorders. *Journal of Autism and Developmental Disorders, 30*, 393–398.

Mundy, P., Sigman, M., Ungerer, J., & Sherman, T. (1986). Defining the social deficits of autism: The contribution of non-verbal communication measures. *Journal of Child Psychology and Psychiatry, 27*, 657–669.

Ricks, D. N., & Wing, L. (1975). Language, communication, and symbols in normal and autistic children. *Journal of Autism and Childhood Schizophrenia, 5*, 191–222.

Rogers, S. J. (2000). Interventions that facilitate socialization in children with autism. *Journal of Autism and Developmental Disorders, 30*, 399–409.

Rogers, S. J. (2001). Diagnosis of autism before the age of 3. *International Review of Mental Retardation, 23*, 1–31.

Rutter, M. (1970). Autistic children: Infancy to adulthood. *Seminars in Psychiatry, 2*, 435–450.

Stone, W. L. (1997). Autism in infancy and early childhood. In D. J. Cohen & F. R. Volkmar (Eds.), *Handbook of autism and pervasive developmental disorders* (2nd ed., pp. 266–282). New York: Wiley.

Stone, W. L., Hoffman, E. L., Lewis, S. E., & Ousley, O. Y. (1994). Early recognition of autism: Parental reports vs. clinical observation. *Archives of Pediatrics and Adolescent Medicine, 148*, 174–179.

Tomasello, M., Carpenter, M., Call, J., Behne, T., & Moll, H. (2005). Understanding and sharing intentions: the origins of cultural cognition. *Behavioral and Brain Sciences, 28*, 675–735.

Wetherby, A. M. (1986). Ontogeny of communicative functions in autism. *Journal of Autism and Developmental Disorders, 16*, 295–316.

Wetherby, A. M., & Prutting, C. (1984). Profiles of communicative and cognitive–social abilities in autistic children. *Journal of Speech and Hearing Research, 27*, 364–377.

Whalen, C., & Schreibman, L. (2003). Joint attention training for children with autism using behavior modification procedures. *Journal of Child Psychology and Psychiatry, 44*, 456–468.

Wing, L., & Gould, J. (1979). Severe impairments of social interaction and associated abnormalities in children: Epidemiology and classification. *Journal of Autism and Childhood Schizophrenia, 9*, 11–29.

Acknowledgments

We would like to extend our gratitude to our "partners" at The Guilford Press, in particular our editor, Rochelle Serwator, for her vision and enthusiasm for this volume and her support throughout its development. Thanks also to Katherine Lieber and Anna Nelson for making the transition from manuscript to final publication so smooth.

We are deeply indebted to the contributors who not only took time from their busy schedules to contribute to this volume but also made the editing job much easier than we know it should have been. We also thank our colleagues and mentors who taught us so much about children with autism and inspired us to do the work we now do—this book would not have been possible without them.

And finally, our deepest appreciation goes to the children and families whose journey into the world of socialization and communication, fast and slow, serves as an inspiration and motivation for us to continue this work into the future.

Contents

SOCIAL AND COMMUNICATION DEVELOPMENT IN AUTISM SPECTRUM DISORDERS

PART I

Assessment and Diagnosis

This section highlights the critical role of understanding typical and atypical development of early social-communicative behaviors in the assessment and diagnosis of young children with autism spectrum disorder (ASD). Instruments to assess skills such as imitation, play, social responsiveness, and other prelinguistic nonverbal behaviors are reviewed, and issues pertinent to the diagnosis of ASD in young preschool children, including stability of diagnosis and ability to indicate prognosis at an early age, are considered.

Wetherby (Chapter 1) contrasts the development of joint attention and symbol use in typical children with the distinctive profile of social-communicative behaviors observed in children with ASD. She highlights several important issues in the measurement of social-communicative behaviors, such as the assessment context and the type of scale employed. Examples of approaches and instruments that can be used to assess and describe social-communicative behaviors in young children (e.g., Early Social Communication Scales, Communication and Symbolic Behavior Scales) are presented, and findings from recent prospective studies of the development of early social-communication skills are described. The importance of measuring change in early social-communicative behaviors in response to treatment is addressed, and examples of recent early intervention studies are summarized.

Lord and Richler (Chapter 2) address issues related to the early diagnosis of young children with ASD, including the application of the standard classification systems to toddlers and preschoolers. Diagnostic instruments that measure social-communication behaviors, as well as repetitive behaviors, are described, with attention to issues of interobserver reliability and the stability of early diagnoses. The authors consider the impact of individual differences in language skills on the diagnostic process and interpretation of results. A framework for understanding the developmental trajectories seen in young children with ASD, including the phenomenon of regression, is employed to inform the diagnostic process and potential interventions, as well as to help us understand emerging evidence at a neurodevelopmental level. Limitations of current diagnostic methods for young children and the need to develop measures to quantify symptom severity are discussed.

1

Understanding and Measuring Social Communication in Children with Autism Spectrum Disorders

AMY M. WETHERBY

Major advances have been made over the past two decades in understanding the social-communication difficulties of children with autism spectrum disorders (ASD), resulting in a greater emphasis on early social-communication features in the diagnostic criteria (American Psychiatric Association, 1994). Research has identified social-communication deficits in children with ASD that can be organized into two major areas: (1) the capacity for joint attention, which reflects difficulty coordinating attention between people and objects; and (2) the capacity for symbol use, which reflects difficulty learning conventional or shared meanings for symbols and is evident in acquiring gestures, words, imitation, and play. This chapter provides an overview of the emergence of social-communication skills in typical development and explores research that characterizes the capacity for joint attention and symbol use in children with ASD. Issues in measurement and approaches to assessment of social communication in children with ASD are described. Implications for early identification of ASD and meaningful outcome measures are underscored.

OVERVIEW OF TYPICAL DEVELOPMENT
OF SOCIAL COMMUNICATION

By the end of the first year, most children are not yet producing true words, but they are able to coordinate attention between people and objects, engage in social exchanges, and communicate intentionally or deliberately with caregivers using conventional gestures and sounds that have shared meanings (Bates, O'Connell, & Shore, 1987). The skills that contribute to social-communication competence in typical development are delineated in this section for the capacities of joint attention and symbol use.

The Emergence of Joint Attention

Children acquire three developmental achievements that contribute to the capacity for joint attention and enable them to be active social partners in learning to talk: (1) sharing attention, (2) sharing affect, and (3) sharing intentions (Stern, 1985). Longitudinal and cross-sectional research on typically developing children has documented a developmental sequence of emergence of these skills over the first year of life (Carpenter, Nagell, & Tomasello, 1998; Wetherby & Prizant, 1993, 2002).

The ability to *share attention* typically begins at birth and continues to develop over the first year of life. It begins in the first few months, with an infant and caregiver sharing attention in dyadic interaction and with the caregiver monitoring what the child is looking at. By 9 months of age, the child actively observes others and has learned to shift gaze between people and objects in order to check and see if the caregiver is attending to the child's focus of interest (Bakeman & Adamson, 1984). This process is also referred to as *coordinated joint engagement* or *social referencing*. Gaze shifts play an important role in regulating social interactions in that they signal attention and social interest to the partner. By the end of the first year of life, the child follows the caregiver's attentional focus when looking at and/or pointing to something of interest (Butterworth, 1995), a process referred to as *gaze/point following* or *responding to joint attention*; this is the basis for the ability to figure out another's visual perspective and intentions.

The ability to *share affect* in expressing emotional states to others is evident when a child displays pleasure and directs gaze to the caregiver to share this positive experience or when the child directs signals of discomfort or distress to a caregiver in order to seek comfort. By sharing affect with caregivers, children also learn to interpret emotional states of others as they experience caregivers responding to their emotional expressions.

Stern (1985) refers to this process of caregivers mirroring their child's emotional tone and pace as *affect attunement*.

The ability to *share intentions* refers to being able to signal or direct behaviors to others in order to achieve specific goals. At about 9–10 months of age, a child begins to use sounds, gestures, and other behaviors to communicate intentionally—that is, the child deliberately uses a particular signal to seek a goal (Bates, 1979). In this early period of development, sharing intentions involves coordinating shared attention and/or affect with the use of gestures and sounds to express intentions to another person. Children communicate to express three major intentions by the end of the first year, and these are expressed later through language as words emerge (Bruner, 1981; Wetherby & Prizant, 1993):

1. *Behavioral regulation*, which uses signals to regulate another person's behavior for purposes of requesting objects or actions or protesting objects or another person's behavior (e.g., pointing to request food; pushing object away to protest it).
2. *Social interaction*, which uses signals to draw another's attention to oneself for affiliative purposes, such as greeting, calling, requesting social routines, and requesting comfort (e.g., waving "bye-bye"; reaching to be comforted).
3. *Joint attention*, which uses signals to direct another's attention to interesting objects and events for the purpose of sharing them with others (e.g., showing interesting objects to others, pointing at an object to bring it to someone's attention).

It is the combination of achievements in sharing attention, affect, and intentions that culminates in the broader developing capacity to share experiences (Stern, 1985). The child begins to understand that other people have their own distinct and unique minds and that thoughts and feelings, the "subject matter" of a person's mind, can be shared with others through communication. This understanding has been referred to as *intersubjectivity*, or the sharing of subjective experience, which underlies a child's deliberate and spontaneous attempts to share experiences with caregivers (Stern, 1985; Trevarthen & Hubley, 1978). Intersubjectivity requires a framework of shared meanings for gestures, facial expressions, intonation, and, ultimately, language. The capacity to share experiences underlies reciprocal social interaction in that the child's behavior becomes more finely contingent on the behavior and goals of others. The caregiver and child coconstruct social "dialogues" by taking turns initiating and responding to communicative bids, grounded in a shared focus of attention in reciprocal exchanges.

The Emergence of Symbol Use

Before using words, children acquire a repertoire of conventional sounds and gestures to express intentions, which reflects their growing knowledge of *shared meanings* (Bates, 1979). Conventional communication develops from the ritualization of functional actions, such as reaching, grasping, and pulling the head away, and, later, from the imitation of new behaviors that have either generally agreed-on meanings, such as waving, showing, and pointing, or private meanings in ritualized exchanges with caregivers (Bates, 1979). Early intentional gestures and sounds are presymbolic communication and are the foundation for the emergence of first words and the transition to symbolic communication. Between 1 and 2 years of age, children develop the capacity to symbolize (i.e., make one thing stand for or represent something else), as is evident in the ability to imitate new behaviors (see Nadel & Aouka, Chapter 8, this volume), to pretend with objects in play (see Wolfberg & Schuler, Chapter 7, this volume), and to use and understand words to refer to objects and events.

The capacity to acquire conventional behaviors is triggered by children's use of active learning strategies that involve exploring objects, observing others, listening to others, and learning from others (McLean & Snyder-McLean, 1999). Over the first year of life, children actively manipulate and explore properties of objects and learn to take turns in social interaction. Usually by 6–9 months of age, the child is able to imitate familiar actions or sounds immediately after the caregiver (i.e., *immediate imitation*). By 12–14 months, the child is able to spontaneously imitate a growing repertoire of familiar actions or sounds at a later time than first observed (i.e., *deferred or delayed imitation*; Barnat, Klein, & Meltzoff, 1996). Thus, shortly after their first birthdays, children have a set of active learning strategies that enable them to establish shared meaning through production and comprehension of conventional signals in social exchange (Bates, 1979).

The emerging capacity to actively explore objects and to imitate people leads to the ability to use familiar objects functionally and conventionally, an important precursor to symbolic play. By 6–9 months of age, children are actively exploring a variety of objects using actions such as grasping, banging, mouthing, and dropping. By 12 months, children are able to use a variety of familiar objects conventionally, such as drinking with a bottle, eating with a spoon, and wiping with a washcloth. These acts of deferred imitation reflect a child's underlying cognitive knowledge, as well as social awareness, of events they have experienced and form the foundation for learning conventional symbols (Bates, 1979).

The roots of language comprehension also are apparent from birth and reflect the capacity to symbolize in parallel with growing achievements in speech perception. Comprehension involves understanding nonverbal and verbal communicative signals used by others and determining meaning based on the context. Early in development, infants orient to sounds and speech in the environment and recognize familiar voices, and, by 4 months, they become proficient at localizing auditory stimuli. There is increasing evidence that the infant's auditory system is specially equipped to perceive acoustic features of speech, especially categorical perception of consonant distinctions and prosody, which aids in recognition of familiar voices and discrimination of speech sounds (Eimas, 1996; Lieberman, 1996). Infants at 4–6 months of age can make fine phonetic discriminations that distinguish consonants and vowels in syllables used in both their native and unfamiliar languages. Experience influences speech perception during the first year of life, as evidenced by infants at 10–12 months who are able to discriminate phonetic variations used only in their native language (Stager & Werker, 1997; Werker & Tees, 1999). Measures of speech perception at 6 months have been found to predict the number of words used at 16 and 24 months (Tsao, Liu, & Kuhl, 2004), highlighting the important role of speech perception in language development.

In spite of relatively sophisticated speech perception skills in infancy, children do not attend to fine phonetic detail when first learning word meanings (Werker & Tees, 1999). By 9–12 months of age, children demonstrate nonverbal comprehension by responding to nonverbal cues such as *gestural cues* (e.g., pointing to the ball and saying "get the ball"; extending the hand and saying "give it to me"), *situational cues* (e.g., standing in front of the sink and saying "wash hands"; saying "put in" after putting several objects in a container to clean up), and *intonation cues* (e.g., saying "stop it" with a firm tone or "I'm gonna get you" with a playful tone). By responding to this rich array of cues, a child may give the appearance of fairly sophisticated language comprehension but yet not understand actual spoken words. Comprehension becomes decontextualized between 12 and 18 months as children recognize the meaning of words outside familiar contexts (Wetherby, Reichle, & Pierce, 1998). However, children do not make fine phonetic discriminations in word learning until 18–24 months (Tsao et al., 2004; Werker & Tees, 1999), which suggests that an organizational shift occurs in processing language, from discriminating syllables in infancy to associating meaning with words over the second year of life.

The discovery that things have names begins to unfold at about 12–13 months of age (Bates, 1979). First-word acquisition has been described as situation specific, tied to the context, or event bound in that, initially, words may be used only with a narrow meaning in a highly specific context or situation (e.g., "up" refers only to being picked up out of a crib; "dog" is only the family pet). Later in development, words are used to refer to generalized concepts of actions or objects (e.g., "up" refers to any action involving movement upward; "dog" refers to any small four-legged animal that barks). Children learn to "free up" their understanding and use of words from very specific events to a wider variety of contexts by hearing the same word in different events and hearing different words in similar situations (Bloom, 1993). Vocabulary increases slowly and steadily until about 18–21 months, when there is an acceleration in the rate of new word acquisition, known as the *vocabulary burst*.

The vocabulary burst defines a quantitative change in vocabulary growth, with a number of corresponding qualitative changes in language abilities that indicate movement to generative language. Shortly after children go through the vocabulary burst, they begin to combine two or more words in novel combinations, and hence have truly acquired a productive language system (Bates et al., 1987; Bloom, 1993). By their second birthdays, most children can use and understand hundreds of words and can combine words into simple sentences (Bates, 1979; Wetherby, Reichle, & Pierce, 1998). The dramatic growth rate in word learning that follows the vocabulary burst triggers the transition to a language system that is categorical, combinatorial, rule governed, and generative.

The developmental interaction of joint-attention and symbol-use capacities enables children to become active partners in the intricate "dance" of *reciprocal social communication*. These emerging capacities form the developmental underpinnings needed to engage in conversation, as children learn to consider the experience, knowledge, and perspective of the social partner, to connect sentences in a cohesive manner, and to negotiate meaning. These capacities are essential to acquiring conversational competence, which entails knowing what to say, how much to say, how to say it, how to interpret what others say, and how to participate in a reciprocal social exchange, depending on who you are talking to and what you are talking about.

SOCIAL-COMMUNICATION PATTERNS OF CHILDREN WITH ASD

There is great heterogeneity in language abilities of children with ASD, ranging from failure to develop any functional speech to the development of functional but idiosyncratic use of spontaneous speech. It has been estimated that between one-third (Bryson, 1996) and one-half (Lord & Paul, 1997) of children and adults with autism have no speech. However, in more recent literature, the proportion of nonverbal children with ASD is much smaller among those who received very early intervention. For example, Lord, Risi, and Pickles (2004) followed children who were initially diagnosed with ASD at age 2 and who received early intervention and reported that 14–20% of this sample was nonverbal (i.e., using less than five words on a daily basis) at age 9. Kjelgaard and Tager-Flusberg (2001) identified subgroups of verbal children with ASD based on language measures; some children showed no linguistic deficits, and other children showed language impairments in grammatical skills with relatively spared vocabulary skills similar to those of children with specific language impairment. In spite of the heterogeneity of language abilities in children with ASD, social-communication or pragmatic impairments are universal across all ages and ability levels (Tager-Flusberg, Joseph, & Folstein, 2001) and are defining features of the clinical disorder (Lord & Paul, 1997; Wetherby, Schuler, & Prizant, 1997). A large body of research over the past two decades has characterized the social-communication deficits of children with ASD, with most children studied being of preschool age. This section reviews research exploring the social-communication skills of children with ASD for the capacities of joint attention and symbol use.

Deficit in the Capacity for Joint Attention

A deficit in joint attention is a core feature of ASD in the diagnostic criteria of DSM-IV (American Psychiatric Association, 1994) and includes a lack of spontaneous seeking to share enjoyment, interests, or achievements with other people. It is not that children with ASD do not communicate but rather that they do not readily communicate for social goals or purposes. Research has documented that children with ASD communicate predominantly or exclusively to regulate the behavior of others to request or protest something and show a deficit in or absence of communication aimed at drawing another's attention to an object or event to label it or comment about it (Sigman, Mundy, Sherman, & Ungerer, 1986; Stone, Ousley, Yoder, Hogan, & Hepburn, 1997; Wetherby, Prizant, & Hutchinson, 1998; Wetherby & Prutting, 1984; Wetherby, Yonclas, & Bryan, 1989). This pattern of deficit in initiating communication for joint attention appears to be a hallmark of ASD and is not characteristic of children with specific language impairments or general developmental delays. Because the ability to communicate for joint attention emerges before words in typical development, a deficit in initiating communication for joint attention may represent a fundamental or core impairment of ASD (Mundy, Sigman, & Kasari, 1990), particularly given that it is evident in very young children with ASD (Charman et al., 1997; Wetherby, Prizant, & Hutchinson, 1998; Wetherby et al., 2004).

Children with ASD also show deficits in joint-attention skills that emerge before initiating joint attention. Compared with children with developmental delays, children with ASD display fewer gaze shifts, spend less time in joint engagement, and have more difficulty following another person's attentional focus by looking where they are looking or pointing (Sigman et al., 1986; Stone, Ousley, Yoder, et al., 1997; Wetherby, Prizant, & Hutchinson, 1998). Preliminary data on a group of 12 preschool children with ASD suggests that the developmental sequence of emergence of joint-attention skills from gaze shifting to gaze/point following to initiating joint attention with gestures is also found in children with ASD (Carpenter, Pennington, & Rogers, 2002). In other words, children with ASD who do not shift gaze also do not follow gaze or point cues or initiate joint attention.

Leekam, Lopez, and Moore (2000) conducted a series of experiments to examine the role of attention in difficulties that preschool children with ASD have in responding to joint attention compared with those of children with developmental delay, matched on nonverbal mental age (MA). They found that children with ASD had more difficulty orienting to attention bids and following a head-turn cue than the control-group children. In contrast, they were as accurate as control-group children in their ability to shift attention to a peripheral target and were faster in responding. These results indicate that children with ASD do not have difficulty shifting attention from a central stimulus and orienting attention to peripheral targets. Rather, children with ASD had difficulty orienting to another person's bid for attention and following another person's gaze and head-turn cue to a peripheral target. Children with ASD were found to show deficits in orienting to social stimuli (their names being called; hands clapping) but not nonsocial stimuli (rattle; musical jack-in-the box) compared with MA-matched controls with Down syndrome and typical development (Dawson, Meltzoff, Osterling, Rinaldi, & Brown, 1998). Responding to joint attention was correlated with orienting to social stimuli but not to nonsocial stimuli, suggesting a core social orientation deficit.

Research has examined contributions of social-affective mechanisms to the joint-attention deficits in ASD. Clinical descriptions of children with ASD include pronounced deficits in the ability to share affective states (American Psychiatric Association, 1994; Dawson, Hill, Spencer, Galpert, & Watson, 1990). Children with ASD have been found to display less gaze directed to people and positive affect during interactions with unfamiliar adults (Snow, Hertzig, & Shapiro, 1987). Dawson and colleagues (1990) found that children with ASD showed significantly less positive affect coordinated with gaze and were much less likely to respond to their mothers' smiles than typical children. The frequency of gaze directed to their mothers was significantly correlated with receptive and expressive language for the children with ASD. Furthermore, evidence suggests that the deficit in the capacity for sharing positive affect among children with ASD may be associated with the deficit in initiating and responding to joint attention. Deficits in joint attention and shared affect both involve the allocation of attention between people and objects. Kasari, Sigman, Mundy, and Yirmiya (1990) compared affect displays of children who were communicating for joint attention versus behavior regulation. They found that typically developing children were more likely to share positive affect during episodes of sharing attention on objects or events, whereas children with ASD showed lower levels of shared affect and did not show this integration of shared affect and joint attention.

Deficits in initiating and responding to joint attention would likely have a cascading effect on language development, because language learning occurs within the context of the modeling by the caregiver of words that refer to objects and events that are jointly regarded. McArthur and Adamson (1996) found that when children with ASD interacted with adults who were calling the children's attention to an object or event to establish shared attention, episodes of joint attention were rare. During these adult-initiated episodes of joint attention, the children with ASD displayed significantly less attention directed to the adult partner, as well as to the objects of reference, than did children with developmental language disorders matched on chronological and nonverbal MA. The authors concluded that for children with ASD, the lack of ability to allocate attention between people and objects may contribute to difficulties in acquiring shared meanings of cultural conventions. In a word-learning task, Baron-Cohen, Baldwin, and Crowson (1997) found that, unlike children in developmental-delay and typical control groups, children with ASD rarely used the speaker's direction of gaze to learn the meaning of a novel word for a novel object; instead, children with ASD relied on mapping the novel word to the object that they (the listeners) were looking at, which led to a high rate of mapping errors.

A number of longitudinal studies provide evidence of a relationship between joint attention and language outcomes. Mundy and colleagues (1990) found that measures of gestural joint attention (i.e., responding to joint attention and initiating joint attention with gaze, showing, or pointing) at a mean age of 45 months were a significant predictor of language development 13 months later for children with ASD, whereas none of the other nonverbal measures, initial language scores, MA, chronological age (CA), nor IQ were significant predictors. These findings have been substantiated in a longitudinal study measuring joint attention at 20 months of age and predicting language outcomes at 42 months of age (Charman, Baron-Cohen, et al., 2003). These findings have also been substantiated in a long-term follow-up study examining joint-attention skills of 51 children with autism with a mean age of 3 years, 11 months (Sigman & Ruskin, 1999). Initial joint-attention skills predicted gains in expressive language at a mean age of 12 years, 10 months.

A joint-attentional state during which the child and partner share a site of interest can be achieved in the following ways, which vary in how active the child's role is in establishing shared attention: (1) the partner looks at the site that the child is looking at; (2) the child looks at the site that the partner is looking at; (3) the child shifts gaze between the site and the partner to check that the partner is looking at the site; (4) the child follows the partner's attentional cue (i.e., gaze, show, or point) to look at the site; and (5) the child uses a communicative gesture or vocalization to draw the partner's attention to the site. This coordination of attention provides a critical moment for language learning when the caregiver models language that interprets and relates the child's experience and focus of attention.

The caregiver may be able to compensate for a child's deficits in joint attention by ensuring a common focus of attention when modeling language. In a longitudinal study of 25 children with ASD, Siller and Sigman (2002) investigated whether caregivers followed the child's focus of attention and toy engagement during play and the extent to which this predicted language outcomes. Play samples were initially gathered when the children with ASD were a mean of 50 months of age. The caregivers of children with ASD synchronized their behaviors to their children's attention and activities as much as did caregivers of typically developing children matched on language abilities. However, the children with ASD whose caregivers showed higher levels of synchronization during initial play samples developed better joint-attention skills 1 year later and better language outcomes 10 and 16 years later compared with children of caregivers who showed lower levels of synchronization initially. The strongest predictor of the child's increase in initiating joint attention was the caregiver's initiation of joint attention that is synchronized to the child's attentional focus. The strongest predictor of gain in language was caregiver utterances that follow the child's attentional focus and allow the child to continue the ongoing toy engagement. These findings have important implications for targeting joint-attention skills in intervention by enhancing the child's skills, as well as the partner's ability to support shared attention, and intervening early to establish or enhance synchronization by caregivers as soon as possible.

Deficit in the Capacity for Symbol Use

Many factors may contribute to the language difficulties of children with ASD in addition to joint-attention deficits. Children with ASD may show specific deficits in acquiring conventional communication or more general deficits that affect cognitive and symbolic functioning. This section examines research on deficits in the capacity for symbol use in children with ASD, including language, gestures, imitation, and play.

Children with ASD have varying degrees of difficulty with language production and comprehension, which may be associated with general cognitive impairment. Although a small subgroup of children with ASD have normal aspects of language skills (Kjelgaard & Tager-Flusberg, 2001), preschool children with ASD have been found to have more severe language comprehension and production deficits than nonverbal MA-matched children with developmental delays (Lord & Paul, 1997). The presence of fluent speech, defined as using multiword combinations spontaneously, communicatively, and regularly, before the age of 5 continues to be a good prognostic indicator of IQ, language measures, adaptive skills, and academic achievement in adolescence (Venter, Lord, & Schopler, 1992). Nonverbal IQ has generally been found to be higher than verbal IQ in groups of children with ASD, but there is individual variation in this profile, and the reverse profile has been associated with Asperger syndrome (Joseph, Tager-Flusberg, & Lord, 2002; Klin, Volkmar, Sparrow, Cicchetti, & Rourke, 1995). Verbal–nonverbal discrepancies have been found to lessen with age because of improvements in language functioning. However, relatively poorer verbal than nonverbal IQ at school age is associated with increased social and communication impairment on the Autism Diagnostic Observation Schedule (ADOS; Joseph et al., 2002).

Children with ASD have difficulty acquiring conventional and symbolic aspects of communication. The quantity and quality of gesture use is limited in children with ASD. Unlike children with language or hearing impairments, children with ASD do not compensate for their lack of speech by using other modalities, such as gestures. Children with ASD predominantly use primitive contact gestures (i.e., leading, pulling, or manipulating another's hand) to communicate and lack the use of many conventional gestures, such as showing, waving, and pointing, as well as symbolic gestures, such as nodding the head and depicting actions (Loveland & Landry, 1986; McHale, Simeonsson, Marcus, & Olley, 1980; Stone & Caro-Martinez, 1990; Wetherby, Prizant, & Hutchinson, 1998; Wetherby et al., 1989). In lieu of conventional means of communicating, children with ASD may develop unconventional or inappropriate behaviors to communicate, such as self-injurious behavior, aggression, or tantrums.

Whereas deficits in gestural communication are characteristic of children with ASD, there is much variability in the use of speech. Some children with ASD have been found to use a limited consonant inventory and less complex syllabic structure, whereas others show adequate complexity of vocalizations (McHale et al., 1980; Stone & Caro-Martinez, 1990; Wetherby et al., 1989; Wetherby, Prizant, & Hutchinson, 1998). In a study of vocal behavior of preschool children who had few or no words, Sheinkopf, Mundy, Oller, and Steffens (2000) found that, compared with children with developmental delays, children with ASD used a comparable proportion of syllables containing consonants but a significantly greater proportion of syllables with atypical phonation, such as squeals, growls, and yells. The vocal atypicalities were independent of joint-attention deficits in this small sample but were negatively correlated with MA, suggesting that the joint-attention and vocal deficits arise from different pathological processes. Vocal deficits may reflect difficulties in the symbolic capacity and/or motor control of the speech mechanism.

The vast majority of those who do learn to talk go through a period of using echolalia, the imitation of speech of others, either immediately or at some time later (Prizant, Schuler, Wetherby, & Rydell, 1997). An echolalic utterance may be equivalent to a single word or a label for a situation or event. Current understanding of echolalia indicates that it may serve a variety of communicative and cognitive functions (Prizant & Rydell, 1993; Prizant et al., 1997) and may be a productive language-learning strategy for many children with ASD, not unlike imitation for typically developing children. The way echolalic children learn to talk is by imitating phrases associated with situations or emotional states, then learning meanings by trying out these phrases and seeing how they work. Although echolalic children produce phrases or sentences, they may be functioning in the one-word stage if all of their utterances are imitated chunks. Children with ASD may have difficulty making the shift from processing language at the syllable level, in other words as a string of syllables, to associating conventional meaning at the word level. Over time, many verbal children learn to use these chunks purposefully in communicative interactions, and eventually they are able to break down the echolalic chunks into smaller meaningful units as part of the process of transitioning to a rule-governed, generative language system. Pronoun reversals are a by-product of echolalia because the child repeats the pronoun heard, thus reversing the pronouns used in reference to self and other. For example, a child may use the echolalic utterance "Do you want a piece of candy" as a way to request the candy, although it sounds like the child is offering it. Thus echolalia can give the appearance of sophisticated language, but careful examination of how a child uses echolalic chunks or creative combinations of words or phrases can reveal a child's true language level and patterns of language development.

Both the use of echolalia and the reliance on primitive contact gestures may reflect a reenactment strategy in the face of difficulties learning symbolic communication (Schuler & Prizant, 1985; Prizant & Wetherby, 1987; Wetherby, 1986). Reenactment involves repeating an aspect of a situation to make the situation recur, such as putting an adult's hand on the door handle to request to go out, getting the car keys to ask to go for a ride, making sounds or movements used during a tickling game to request to be tickled, or repeating a memorized portion of a song as a request to have someone sing the song. Reenactments occur at early stages of typical communication development and are regarded as *indexical* communication rather than symbolic communication (McLean & Snyder-McLean, 1999).

In symbolic communication, the symbol stands for and is separate from its referent. Repeating an action or phrase that is part of the referent or goal is indexical rather than symbolic because it is an index of, or associated with, the goal (Werner & Kaplan, 1963). Children with ASD may need to acquire a large set of communicative signals at a reenactment level before moving on to become symbol users.

Children with ASD who progress beyond echolalia may acquire a large vocabulary and more advanced aspects of grammar. Most verbal children develop grammatical skills in the same general progression as typically developing children do, but they show persisting problems with conversational rules (Baltaxe, 1977; Tager-Flusberg, 1996), which are pragmatic aspects of language. Some verbal children have difficulties with grammatical aspects of language similar to those of children with specific language impairment (Kjelgaard & Tager-Flusberg, 2001).

Another line of research that elucidates the symbolic deficit in ASD is the study of imitation. Numerous studies have documented that children with ASD have difficulty on tasks of body imitation involving simple hand and facial movements, symbolic pantomimes, and actions with objects, compared with CA- and MA-matched control groups (Rogers, Hepburn, Stackhouse, & Wehner, 2003; Stone, Ousley, & Littleford, 1997; Williams, Whiten, & Singh, 2004); however, there is variation in the pattern of imitation deficit. Stone, Ousley, and Littleford (1997) found that in children with ASD, imitation of facial and body movements showed concurrent and predictive associations with expressive language skills, whereas imitation of actions with objects showed concurrent associations with play skills. However, Rogers et al. (2003) did not replicate these relations when controlling for developmental level. Rogers et al. (2003) found that oral–facial imitation and object imitation correlated with dyadic and triadic social responsivity and overall developmental level. Imitation skills were not related to expressive language, play, visual–spatial abilities, or adaptive behavior when controlling for developmental functioning. The children with ASD performed as well as controls on a praxis battery, and imitation was correlated with fine motor skills, not praxis, indicating that general motor dyspraxia did not account for the imitation deficits. They found that developmental functioning accounted for 53% of the variance in imitation, and neither fine-motor skills nor social responsivity added additional predictive value. These findings support the relation between the imitation deficit in children with ASD and both general developmental functioning and a social impairment in dyadic and triadic engagement. However, research on imitation in children with ASD has been restricted to tasks that elicit imitation in a clinical setting. Other than research documenting the use of echolalia, little is known about the spontaneous use of immediate or deferred imitation as an active learning strategy in natural contexts by children with ASD.

Further evidence of a deficit in the symbolic capacity in ASD is the limited ability to develop symbolic or pretend play. It is noteworthy that a lack of varied, spontaneous make-believe play is one of the four diagnostic features of the impairment in communication in DSM-IV (American Psychiatric Association, 1994). Children with ASD show significant deficits in symbolic play (i.e., using pretend actions with objects) and limited abilities in functional play (i.e., using objects functionally; Dawson & Adams, 1984; Sigman & Ungerer, 1984; Wetherby & Prutting, 1984; Williams, Reddy, & Costall, 2001; Wing, Gould, Yeates, & Brierley, 1977). Functional and symbolic play skills have been found to be significantly correlated with receptive and expressive language (Mundy, Sigman, Ungerer, & Sherman, 1987). In their longitudinal study, Sigman and Ruskin (1999) found that the number of different functional play actions predicted expressive language gains, even when controlling for initial language level. When Sigman and Ruskin (1999) compared the predictive value of play and joint attention, a regression analysis revealed that a significant amount of variance in expressive language was accounted for by both functional play and response to joint attention, suggesting that these may reflect separate sources of deficits.

In contrast to deficits in functional object use and symbolic play, children with ASD perform at similar or higher levels on constructive play (e.g., using objects relationally in combination to create a product, such as stacking blocks, nesting cups, or putting puzzles together) compared with typically developing children and children with developmental delays at the same expressive language stage (Wetherby & Prutting, 1984; Wetherby, Prizant, & Hutchinson, 1998). Bates (1979) suggested that symbolic play is acquired through observational learning and that constructive or combinatorial play can be acquired either through observational learning or trial-and-error problem solving. Children with ASD seem to excel at behaviors learned through trial and error. Many of the gestures used by children with ASD (e.g., taking another's hand and leading the person to a goal) are contextually restricted and can emerge naturally from exploration with the child's own body through trial-and-error learning strategies. Similarly, constructive play can be learned through trial and error. The acquisition of conventional gestures, conventional meanings for words, deferred imitation, and conventional use of objects can be learned only through observation. This learning entails observing and imitating the behavior of others from a stream of behaviors and then decontextualizing the behavior to new contexts (Carpenter & Tomasello, 2000). Learning shared meanings, imitating and using conventional behaviors, and being able to decontextualize meaning from the context constitute the symbolic deficits in children with ASD (Wetherby, Prizant, & Schuler, 2000).

It is possible that the joint-attention deficits underlie or contribute to the symbolic deficits in children with ASD in that difficulties coordinating attention may interfere with learning shared meanings. Wetherby, Prizant, and Hutchinson (1998) examined the social-communication profiles of 22 children with ASD compared with 22 children with developmental delays at the same expressive language level. The children with ASD displayed significantly poorer scores with large effect sizes on the following social-communication measures: gaze shifts, shared positive affect, initiating communication for joint attention, inventory of conventional gestures, use of distal gestures, coordination of gestures and vocalizations, language comprehension, and inventory and complexity of actions in symbolic play. However, they displayed comparable scores in initiating communication for behavior regulation, inventory of consonants, and level of constructive play. These findings support other research that indicates that the profiles of children with ASD are characterized by a distinct constellation of strengths and weaknesses in parameters of social communication. Correlational findings from this study showed that expressive language and language comprehension were not correlated with each other in these children with ASD and that different constellations of social-communication skills were correlated with expressive language versus language comprehension. Expressive language showed large correlations with initiating joint attention and measures of vocal communication, including inventory of consonants. Language comprehension showed moderate correlations with initiating joint attention, inventory of conventional gestures, gaze shifts, and shared positive affect and a large correlation with complexity of actions in symbolic play. These findings support an association between measures of sharing attention and sharing meanings in children with ASD, but further research with larger samples is needed to examine the causal relations among these constructs.

EXPLANATORY HYPOTHESES OF THE SOCIAL-COMMUNICATION DEFICITS OF CHILDREN WITH ASD

Bates (1979) hypothesized that the human symbolic capacity evolved in phylogeny as a "new product" built from the interaction of available "old parts" through the process of "heterochrony," which refers to changes in the developmental timing and rate of maturation of preexisting capacities. Quantitative variations in timing led to a qualitatively new capacity. Bates applied this concept to the ontogenetic development of symbol use. When the relative proportion of available social–cognitive component skills (i.e., communicative intent, tool use, imitation) reaches a certain threshold level in development, new interactions among the components result, creating a new capacity for symbols.

The process of heterochrony may explain the core deficits in social communication, as well as individual variation, in children with ASD (Wetherby & Prutting, 1984; Wetherby, 1991). The relative proportions of component skills available at varying times in development may influence the child's social-communication profile. Slight variations in the developmental timing of individual components may have developmental consequences that are cumulative and pervasive in later stages. The particular combination of skills and experiences available to a child with ASD is not seen at any point in typical development and may lead to distinct profiles of social communication because of the interplay among the available components and interaction with the learning environment. However, the child's skills within specific domains may follow typical developmental progressions. Heterochrony may be the mechanism that operates to produce discrepancies in a child's profile and may be caused by individual variation in or disruption of the precise orchestration of events that unfold during neural maturation.

MEASUREMENT OF SOCIAL COMMUNICATION

Exploring developmental profiles of social-communication skills has contributed to distinguishing children with ASD from children with other developmental delays and to elucidating the core deficits of ASD. Measurement of social communication can address a broad array of skills, including the many facets of joint attention and symbol use reviewed in this chapter. Because of the heterogeneity in children with ASD, it is critical to characterize the nature and extent of deficits in joint attention and symbol use, because these deficits have important implications for language outcomes. This section first discusses psychometric issues that need to be considered in the measurement of social communication and then provides an overview of different approaches to measurement of social communication in children with ASD.

Psychometric Issues in the Measurement of Social Communication

Efforts to better understand and enhance social-communication skills of children with ASD hinge on our ability to accurately quantify social communication. Measurement of social communication poses challenges because it is influenced by many variables, including the social partner, the interactive context, the source of information, and psychometric features of the measurement scale. The challenge is how to gather meaningful and accurate measures of social communication efficiently. The following questions are important to consider in making decisions about measurement of social communication for children with ASD.

• *How is the information gathered?* Measures of social communication can be gathered from observation in the natural environment, from interactive sampling in a laboratory or clinical setting, or from information reported by parents or teachers familiar with the child. Each of these procedures has strengths and limitations. Naturalistic observations of a child interacting with a variety of partners over an extended period of time may capture the child's repertoire of skills and how ecological variables influence the child's social communication, but this outcome is dependent on the child's having adequate natural opportunities to use social communication. Furthermore, quantifying the child's behavior from naturalistic observation is challenging, and sound psychometric methods must be ensured. Measures based on reported information capitalize on the knowledge of a familiar person who interacts with the child on a daily basis. However, parents or teachers may over- or underestimate the child's abilities. It is also challenging to secure accurate measures from children by using interactive sampling procedures. Many factors may influence children's performance, including attention, interest, fatigue, comfort level, and experience in unfamiliar settings. Interactive sampling procedures can range from unstructured play to semistructured opportunities or staged situations designed to encourage or elicit social communication. The person interacting with the child during the sampling may be an unfamiliar experimenter or a familiar person, such as a parent, teacher, sibling, or peer. The accuracy of the information gathered from any of these sources of information needs to be documented.

• *What social communication behaviors will be measured?* Social communication consists of a number of different theoretical constructs, such as shared or coordinated attention, intentionality, and reciprocity, that may be reflected best as latent variables that are not directly observable. Individual items or behaviors to be measured should be selected based on their relationship to a latent variable or underlying construct. In other words, a good measure is an accurate estimate of the magnitude of a latent variable. Because a latent variable cannot be directly measured and observed, the accuracy of the item or behavior measured is inferred by relationships among different items or measures that are assumed to have a causal relationship with the latent variable (DeVellis, 2003). Because the study of social communication is relatively new, the field is in its infancy in determining what the latent variables are and what are good items to measure the latent variables. For example, is joint attention one latent variable, or are initiating and responding to joint attention separate latent variables? Are gaze shifts and drawing attention to objects with a point or show gesture or a word separate skills but correlated measures that reflect a single construct of initiating joint attention? Or are these separate variables that have different developmental trajectories?

• *What measurement scale will be used?* Items or measures can be categorical or continuous variables. Categorical variables measure values that change in steps and may be dichotomous (e.g., gender) or may take on a small or finite number of values (e.g., seasons, days of the week). Categorical variables can represent quantitative attributes in which the categories stand for ranges or degrees of values (e.g., *rarely, sometimes, often*). Continuous variables measure values that change smoothly, such as age and height. Measures of social communication may be continuous, such as frequency counts and rates of behavior, or categorical, such as the rating scale for the ADOS. Categorical variables may be sufficient to differentiate children with ASD from other populations and thus are useful as screening and diagnostic tools. The advantage of continuous variables is that they provide more precise information to characterize individual variation, allowing for larger variance and greater potential for documenting relationships among variables measured. However, ceiling or floor effects may restrict the range of continuous variables and hence obscure relationships studied.

• *Are the items that constitute the measure homogenous?* The homogeneity or consistency across items or behaviors selected to measure a construct is an important aspect of reliability (DeVellis, 2003). Internal consistency, most commonly measured with Cronbach's coefficient alpha, expresses the degree to which the parts or individual items measure the same underlying construct. High correlations among items suggest that they are all measuring the same thing and hence are presumed to be strongly linked with the latent variable. Thus a good measure of any construct of social communication would be one with multiple items or behaviors that have high internal consistency. Measures with higher internal consistency increase statistical power and the ability to demonstrate relationships among variables.

• *Is a child's performance on the measure judged similarly by different raters?* Because measures of social communication require ongoing judgments about the occurrence or nonoccurrence of behaviors, interrater agreement should be documented by comparing the measures obtained by at least two independent raters.

• *Is the measure stable from test to retest?* Another aspect of reliability is whether the measure is stable from one point in time to another when development or learning has had little or no effect on the child's relative standing in the group. The stability of scores, reflected in high correlations from test to retest, may indicate minimal measurement error.

• *Does the measure capture growth or change in this construct?* Although we want a measure to be stable over time when no learning or development has occurred, we also want it to detect change over time when development or learning has occurred. Thus we want to know if a measure of social communication is sensitive to change over time. In research on children with typical development, we want to know the age range over which the measure captures growth and the smallest time interval over which the measure is able to detect change. In research on children with ASD, we want to know whether the measure is able to capture change over time that may reflect development or treatment effects.

• *Does the measure have an empirical association with some criterion measure?* We want to know whether the measure is related to a different measure that has been designated as important or as a "gold standard" for this construct. This is referred to as criterion-related validity, which may be measured at the same point in time (concurrent validity) or at a later point in time (predictive validity). Social-communication measures are often explored in relation to language.

• *Does the measure differentiate children with ASD from other populations?* It is important to know whether a measure of social communication can differentiate children with ASD from other populations. This is referred to as known-groups validation and is accomplished in one of two ways. First, comparisons of the measure in two or more groups of children can reveal whether there are statistical differences. Second, the predictive accuracy of the measure can be examined by classifying the predictor and the criterion measure into dichotomous categories (e.g., pass/fail; low/high) and examining the "hit rate" for correctly classifying children.

• *Does the measure actually measure the construct it purports to measure?* It is important to know that the measure is positively correlated with other measures that are theoretically related and uncorrelated with measures that would not be expected to be related. This is referred to as construct validity, and correlations among constructs should be demonstrated above and beyond the measurement method (e.g., interviewing vs. sampling).

Approaches to Measurement of Social Communication

The most common approach to measuring social communication in research on children with ASD is interactive sampling. This section describes two formal sampling procedures, the Early Social Communication Scales (ESCS) and the Communication and Symbolic Behavior Scales (CSBS), and informal sampling procedures of parent–child interaction that have been used to measure social communication. Additionally, the recent use of parent-report tools to measure social communication is described. Psychometric features of each of these approaches are presented.

Early Social Communication Scales

The ESCS is a structured observation tool designed to measure nonverbal communication skills in a laboratory setting (Seibert, Hogan, & Mundy, 1982; Mundy, Hogan & Doehring, 1996). The ESCS sample takes 15–25 minutes to administer and is videotaped for later scoring. It consists of a set of semistructured eliciting situations designed to encourage specific nonverbal behaviors between the examiner and the child and measures low- and high-level behaviors for both initiating and responding to joint attention, requesting, and social interaction. For example, for initiating joint attention, low-level behavior includes eye contact and alternating gaze, and high-level behavior includes showing and pointing gestures. For responding to joint attention, low-level behavior consists of following a proximal point or touch, and high-level behavior consists of following a line of regard of a distal point.

Numerous research studies have documented aspects of reliability and validity of the ESCS in children with ASD, Down syndrome, and typical development (Mundy et al., 1996). High interrater agreement for the ESCS has been well documented. Test–retest stability of initiating and responding to joint attention from 14 to 17 months and concurrent relations with language outcomes were demonstrated with typically developing children (Mundy & Gomes, 1998). Studies using the ESCS have documented the predictive validity of initiating and responding to joint attention and requesting in relation to language outcomes in children with typical development (Morales, Mundy, & Rojas, 1998; Mundy & Gomes, 1998), Down syndrome (Mundy, Kasari, Sigman, & Ruskin, 1995), and ASD (Mundy et al., 1990; Rogers et al., 2003; Sigman & Ruskin, 1999) and significant group differences between children with typical development, Down syndrome (Mundy et al., 1995), and ASD (Mundy et al., 1990).

Measures of internal consistency have not been reported for the ESCS, which limits our ability to interpret correlations or lack of correlations with other measures. For instance, we do not know whether measures of responding to joint attention have higher internal consistency than measures of initiating joint attention. If this were the case, this would be one explanation for measures of responding to joint attention having stronger predictive correlations (e.g., Sigman & Ruskin, 1999). Correlational data among the six social-communication skills measured with the ESCS and receptive and expressive language have been published and support criterion-related validity. However, further research using factor analysis is needed to determine the latent variables that underlie individual items measured on the ESCS (e.g., low vs. high level of initiating and responding to joint attention) and separate or shared constructs measured.

Communication and Symbolic Behavior Scales Developmental Profile

The CSBS Developmental Profile (CSBS-DP; Wetherby & Prizant, 2002) is a standardized tool designed for screening and evaluation of communication and symbolic abilities of children from 6 to 24 months of age. It was recently developed based on the CSBS (Wetherby & Prizant, 1993), which is a more in-depth tool designed for program planning. The CSBS-DP behavior sample is a face-to-face evaluation of the child interacting with a parent and clinician that takes about 25 minutes to administer and that is videotaped for later analysis. The sample consists of systematic procedures designed to entice or tempt the child to communicate and to encourage spontaneous play. It measures the following social-communication skills organized into three composites:

1. *Social:* gaze shifts; shared positive affect; gaze/point following; rate of communication; initiating communication for behavior regulation, social interaction, and joint attention; inventory of conventional gestures; and distal gestures.
2. *Speech:* syllables with consonants, inventory of consonants, inventory of words, and inventory of word combinations.
3. *Symbolic:* comprehension of object names, person names, and body parts, inventory and complexity of actions in symbolic play, and constructive play with blocks.

The CSBS-DP has been nationally field tested, and standard scores and percentiles can be calculated based on a normative sample (Wetherby & Prizant, 2002). Information about the psychometric features of the CSBS-DP has been reported in Wetherby, Allen, Cleary, Kublin, and Goldstein (2002); Wetherby, Goldstein, Cleary, Allen, and Kublin (2003); and Wetherby and Prizant (2002). The behavior sample has a high degree of internal consistency (alpha coefficients ranging from .86 to .92), very good interrater reliability, and good test–retest reliability for standard scores over a 4-month interval, with significant increases in raw scores, providing evidence that it detects growth over short periods but produces relatively stable rankings of children. Construct validity has been supported by the developmental progression of scores from 6 to 24 months of age and by intercorrelations among cluster and composite scores. A principal-component analysis of the items was used to form the seven clusters and three composites of the behavior sample (Wetherby & Prizant, 2002). More variables are measured with the CSBS-DP than with the ESCS, with some overlap, and they are organized differently. For example, on the CSBS-DP, gaze shifts, shared positive affect, and gaze/point following are grouped in the Emotion and Eye Gaze cluster, and initiating joint attention is grouped with social interaction and behavior regulation in the Communication cluster. The ESCS provides more precise ratings of the six skills measured. Moderate to large correlations were found between the behavior sample gathered between 12 and 21 months and outcomes on standardized language tests at 2 and 3 years of age (Wetherby et al., 2002, 2003), supporting the predictive validity of the CSBS-DP and the value of measuring social-communication skills to predict later language. The CSBS (Wetherby, Prizant, & Hutchinson, 1998) and the CSBS-DP (Wetherby et al., 2004) have been found to show significant group differences in social-communication skills of children with typical development, developmental delays, and ASD.

Parent–Child Interaction Measures of Social Communication

Sampling procedures that gather parent–child interactions to measure social communication have been reported; however, little is known about the psychometric features of these procedures. Unstructured parent–child play samples have yielded limited spontaneous communication, and, therefore, researchers have added structure to the sampling procedures, as done in the ESCS and CSBS. For example, Yoder and Warren (1998) found that child initiations were rare in unstructured play samples of mother–child interaction with 58 prelinguistic children with developmental disabilities, and they added structured requesting opportunities. Virtually no research is available on the psychometric features of measures of social communication gathered from parent–child interactions in natural environments. The ecological validity of measuring social communication from naturalistic parent–child interaction underscores the critical need for research in this area.

Parent-Report Measures of Social Communication

Another method for measuring a child's social communication is to use reported information from significant others familiar with the subtle nuances of the child's social communication in natural environments. Research on parent report of early language skills has demonstrated that parents can be very accurate in reporting about current and emerging behaviors, as opposed to giving retrospective accounts of past milestones (Fenson et al., 1993). Furthermore, accuracy is greater when a recognition format or checklist is used instead of free-form reports or diary methods. Numerous studies indicate that parent report using the MacArthur Communicative Development Inventory (CDI; Dale, Bates, Reznick, & Morisset, 1989; Fenson et al., 1993, 1994; Miller, Sedey, & Miolo, 1995; Thal, O'Hanlon, Clemmons, & Fralin, 1999) and the Language Development Survey (Rescorla & Alley, 2001) are reliable and valid measures of communication development in children with typical development, specific language impairment, and Down syndrome and sensitive indicators of language delays in young children. The CDI has been used with a small sample of children with ASD, and the number of words produced based on parent report showed a large correlation with standardized measures of language production; in contrast, the number of words comprehended based on parent report were not correlated with standardized measures of language comprehension (Charman, Drew, Baird, & Baird, 2003). These findings are preliminary but suggest that either parent report or standardized language comprehension measures may be inaccurate for children with ASD.

In addition to the behavior sample, the CSBS-DP includes two parent-report tools, a one-page 24-item Infant–Toddler Checklist that is completed quickly at a physician's office or child-care center for screening and a four-page follow-up Caregiver Questionnaire, both of which measure the same social-communication skills as the behavior sample. The psychometric features of these parent-report tools have been reported by Wetherby and colleagues (Wetherby et al., 2002, 2003; Wetherby & Prizant, 2002). The Checklist and Caregiver Questionnaire have large concurrent correlations with each other, moderate correlations with the behavior sample on the Social composite, and large correlations with the behavior sample on the Speech and Symbolic composites (Wetherby & Prizant, 2002). The accuracy of the Checklist has been compared to standardized language measures at 2 years. Sensitivity was 87.4%, and specificity was 75.2% using the bottom 10th percentile, or 1.25 standard deviations below the mean, as criterion for risk. A regression analysis indicated that the Checklist and behavior sample were a significant predictor of receptive and expressive language outcomes at 2 and 3 years of age but that the behavior sample explained a significant amount of unique variance in language outcomes beyond the Checklist (Wetherby et al., 2003). Preliminary findings using the Infant–Toddler Checklist on a general population screen of more than 3,000 children between 12 and 24 months indicate that sensitivity was 89% for children identified with developmental delay and ASD combined and increased to 94% for children later identified with ASD (Wetherby et al., 2004). These findings indicate that parent report is a valuable measure of social communication and suggest that combining it with interactive sampling may improve accuracy. However, further research is needed to examine the accuracy of parent-report tools of social communication for children with ASD. For now, caution is needed, because adding an inaccurate measure to an accurate measure or adding two inaccurate measures together will not improve accuracy.

A number of diagnostic and screening tools also measure social-communication skills, and these are reviewed in detail in other chapters in this volume (Charman & Baron-Cohen, Chapter 3, Lord & Richler, Chapter 2; Zwaigenbaum & Stone, Chapter 4).

Implications for Earlier Identification of ASD

The diagnostic features of ASD should be evident in very young children, because they involve abilities that typically develop in the first few years of life. The literature reviewed suggests that there is a constellation of social-communication parameters that are important early indicators of ASD. The lack of language and limitations in communication development may be among the first symptoms that are evident to parents and professionals.

Wetherby et al. (2004) conducted a prospective longitudinal study to identify red flags for ASD from videotapes collected during the second year of life. Three groups of 18 children were identified: one with ASD, one with developmental delays in which ASD was ruled out (DD), and one with typical development (TD) who were screened under 24 months of age. Significant group differences were found between the ASD and both the DD and TD groups on the following nine red flags observed in the behavior sample: (1) lack of appropriate gaze; (2) lack of warm, joyful expressions with gaze; (3) lack of sharing enjoyment or interest; (4) lack of response to name; (5) lack of coordination of gaze, facial expression, gesture, and sound; (6) lack of showing; (7) unusual prosody; (8) repetitive movements or posturing of body, arms, hands, or fingers; and (9) repetitive movements with objects. Significant differences were found between the ASD and TD groups, but not the ASD and DD groups, on the following four red flags: (1) lack of response to contextual cues; (2) lack of pointing; (3) lack of vocalizations with consonants; and (4) lack of playing with a variety of toys conventionally. These findings indicate that children with ASD can be distinguished from those with DD and TD in the second year of life on a combination of lack of typical behaviors and presence of atypical behaviors, and they underscore the importance of social communication in earlier identification of ASD.

Social-Communication Outcome Measures in Intervention Research

Although a large number of studies delineate the core social-communication deficits associated with ASD, very few studies have documented intervention effects on these core skills. The most widely used outcome measures in group intervention studies with children with ASD are changes in IQ and percentage of children with posttreatment placement in regular classrooms (National Research Council, 2001). Considering the heterogeneity in the social-communication skills of children with ASD, it is important to measure these skills in intervention research in order to adequately describe participants being studied and to document how children with different characteristics respond to different treatments. There have been several studies using single-subject design that have provided systematic evidence of naturalistic behavioral teaching techniques to improve social-communication skills in children with ASD (e.g., Buffington, Krantz, McClannahan, & Poulson, 1998; Hancock & Kaiser, 2002; Hwang & Hughes, 2000; Whalen & Schriebman, 2003) and a recent randomized group design (Aldred, Green, & Adams, 2004). Although it is beyond the scope of this chapter to review intervention research, two recent studies are discussed in detail, one single-subject and one group design, to examine the social-communication measures utilized.

Whalen and Schreibman (2003) implemented a multiple-baseline design study across participants using pivotal response training to target initiating and responding to joint attention in 5 children with ASD ranging from 49 to 52 months of age. They measured social communication in three contexts: (1) unstructured play sample with an experimenter presenting joint-attention probes (showing objects, pointing, shifting gaze) every 30 seconds; (2) structured joint-attention sample with an experimenter using procedures from the ESCS with an adapted scale (*significantly*, *somewhat*, and *not impaired*); and (3) structured laboratory observations with an untrained experimenter and with the caregiver in a generalization setting. Phase 1 of treatment was response training to teach responding to joint-attention bids of the experimenter, and Phase 2 was initiation training to teach initiating joint attention with gaze shifting and pointing. Four assessments were carried out: at baseline, after Phase 1 of treatment, posttreatment, and 3 months following treatment. Response training was effective for all 5 participants, and initiation training was effective for 4 of the 5 participants. It is noteworthy that all of the participants showed some response to joint attention at baseline but minimal or no initiating of joint attention. Response training did not lead to changes in initiation of joint attention. All participants maintained responding to joint attention but decreased initiating joint attention from posttreatment to follow-up. This study demonstrated that changes in joint-attention skills can be systematically taught and documented in children with ASD using structured sampling procedures.

Aldred et al. (2004) implemented a randomized group design with 14 children each in the treatment and control groups ranging from 29 to 60 months of age. Parents of children in the treatment group attended monthly sessions focused on facilitating the children's communication and were asked to spend 30 minutes daily practicing these strategies with their children. The pre- and posttreatment measures included the ADOS, the Vineland Adaptive Behavior Scales, the CDI, the Parenting Stress Index, and a parent–child interaction sample. The sample was a 30-minute unstructured play sample videotaped to measure child communication acts, asynchronous and synchronous parental communication, and shared attention. They found significantly lower ADOS scores in the treatment group, covarying for baseline ADOS score. The treatment group showed higher scores on the Vineland, but this was nonsignificant when covaried for baseline score. The treatment group showed significantly greater improvement on expressive language measured on the CDI, but no difference from the controls in language comprehension. The treatment group showed significantly better outcomes in parental positive synchronous communication and in child communicative acts. There was no significant difference between groups in level of shared attention. This study suggests that significant gains in social communication can be documented by teaching parents how to enhance their children's communication in a cost-effective treatment.

Future research should strive to document meaningful changes that reflect the core social-communication deficits in children with ASD. The research reviewed in this chapter suggests that multiple aspects of joint attention and symbol use should be measured, both to describe the participants and to be used as possible treatment outcomes. Even the most effective treatment studies of children with ASD show variable outcomes (National Research Council, 2001), and a child's social-communication skills before treatment may influence the response to treatment. For example, Bono, Daley, and Sigman (2004) found that the relation between amount of intervention and amount of gain in language for children with ASD depended on their ability to respond to joint attention from others, as well as initial language skills. Systematic measurement of social communication will contribute to our understanding of interactions between treatment and child characteristics. For example, treatments that use adult-directed teaching strategies may be more effective with children who have better skills in responding to joint attention or in language comprehension than with children who are deficient in those skills. Treatments in which the adult synchronizes with the child's attentional focus may be more effective than more directive approaches for children who have limited skills in responding to or initiating joint attention. As we work with younger and younger children, targeting and documenting progress in social-communication skills becomes even more essential, because these skills form the underpinnings of later social competence and enable children to participate more actively and successfully in a variety of learning contexts.

REFERENCES

Aldred, C., Green, J., & Adams, C. (2004). A new social communication intervention for children with autism: Pilot randomized controlled treatment study suggesting effectiveness. *Journal of Child Psychology and Psychiatry, 45,* 1420–1430.

American Psychiatric Association. (1994). *Diagnostic and statistical manual of mental disorders* (4th ed.). Washington, DC: Author.

Bakeman, R., & Adamson, L. (1984). Coordinating attention to people and objects in mother–infant and peer–infant interaction. *Child Development, 55*, 1278–1289.

Baltaxe, C. (1977). Pragmatic deficits in the language of autistic adolescents. *Journal of Pediatric Psychology, 2*, 176–180.

Barnat, S., Klein, P., & Meltzoff, A. (1996). Deferred imitation across changes in context and object: Memory and generalization in 14–month-old infants. *Infant Behavior and Development, 19*, 241–251.

Baron-Cohen, S., Baldwin, D., & Crowson, M. (1997). Do children with autism use the speaker's direction of gaze to crack the code of language? *Child Development, 68*, 48–57.

Bates, E. (1976). *Language and context: The acquisition of pragmatics.* New York: Academic Press.

Bates, E. (1979). *The emergence of symbols: Cognition and communication in infancy.* New York: Academic Press.

Bates, E., O'Connell, B., & Shore, C. (1987). Language and communication in infancy. In J. Osofsky (Ed.), *Handbook of infant development* (pp. 149–203). New York: Wiley.

Bloom, L. (1993). *The transition from infancy to language.* New York: Cambridge University Press.

Bono, M., Daley, T., & Sigman, M. (2004). Relations among joint attention, amount of intervention and language gain in autism. *Journal of Autism and Developmental Disorders, 34*, 495–505.

Bruner, J. (1981). The social context of language acquisition. *Language and Communication, 1*, 155–178.

Bryson, S. (1996). Brief report: Epidemiology of autism. *Journal of Autism and Developmental Disorders, 26*, 165–167.

Buffington, D., Krantz, P., McClannahan, L., & Poulson, C. (1998). Procedures for teaching appropriate gestural communication skills to children with autism. *Journal of Autism and Developmental Disorders, 28*, 535–545.

Butterworth, G. (1995). Origins of mind in perception and action. In C. Moore & P. Dunham (Eds.), *Joint attention: Its origins and role in development* (pp. 29–40). Hillsdale, NJ: Erlbaum.

Carpenter, M., Nagell, K., & Tomasello, M. (1998). Social cognition, joint attention, and communicative competence from 9 to 15 months of age. *Monographs of the Society for Research in Child Development, 63*(4, Serial No. 255).

Carpenter, M., Pennington, B., & Rogers, S. (2002). Interrelations among social-cognitive skills in young children with autism. *Journal of Autism and Developmental Disorders, 32*, 91–106.

Carpenter, M., & Tomasello, M. (2000). Joint attention, cultural learning, and language acquisition: Implications for children with autism. In A. Wetherby & B. Prizant (Eds.), *Autism spectrum disorders: A transactional developmental perspective* (pp. 31–54). Baltimore: Brookes.

Charman, T., Baron-Cohen, S., Swettenham, J., Baird, G., Drew, A., & Cox, A. (2003). Predicting language outcome in infants with autism and pervasive developmental disorder. *International Journal of Language and Communication Disorders, 3*, 265–285.

Charman, T., Drew, A., Baird, C., & Baird, G. (2003). Measuring early language development in preschool children with autism spectrum disorder using the MacArthur Communicative Development Inventory (Infant Form). *Journal of Child Language, 30,* 213–236.

Charman, T., Swettenham, J., Baron-Cohen, S., Cox, A., Baird, G., & Drew, A. (1997). Infants with autism: An investigation of empathy, pretend play, joint attention, and imitation. *Developmental Psychology, 33,* 781–789.

Dale, P., Bates, E., Reznick, J., & Morisset, C. (1989). The validity of a parent report instrument of child language at 20 months. *Journal of Child Language, 16,* 239–249.

Dawson, G., & Adams, A. (1984). Imitation and social responsiveness in autistic children. *Journal of Abnormal Child Psychology, 12,* 209–226.

Dawson, G., Hill, D., Spencer, A., Galpert, L., & Watson, L. (1990). Affective exchanges between young autistic children and their mothers. *Journal of Abnormal Child Psychology, 18,* 335–345.

Dawson, G., Meltzoff, A., Osterling, J., Rinaldi, J., & Brown, E. (1998). Children with autism fail to orient to naturally occurring social stimuli. *Journal of Autism and Developmental Disorders, 28,* 355–379.

DeVellis, R. (2003). *Scale development: Theory and applications* (2nd ed.). Thousand Oaks, CA: Sage.

Eimas, P. (1996). The perception and representation of speech by infants. In J. Morgan & K. Demuth (Eds.), *Signal to syntax: Bootstrapping from speech to grammar in early acquisition* (pp. 25–39). Mahwah, NJ: Erlbaum.

Fenson, L., Dale, P. S., Reznick, J. S., Bates, E., Thal, D., & Pethick, S. J. (1994). Variability in early communicative development. *Monographs of the Society for Research in Child Development, 59*(5), 1–173.

Fenson, L., Dale, P., Reznick, S., Thal, D., Bates, E., Hartung, J., et al. (1993). *MacArthur Communicative Development Inventories: User's guide and technical manual.* San Diego, CA: Singular.

Hancock, T., & Kaiser, A. (2002). The effects of trainer-implemented enhanced milieu teaching on the social communication of children with autism. *Topics in Early Childhood Special Education, 22,* 39–54.

Hwang, B., & Hughes, C. (2000). Increasing early social-communicative skills of preverbal children with autism through social interactive training. *Journal of the Association for Persons with Severe Handicaps, 25,* 18–28.

Joseph, R., Tager-Flusberg, H., & Lord, C. (2002). Cognitive profiles and social-communicative functioning in children with autism spectrum disorder. *Journal of Child Psychology and Psychiatry, 43,* 807–821.

Kasari, C., Sigman, M., Mundy, P., & Yirmiya, N. (1990). Affective sharing in the context of joint attention. *Journal of Autism and Developmental Disorders, 20,* 87–100.

Kjelgaard, M., & Tager-Flusberg, H. (2001). An investigation of language impairment in autism: Implications for genetic subgroups. *Language and Cognitive Processes, 16,* 287–308.

Klin, A., Volkmar, F., Sparrow, S., Cicchetti, D., & Rourke, B. (1995). Validity and neuropsychological characterization of Asperger syndrome. *Journal of Child Psychology and Psychiatry, 36,* 1127–1140.

Leekam, S., Lopez, B., & Moore, C. (2000). Attention and joint attention in preschool children with autism. *Developmental Psychology, 36,* 261–273.

Lieberman, P. (1996). Some biological constraints on the analysis of prosody. In J. Morgan & K. Demuth (Eds.), *Signal to syntax: Bootstrapping from speech to grammar in early acquisition* (pp. 25–39). Mahwah, NJ: Erlbaum.

Lord, C., & Paul, R. (1997). Language and communication in autism. In D. Cohen & F. Volkmar (Eds.), *Handbook of autism and pervasive developmental disorders* (2nd ed., pp. 195–225). New York: Wiley.

Lord, C., Risi, S., & Pickles, A. (2004). Trajectory of language development in autism spectrum disorders. In M. Rice & S. Warren (Eds.), *Developmental language disorders: From phenotypes to etiologies* (pp. 7–29). Mahwah, NJ: Erlbaum.

Loveland, K., & Landry, S. (1986). Joint attention and language in autism and developmental language delay. *Journal of Autism and Developmental Disorders, 16,* 335–349.

McArthur, D., & Adamson, L. B. (1996). Joint attention in preverbal children: Autism and developmental language disorders. *Journal of Autism and Developmental Disorders, 26,* 481–496.

McHale, S., Simeonsson, R., Marcus, L., & Olley, J. (1980). The social and symbolic quality of autistic children's communication. *Journal of Autism and Developmental Disorders, 10,* 299–310.

McLean, J., & Snyder-McLean, L. (1999). *How children learn language.* San Diego, CA: Singular.

Miller, J. F., Sedey, A. L., & Miolo, G. (1995). Validity of parent report measures of vocabulary development for children with Down syndrome. *Journal of Speech and Hearing Research, 38,* 1037–1044.

Morales, M., Mundy, P., & Rojas, J. (1998). Following the direction of gaze and language development in 6-month-olds. *Infant Behavior and Development, 21,* 373–377.

Mundy, P., & Gomes, A. (1998). Individual differences in joint attention skill development in the second year. *Infant Behavior and Development, 21,* 469–482.

Mundy, P., Hogan, A., & Doehring, P. (1996). *A preliminary manual for the Abridged Early Social Communication Scales.* Unpublished manuscript.

Mundy, P., Kasari, C., Sigman, M., & Ruskin, E. (1995). Nonverbal communication and early language acquisition in children with Down syndrome and in normally developing children. *Journal of Speech and Hearing Research, 38,* 157–167.

Mundy, P., Sigman, M., & Kasari, C. (1990). A longitudinal study of joint attention and language development in autistic children. *Journal of Autism and Developmental Disorders, 20,* 115–128.

Mundy, P., Sigman, M., Ungerer, J., & Sherman, T. (1987). Nonverbal communication and play correlates of language development in autistic children. *Journal of Autism and Developmental Disorders, 17,* 349–364.

National Research Council, Committee on Educational Interventions for Children with Autism. (2001). *Educating children with autism.* Washington, DC: National Academies Press.

Prizant, B. M., & Rydell, P. J. (1993). Assessment and intervention considerations for unconventional verbal behavior. In J. Reichle & D. Wacker (Eds.), *Communica-*

tive alternatives to challenging behavior: Integrating functional assessment and intervention strategies (pp. 263–297). Baltimore: Brookes.

Prizant, B. M., Schuler, A. L., Wetherby, A. M., & Rydell, P. R. (1997). Enhancing language and communication: Language approaches. In D. Cohen & F. Volkmar (Eds.), *Handbook of autism and pervasive developmental disorders* (2nd ed., pp. 572–605). New York: Wiley.

Prizant, B. M., & Wetherby, A. M. (1987). Communicative intent: A framework for understanding social-communicative behavior in autism. *Journal of the American Academy of Child Psychiatry, 26,* 472–479.

Rescorla, L., & Alley, A. (2001). Validation of the Language Development Survey (LDS): A parent report tool for identifying language delay in toddlers. *Journal of Speech, Language, and Hearing Research, 44,* 434–445.

Rogers, S., Hepburn, S., Stackhouse, T., & Wehner, E. (2003). Imitation performance in toddlers with autism and those with other developmental disorders. *Journal of Child Psychology and Psychiatry, 44,* 763–781.

Schuler, A. L., & Prizant, B. (1985). Echolalia. In E. Schopler & G. Mesibov (Eds.), *Communication problems in autism* (p. 163–184). New York: Plenum Press.

Seibert, J., Hogan, A., & Mundy, P. (1982). Assessing interactional competencies: The Early Social Communication Scales. *Infant Mental Health Journal, 3,* 244–245.

Sheinkopf, S., Mundy, P., Oller, D. K., & Steffens, M. (2000). Vocal atypicalities of preverbal autistic children. *Journal of Autism and Developmental Disorders, 30,* 345–354.

Sigman, M., Mundy, P., Sherman, T., & Ungerer, J. (1986). Social interactions of autistic, mentally retarded, and normal children and their caregivers. *Journal of Child Psychology and Psychiatry, 27,* 647–656.

Sigman, M., & Ruskin, E. (1999). Continuity and change in the social competence of children with autism, Down syndrome, and developmental delays. *Monographs of the Society for Research in Child Development, 64.*

Sigman, M., & Ungerer, J. (1984). Cognitive and language skills in autistic, mentally retarded and normal children. *Developmental Psychology, 20,* 293–302.

Siller, M., & Sigman, M. (2002). The behaviors of parents of children with autism predict the subsequent development of their children's communication. *Journal of Autism and Developmental Disorders, 32,* 77–89.

Snow, M. E., Hertzig, M. E., & Shapiro, T. (1987). Expressions of emotion in young autistic children. *Journal of the American Academy of Child and Adolescent Psychiatry, 27,* 647–655.

Stager, C., & Werker, J. (1997). Infants listen for more phonetic detail in speech perception than in word-learning tasks. *Nature, 388,* 381–382.

Stern, D. (1985). *The interpersonal world of the infant.* New York: Basic Books.

Stone, W. L., & Caro-Martinez, L. M. (1990). Naturalistic observations of spontaneous communication in autistic children. *Journal of Autism and Developmental Disorders, 20,* 437–453.

Stone, W., Ousley, O., & Littleford, C. (1997). Motor imitation in young children with autism: What's the object? *Journal of Abnormal Child Psychology, 25,* 475–485.

Stone, W., Ousley, O., Yoder, P., Hogan, K., & Hepburn, S. (1997). Nonverbal communication in 2– and 3–year old children with autism. *Journal of Autism and Developmental Disorders, 27,* 677–696.

Tager-Flusberg, H. (1996). Brief report: Current theory and research on language and communication in autism. *Journal of Autism and Developmental Disorders, 26,* 169–178.

Tager-Flusberg, H., Joseph, R., & Folstein, S. (2001). Current directions in research on autism. *Mental Retardation and Developmental Disabilities Research Reviews, 7,* 21–29.

Thal, D. J., O'Hanlon, L., Clemmons, M., & Fralin, L. (1999). Validity of a parent report measure of vocabulary and syntax for preschool children with language impairment. *Journal of Speech, Language, and Hearing Research, 42,* 482–496.

Trevarthen, C., & Hubley, P. (1978). Secondary intersubjectivity: Confidence, confiding and acts of meaning in the first year. In A. Lock (Ed.), *Action, gesture, and symbol: The emergence of language* (pp. 183–229). New York: Academic Press.

Tsao, F., Liu, I I., & Kuhl, P. (2004). Speech perception in infancy predicts language development in the second year of life: A longitudinal study. *Child Development, 75,* 1067–1084.

Venter, A., Lord, C., & Schopler, E. (1992). A follow-up study of high-functioning autistic children. *Journal of Child Psychology and Psychiatry, 33,* 489–507.

Werker, J., & Tees, R. (1999). Influences on infant speech processing: Toward a new synthesis. *Annual Review of Psychology, 50,* 509–535.

Werner, H., & Kaplan, B. (1963). *Symbol formation: An organismic-developmental approach to language and the expression of thought.* New York: Wiley.

Wetherby, A. (1986). The ontogeny of communicative functions in autism. *Journal of Autism and Developmental Disorders, 16,* 295–316.

Wetherby, A. (1991). Profiling pragmatic abilities in children's emerging language. In T. Gallagher (Ed.), *Pragmatics of language* (pp. 249–281). San Diego, CA: College Hill Press.

Wetherby, A , Allen, L , Cleary, J , Kublin, K , & Goldstein, H. (2002). Validity and reliability of the Communication and Symbolic Behavior Scales Developmental Profile with very young children. *Journal of Speech, Language, and Hearing Research, 45,* 1202–1218.

Wetherby, A., Goldstein, H., Cleary, J., Allen, L., & Kublin, K. (2003). Early identification of children with communication disorders: Concurrent and predictive validity of the CSBS Developmental Profile. *Infants and Young Children, 16*(2), 161–174.

Wetherby, A., & Prizant, B. (1993). *Communication and Symbolic Behavior Scales—Normed Edition.* Baltimore: Brookes.

Wetherby, A., & Prizant, B. (2002). *Communication and Symbolic Behavior Scales Developmental Profile—First Normed Edition.* Baltimore: Brookes.

Wetherby, A. M., Prizant, B. M., & Hutchinson, T. (1998). Communicative, socialaffective, and symbolic profiles of young children with autism and pervasive developmental disorder. *American Journal of Speech-Language Pathology, 7,* 79–91.

Wetherby, A., Prizant, B., & Schuler, A. (2000). Understanding the nature of the communication and language impairments. In A. Wetherby & B. Prizant (Eds.), *Autism spectrum disorders: A transactional developmental perspective* (pp. 109–141). Baltimore: Brookes.

Wetherby, A., & Prutting, C. (1984). Profiles of communicative and cognitive-social abilities in autistic children. *Journal of Speech and Hearing Research, 27*, 364–377.

Wetherby, A., Reichle, J., & Pierce, P. (1998). The transition to symbolic communication. In A. Wetherby, S. Warren, & J. Reichle (Eds.), *Transitions in prelinguistic communication* (pp. 197–230). Baltimore: Brookes.

Wetherby, A., Schuler, A., & Prizant, B. (1997). Enhancing language and communication: Theoretical foundations. In D. Cohen & F. Volkmar (Eds.), *Handbook of autism and pervasive developmental disorders* (2nd ed., pp. 513–538). New York: Wiley.

Wetherby, A., Woods, J., Allen, L., Cleary, J., Dickinson, H., & Lord, C. (2004). Early indicators of autism spectrum disorders in the second year of life. *Journal of Autism and Developmental Disorders, 34*, 473–493.

Wetherby, A., Yonclas, D., & Bryan, A. (1989). Communicative profiles of handicapped preschool children: Implications for early identification. *Journal of Speech and Hearing Disorders, 54*, 148–158.

Whalen, C., & Schreibman, L. (2003). Joint attention training for children with autism using behavior modification procedures. *Journal of Child Psychology and Psychiatry, 44*, 456–468.

Williams, E., Reddy, V., & Costall, A. (2001). Taking a closer look at functional play in children with autism. *Journal of Autism and Developmental Disorders, 31*, 67–77.

Williams, J., Whiten, A., & Singh, T. (2004). A systematic review of action imitation in autism spectrum disorder. *Journal of Autism and Developmental Disorders, 34*, 285–299.

Wing, L., Gould, J., Yeates, R. R., & Brierley, L. M. (1977). Symbolic play in severely mentally retarded and autistic children. *Journal of Child Psychology and Psychiatry, 18*, 167–178.

Yoder, P., & Warren, S. (1998). Maternal responsivity predicts the prelinguistic communication intervention that facilitates generalized intentional communication. *Journal of Speech, Language, and Hearing Research, 41*, 1207–1219.

2

Early Diagnosis of Children with Autism Spectrum Disorders

CATHERINE LORD
JENNIFER RICHLER

BACKGROUND

The preschool years are a time of very rapid development. In the second year of life, children begin walking and become able to manipulate objects with much greater dexterity. There is an enormous increase in language and functional understanding; expressive language moves from the first associative labels to the word "explosion" and the emergence of syntax. Imaginative play, more complex social cognition and, concomitantly, independence and autonomy all result in the beginnings of a much more sophisticated understanding of events and social relationships and give a child many more options to initiate actions and interactions in which he or she is interested. It is during this time, between 2 and 4 years, that most children with autism are now identified as having major deficits in social communication, though many parents have noticed differences even in the first year of life (Luyster et al., 2005).

Because typical development proceeds at such a rapid pace, it is not surprising that parents of children with autism spectrum disorders (ASD) often become concerned so early as they witness their children failing to make the rapid gains that would be expected. However, because of the variability within typical development itself, even when slow development or lack of change is recognized, it is difficult to interpret. Fenson et al. (1994), for instance, found that even among typically developing children, the rate of word acquisition varies considerably.

Parents who are concerned about their child's development early on often seek professional advice and diagnosis at this stage (Siegel, Pliner, Eschler, & Elliott, 1988). In order to make a diagnosis on the autism spectrum, clinicians generally rely on diagnostic instruments, both child observation and parent-report measures. Most instruments currently used to diagnose ASD, however, are not ideally suited to the task of identifying these disorders in very young children. Although the criteria for autism were modified in the revised third edition of *Diagnostic and Statistical Manual of Mental Disorders* (DSM-III-R; American Psychiatric Association, 1987) to be more appropriate for younger children, the current diagnostic instruments are still organized primarily with the skills of slightly older preschool-age children in mind. For example, the Autism Diagnostic Interview—Revised (ADI-R; Le Couteur, Lord, & Rutter, 2003), a parent-report measure, focuses on the period between the child's fourth and fifth birthdays, as this is considered the age at which symptoms of ASD are clearest. Some of the questions, however, are not useful for younger children, such as questions about how the child acts in groups of children.

Researchers are currently working to tailor diagnostic instruments to younger children. In addition, and perhaps as a complement to these efforts, it is important to consider other ways in which a clinician can use information about a child's very early development to predict outcomes and plan appropriate intervention. With very young children, many clinicians and researchers are hesitant about anticipating future development on the basis of observations or reports of behaviors that may not be on predictable trajectories. This reluctance is to be respected, given a well-established literature on the effect of expectations and stigmatization on developmental course (see Rosenthal & Jacobson, 1968; Trivette, Dunst, & Hamby, 2004). However, the steep developmental trajectories seen in typical development, particularly in socialization and language, offer an alternative strategy, which is to consider the trajectory of development from the point of concern to a time in the near future as an important piece of information in making a diagnosis. Because of the rapidity of typical development, meaningful comparisons can be made between a child's behavior at points relatively close in time, such as within a month or two. Thus a child's failure to make progress in very early communication or social skills within a relatively brief period of time may be much more valuable information than knowledge about the same behaviors at only one point in time, even the later one. Repeating an observation or a parent report can eliminate much of the day-to-day variation in many behaviors and provide the beginning of a trajectory or trajectories to be compared with those of typical children or children with other kinds of developmental disorders.

The term *trajectory* can also be applied to a child's development over months or years and to shorter-term changes, such as differences in the level of a particular skill before and after instruction or in a child's behavior from one week to the next in response to behavior plans or introduction to a preschool program (Rogers, Herbison, Lewis, Pantone, & Reis, 1986). In studies of the outcomes of children receiving applied behavior analysis, progress within a 3-month period in elicited vocal imitation is considered a milestone (Lord et al., in press-b). The same time period was recommended by the National Research Council Committee for evaluating progress in response to any specific intervention (National Research Council, 2001). Repeated measures over even briefer intervals may be useful when making working hypotheses about an initial diagnosis with very young children, assuming more comprehensive reevaluations after a longer time.

There has been widespread agreement that diagnostic classifications should be based on information from a variety of different sources, such as parent reports, natural or semistructured observations, and standardized testing (Ozonoff, Goodlin-Jones, & Solomon, 2005). In general, these sources of information involve several different medical and research disciplines, such as psychology, developmental pediatrics, child psychiatry, speech and language pathology, special education, and other areas. Although these disciplines differ in perspectives and knowledge bases, they often share implicit notions of discrepancy. For example, one area of focus involves the difference between the social-communication skills of the child with autism and those of other children the same age. Another form of discrepancy is the difference between a child's social-communication abilities and his or her level of functioning in other areas, such as nonverbal problem-solving skills. Using these sources, the clinician puts together information about the child's trajectory of development to propose a particular classification at a given point in time.

In considering a diagnosis of ASD for a very young child, it is important to consider the nature of development both across and within domains. Across different domains, the trajectories or "slopes" of development can vary significantly. For example, most children who begin walking will soon be able to walk many steps. The difference between walking 2 steps and 10 steps is not as great as the difference between a child speaking 2 words and 10 words, because the "slope" of early word use is not as steep as the "slope" of learning to walk. Slopes of development can also differ within a single domain over time. Using the example of language development again, the rate at which a child acquires new words varies across development; the typical child learns only a few words a week between the ages of 12 and 16 months (Fenson et al., 1994) but learns an average of 3.6 words per *day* between 30 months and 6 years (Anglin, 1993).

In a recent study, Charman et al. (2005) found similar variability across and within domains of development in a sample of children diagnosed with autism at age 2 and reassessed at ages 3 and 7. Because of the variability in development both across and within domains, it is difficult to define succinct diagnostic criteria that are appropriate across developmental levels, particularly from preschool to school age, as well as across areas of skills. Instead, diagnostic frameworks for autism have tended to depend on exemplars (e.g., poor eye contact, not offering comfort to others) rather than on continuous quantitative measures.

PURPOSES OF DIAGNOSIS

For many families, the primary purpose in obtaining a diagnosis for a child in preschool or younger is to gain access to services. In many states in the United States, as well as in other countries, a diagnosis is required before families receive access to special funds or treatment programs. Theoretically, this requirement is justified by the belief that a meaningful diagnosis should predict treatment responses. Yet treatments for ASD have been widely marketed that have not yet been shown to be any more effective than equivalent numbers of hours of attention and encouragement. The most well-researched treatments have been shown to be more effective than very minimal or no special treatment (see Aldred, Green, & Adams, 2004; Eikeseth, Smith, Jahr, & Eldevik, 2002). Because we do not know the "active ingredient" behind successful ASD treatments, there is relatively little understanding of whether certain treatments are better than others and, if so, for whom and when (Kasari, 2002). A diagnosis should, however, have implications for the intensity of treatment, for the areas to be addressed, for the needs for particular features (for example, a one-to-one adult-to-child ratio, a deliberate focus on joint attention), and for ways to measure whether a child has met the short- and long-term goals of treatment. One of the most interesting recent observations (see Lord et al., in press-b) is that, in studies that have contrasted two treatments carried out presumably by equally skilled therapists who believe in their approaches, quite different interventions and/or treatments with different goals can result in equal amounts of improvement that are often similar in quality.

Aside from information about response to treatment, a meaningful diagnosis should provide a family with information about anticipated developmental changes in the disorder. For example, a toddler with the social and communication deficits characteristic of autism who does not show restrictive and repetitive behaviors may begin to exhibit these behaviors between the ages of 2 and 4. A diagnosis should also allow the clinician to discuss associated features that are not part of the criteria for the diagnosis (e.g., risk for epilepsy, recurrence risks in siblings) and to make some statements about prognosis, such as that the likelihood of independence is much greater for children with nonverbal IQs over 70 (Howlin, Mawhood, & Rutter, 2000). For parents, a diagnosis within the autism spectrum can also mean some relief from guilt that they have somehow caused their children's problems. The knowledge that there are other families with children who have similar behaviors and who have responded to treatment can offer hope and practical strategies.

Overall, a diagnosis of ASD can be very helpful in generating working hypotheses about the nature of the disorder and ways that intervention can be used to change its course. For example, a preschool child with ASD who has temper tantrums is likely behaving this way, at least in part, because he is unable to make sense of his environment and to appropriately communicate his resulting frustration. This hypothesis predicts that if the child can be helped to better understand what is going to happen and what is expected of him, and if he is given more options to communicate his preferences, tantrums should decline.

DIAGNOSTIC CRITERIA

A diagnosis of autism is based on symptoms in three areas: difficulties in reciprocal social interaction, difficulties in communication, and the presence of restricted and repetitive behaviors or interests. In addition, a formal diagnosis of autism, according to the *Diagnostic and Statistical Manual of Mental Disorders* (DSM-IV; American Psychiatric Association, 1994) and the *International Classification of Diseases* (World Health Organization, 1992) requires that behaviors in the areas related to autism have been observed prior to age 3. Specific subdomains of difficulty within each major domain are listed in the diagnostic criteria.

It is important to note that the subdomains described in an ASD diagnosis are not independent of each other, nor are they additive; some of them, in fact, could arguably be subsumed into others. For example, within the broad category of social interaction, the subdomains involve nonverbal communication, sharing enjoyment, peer interactions, and social reciprocity, the last of which could include all of the previous other subdomains. There is now a considerable amount of evidence suggesting that many of the features of autism described within the social and communication domains overlap (Constantino et al., 2004; Lord, Leventhal, & Cook, 2001). There may be little use in trying to distinguish nonverbal behaviors that are "social" from those that are "communicative." Similarly, there may be little to be gained in making distinctions between atypical conversational ability (which is a DSM-IV/ICD-10 criterion in the communication domain) and difficulties with reciprocal social interaction (a criterion in the social domain).

In contrast to the move to combine the areas of social reciprocity and communication, researchers have recently argued that the third domain, restricted and repetitive behaviors and interests, may be better broken into at least two other areas: (1) insistence on sameness and (2) repetitive behaviors (Cuccaro et al., 2003; Shao et al., 2002; Silverman et al., 2002; Spiker et al., 1994). Researchers have differed as to where within these factors to include other DSM-IV/ICD-10 subdomains of repetitive and restricted behaviors, such as unusual preoccupations, circumscribed interests, compulsive behaviors, interests in parts of objects, and unusual sensory interests. Although this issue has not been completely resolved, several papers emphasizing concordance among relatives suggest that repetitive behaviors are more closely associated with developmental level and level of cognitive impairment than is insistence on sameness, which may be more related to social-communication measures of autism, independent of IQ and developmental level (see Cuccaro et al., 2003; Silverman et al., 2002).

Our understanding of ASD can be considered within a prototype model of the most well-studied, well-defined disorder within the spectrum, autism. In the case of autism, the major diagnostic systems have required a rather arbitrary number of features, including two of four features in reciprocal social interaction specified in DSM-IV and ICD-10; one feature in communication (which can include being nonverbal and failing to compensate for this by other modes of communication); and one example of restricted or repetitive behavior. These criteria were written primarily with school-age children in mind, because at the time these children made up the majority of research participants and a high proportion of diagnostic referrals. Although the criteria in the DSM-III-R and ICD-9 were deliberately modified to better apply to younger and older children and adults, it is still unclear which features are applicable at different ages. For example, difficulty with peers is one of four social subdomains. Although knowledge about a child's interest in other children and response to other children might influence a diagnosis of autism in a 2-year-old child, these difficulties are far less obvious and impairing (and may be less autism-specific) in a 2-year-old than in a 5-year-old.

Various organizations, including Zero to Three and the American Academy of Pediatrics, have proposed criteria for autism and related disorders using somewhat different systems that can be difficult to incorporate into the ICD-10 and DSM-IV systems for characterizing psychiatric disorders in older children. In particular, in the framework outlined by Zero to Three, different diagnoses contain overlapping symptoms, such that it is difficult to know when the same behavior is being described from a different theoretical perspective and when it truly is a different behavior. Also, a particular skill or absence of skill may be described as a single characteristic, when it might be better understood as a product of many different behaviors. An example would be describing a preschool child as "hyperlexic" because his sight reading is very good and his language comprehension is not, without attending to the child's behavior problems or social behaviors; or describing a child as having a "multisystemic developmental disorder" or a "sensory integration dysfunction" because of her reactions to certain noises or strong kinesthetic input, without attending to her difficulties in social behavior and communication.

Finally, in diagnosing ASD, the assumption is that, although the social deficit is the most common and preeminent feature, knowledge about other behaviors often increases specificity and prognostic value. Particularly for preschool children, several studies have reported that a substantial minority of children who later meet criteria for autism are not described by their parents as having restricted or repetitive behaviors at age 2 (Cox et al., 1999; Lord, 1995; Stone, Coonrod, & Ousley, 2000; Stone et al., 1999). The prevalence of restricted and repetitive behaviors and interests changes quite dramatically between 2 and 3 and between 3 and 4 (Moore & Goodson, 2003), suggesting that the diagnostic criteria for children at age 2 may be more effective at predicting later diagnoses if the restricted and repetitive category is not included. On the other hand, our longitudinal data and studies using the Social Responsiveness Scale (Constantino, 2002) suggest that the inclusion of restricted and repetitive behaviors in an overall "measure of severity" for preschool children substantially increases its ability to distinguish between autism and other communication and social impairments (see Bishop & Norbury, 2002). In our study (Lord et al., in press-a), restricted and repetitive behaviors were not present in all 2-year-olds diagnosed with autism, but when they were, children were more likely to continue to have an autism diagnosis at age 9 than children who did not have these behaviors at age 2. These findings suggest that the presence of restricted and repetitive behaviors at a young age tends to be associated with more severe outcomes on the autism spectrum; however, because some of these behaviors are rarely observed at a very young age, their absence at one time does not necessarily indicate that they will never occur.

ROLE OF LANGUAGE

Whereas social interaction and communication may in the end be a single broad area of deficit, a child's current language level and degree of language impairment are additional, separate issues that must be taken into account in any assessment of symptoms. That is, although language level could be considered an independent factor from ASD in the sense that individuals with ASD may range from being nonverbal to being very verbally fluent, language level affects how symptoms are manifested and often affects severity in terms of degree of impairment (Lord & Pickles, 1996; Tager-Flusberg & Joseph, 2003). For example, a child with ASD who has fluent language might reveal an impairment in communication through poor conversational skills, whereas a child with minimal language would be more likely to exhibit communicative impairment through stereotyped speech and echolalia. Thus language level should be considered an important factor to assess, even though language impairment is neither necessary nor sufficient for a diagnosis on the autism spectrum.

In very young children, language delay is a strong indicator of autism. Although delays in spoken language are often the first concern for parents of children with autism, delays in receptive language tend to be more severe (Charman, Drew, Baird, & Baird, 2003) and may well be more uniquely characteristic of autism than delays in expressive language (Mirrett, Bailey, Roberts, & Hatton, 2004; Philofsky, Hepburn, Hayes, Hagerman, & Rogers, 2004), though they are often not recognized by parents and teachers. To observe a delay in receptive language, situations must arise in which a child is clearly attending to another person's speech and trying to understand it when the context does not provide obvious cues (e.g., listening to his or her father talking about his or her mother going to get a pizza). These situations tend to arise only when a child displays socially directed behavior and complex nonverbal communication, skills that are typically lacking in children with autism. As a result, difficulties with receptive language may be easier for parents to detect in a child who displays typical social behavior. It is also understandably difficult for parents to determine whether their child truly understands specific words or whether he or she has learned to decipher the various other cues parents usually provide (e.g., holding up a blanket and pointing to the crib when they say "Time to go night-night"). In order to assess a child's receptive language level, it is often necessary to conduct specific tests in which understanding of words is teased apart from understanding of other forms of communication.

Later, specific patterns of language development—including the presence of delayed echolalia and pronoun reversal; relatively strong expressive language compared with receptive language, at least on standardized tests; and specific features such as odd intonation—become more associated with autism (Tager-Flusberg, Paul, & Lord, 2005). It has also been argued that by school age, there is a subset of children with ASD who show typical features of specific language impairment (SLI), such as shorter utterances, more variable use of word endings, articulation problems, and difficulty with nonword repetition (Rice, Wexler, & Cleave, 1995; Tager-Flusberg et al., 2001). Children with ASD who have much higher nonverbal than verbal IQs by school age also seem to be somewhat different from other children with autism: They show more severe social deficits, larger head circumferences, and a greater number of affected relatives (Tager-Flusberg & Joseph, 2003). Here again, both language level and level of impairment at the time of testing are important to consider; a 5-year-old who has the vocabulary of a 2-year-old is proportionately more impaired than a 3-year-old with the same vocabulary level. Both degree of language impairment and current language level are factors associated with the severity of other symptoms, particularly social deficits (Lord & Pickles, 1996). Other factors that differentiate preschool children with autism who can talk from those who cannot—at least in terms of the kinds of goals and methods one would use in teaching them—include imagination, the presence of certain kinds of rituals, and "paralinguistic" abnormalities, such as odd intonation, all of which are harder to measure in children who cannot talk.

Our recent analysis of longitudinal data suggests that an important distinction may exist between children who have language fluent enough so that they use five or more words within the context of a 30- to 40-minute observation and children who are completely nonverbal or have only a few words (Gotham, Risi, Pickles, & Lord, 2005). Many social-communicative behaviors, such as the frequency of gesture, were found to be strongly associated with this relatively gross measure of language level.

DIAGNOSTIC INSTRUMENTS

Child Observation Measures

A number of diagnostic instruments exist that can be used to assess ASD in preschool-age children. Probably the most common observational instruments used in clinical assessments are the Childhood Autism Rating Scale (CARS; Schopler, Reichler, & Renner, 1988) and the Autism Diagnostic Observation Schedule (ADOS; Lord et al., 2000). The CARS (Schopler et al., 1988), a well-documented description of autism, is particularly useful in discriminating children with autism who also have mild to moderate retardation from children with other disorders, although having slightly higher thresholds (even as many as 3 points) can produce greater specificity for young preschool children (Lord, 1991).

In general, interrater reliability on these instruments has been as strong for preschool children as for older children. Test–retest data based on small samples have indicated adequate reliability over time. However, particularly with the ADOS, because the instrument attempts to make a distinction between broadly defined ASD and a more narrowly defined autism, the standard error results in shifts over diagnostic lines (from autism to

ASD and vice versa) quite frequently when scores are compared across time or raters. Moreover, because the ADOS uses four modules with different tasks and screening codes to decrease the effect of language level on diagnosis, a child who experiences gains in language will likely advance to a higher module that has more difficult social and communicative demands. If the child's strides in language are not accompanied by similarly large gains in social and communication skills, the child could appear more severely autistic when assessed with the more advanced module. In contrast, a child who shows slow gains in language skills (or no gains at all) will likely not change modules and, as a result, may show a change in diagnostic category, particularly from autism to pervasive developmental disorder not otherwise specified, because of the eventual acquisition of very basic skills.

The Communication and Symbolic Behavior Scales (CSBS; Wetherby & Prizant, 2003), the Early Social Communication Scales (ESCS; Mundy, Hogan, & Doehring, 1996) and the Screening Tool for Autism in Two-Year-Olds (STAT; Stone et al., 2000; Stone, Coonrod, Turner, & Pozdol, 2004) are three scales that assess various aspects of social communication in preschool children. Although all three overlap with the ADOS, the STAT and the CSBS are much easier than the ADOS to administer, and the STAT is easier to score, so that each of these instruments can be very useful in describing social-communicative behavior. However, they are all limited by the "ceiling" effect that the ADOS module system is intended to address. That is, they are not intended to measure ASD severity across a wide span of development, and so they may underestimate deficits in high-functioning preschool children.

Parent-Report Measures

Gathering information from the child's parent(s) or guardian(s) can often be useful to a clinician in making a diagnosis, particularly in getting more information about the child's acquisition of early developmental milestones. The most widely used parent-report measure is the aforementioned Autism Diagnostic Interview—Revised (Le Couteur et al., 2003). The ADI-R is a semistructured parent interview that provides scores in three areas: communication, reciprocal social interaction, and restricted and repetitive behaviors, as well as separate algorithms for verbal and nonverbal children. Although the ADI-R has been found to have good reliability and validity (Le Couteur et al., 2003), the currently used algorithms tend to overdiagnose ASD in children with nonverbal mental ages of less than 2 years or with severe to profound mental retardation.

The Vineland Adaptive Behavior Scales (VABS; Sparrow, Balla, & Cicchetti, 1984; see also Sparrow, Cicchetti, & Balla, 2005) gather information from the parent about the child's everyday adaptive functioning. Although the VABS is not used to diagnose ASD directly, it can be used in conjunction with parent-report measures such as the ADI-R to help the clinician form more specific diagnostic impressions and provide the parent with recommendations for intervention (Paul et al., 2004).

In an attempt to diagnose ASD as early as possible, researchers have also begun to develop instruments designed to screen for ASD in very young children; these include the aforementioned STAT (Stone et al., 2000) and CSBS (Wetherby & Prizant, 2003), the CHecklist for Autism in Toddlers (CHAT; Baird et al., 2000), and the Modified CHecklist for Autism in Toddlers (M-CHAT; Robins, Fein, Barton, & Green, 2001). These instruments are discussed in other chapters in this volume (see Charman & Baron-Cohen, Chapter 3; Zwaigenbaum & Stone, Chapter 4).

Although the items on the instruments described here are generally reliable with young children, even down to toddlers, diagnostic algorithm cutoffs based on data for older preschoolers are not necessarily appropriate for children either at younger ages or at lower stages of development. Thus it has been recommended that children with nonverbal age equivalents of less than 18 or 24 months not be judged by the standard ADI-R algorithm (Le Couteur et al., 2003). Though item scores may be quite reliable and group differences between children with and without autism may be significant, specificity—that is, the extent to which the algorithm identifies children with autism and does not identify children with other disorders—will likely be compromised (Le Couteur et al., 2003; Lord, Storoschuk, Rutter, & Pickles, 1993). Similarly, for the ADOS, it is recommended that the standard algorithms be used only with children who are walking and children who have nonverbal age equivalents of 12 months or more. Again, with children who can walk but whose nonverbal age equivalents are under a year, interrater reliability has been found to be quite good (see Lord et al., 2000), but research has suggested that there is a greater chance of overdiagnosis at younger developmental levels (Philofsky et al., 2004). For example, recent results from several studies have indicated that children with fragile-X syndrome younger than 24 months often met ADOS criteria for ASD, even when clinical diagnoses did not place them within this category (Bailey, Hatton, Skinner, & Mesibov, 2001; Rogers, Wehner, & Hagerman, 2001).

ISSUES IN DIAGNOSING ASD IN VERY YOUNG CHILDREN

There are many issues that affect how a clinician gets information leading to a diagnosis of ASD in preschool children that are different from those relevant to children who are older or have other disorders. Because ASD is defined by social and communication difficulties, it is important that the clinician observe the child in contexts in which some fairly predictable, well-defined social behaviors can be expected. These contexts are not always easily available in an office visit; instead, the child is often observed while his parents are talking to a clinician, or in a waiting room or playroom—situations that may not be sufficiently structured for a clinician to reach any strong conclusions. In order for a clinician to make reasonable judgments about social behavior in a preschool child, the child needs to be engaged in an activity that is fun and creative and that contains opportunities for that child to make initiations, as well as to respond to the examiner. A number of diagnostic and descriptive instruments, including the aforementioned CSBS (Wetherby & Prizant, 2003), the ESCS (Mundy et al., 1986), and the ADOS (Lord et al., 2000), all attempt to do this by including communicative "temptations" (Wetherby & Prizant, 1998) or "presses" (Lord et al., 2000). These situations allow the examiner to assess reciprocal social interaction in "obligatory contexts" for social behavior (e.g., the examiner directs the child's attention to an object of interest) but also to move beyond these structured situations by giving the child the opportunity to initiate and respond to social overtures spontaneously. Trying to establish shared enjoyment is also an important strategy, particularly for older preschool children, who are usually more familiar than toddlers with carrying out tasks with a friendly but unfamiliar adult.

Another critical factor is the duration of the assessment. Without enough time, the examiner may be able to make only a few brief observations and as a result may be unable to observe subtleties in a child's behavior and difficulties that may have greater implications in less structured or more child-centered situations. With too much time, the child may become bored and frustrated. In addition, the child's physical position and activity level can affect his or her social behavior in a number of ways; for example, it is difficult for a toddler to give or show objects to a parent if he or she is seated in a high chair with limited mobility or to play with toys creatively if he or she is in constant motion.

There are aspects of parent-report diagnostic interviews that are also specific to preschool years. In particular, parents of firstborn children may have had relatively little exposure to young children and therefore may not realize that most children behave differently than their child does (De Giacomo & Fombonne, 1998). There are certain prosocial behaviors that are expected by age 2, such as offering comfort and sharing enjoyment, that parents may not be aware of and therefore may not notice. Furthermore, many children who are 3 years of age or younger may not have regular interactions with peers, except perhaps a younger or older sibling. There is also quite a lot of variability in peer interactions in very young typically developing children (see Hartup, 1983). Another issue is that parents may interpret questions about eye contact, facial expression, gestures, and intonation as applying to their child at his or her most communicative. Most preschool children, even the most autistic preschool child, have moments when they truly are indistinguishable from other children. It is important to convey gently to parents that unless otherwise specified, the interview is intended to assess their child's social and communicative behavior on a typical day. Further complicating matters is the fact that parents, particularly those of preschool children who do not have contact with classmates or a school curriculum, may understandably avoid situations in which their child is likely to be upset or unable to cope, so that the parent is unable to describe how the child adjusts to a particular challenge. In addition, the issues about which many parents of children with ASD are concerned, such as sleep, eating, and temper tantrums, are not unique to autism, and so are omitted from many standard diagnostic evaluations, even though they are very important to parents.

Although we can describe the social behavior in children with autism based on observations and interviews, the field has not yet been very good at quantifying the severity of social deficits. Tests that describe themselves as measures of social reciprocity, such as the Social Responsiveness Scale (Constantino, 2002) and the Social Communication Questionnaire (Rutter, Bailey, Lord, & Berument, 2003), often include a number of questions about restricted and repetitive behaviors along with social behavior and have not been used regularly with children under 4. In quantifying abnormalities within social communication, it is often unclear whether one should be calculating the occurrence of normal behaviors, the "frequency" of the absence of such behaviors, the proportion of "normal" versus "abnormal" behaviors, or the probability of a social response in a particular context. How children may compensate for difficulties or "repair" interactions that have not been successful are also important issues for designing treatment programs and for understanding autism. Various strategies for making these codings (e.g., in vivo, on videotapes, through parent questionnaires or interviews) all affect the quality of information available to the clinician or researcher. For example, overall interrater reliability for videotaped ADOS administrations has been found to be as high as for two live observations, but it was reduced for repetitive behaviors, in part because what the observers saw live was somewhat different from what they saw on videotape (Lord, Rutter, DiLavore, & Risi, 1999).

DIFFERENTIAL DIAGNOSIS

Many years ago, it was hoped that disorders on the autism spectrum could be distinguished from other developmental disorders primarily on the basis of deviance from typical development and the presence of behaviors that were not appropriate at any stage of development, with general developmental delay treated as a completely separate dimension. However, many specific studies of particular behaviors have indicated that the absence or limited nature of typical development, particularly in social skills, may be just as important as, if not more important than, the presence of abnormalities such as stereotyped movements or unusual repetitive behaviors in distinguishing autism from other developmental disorders (Charman & Baird, 2002; Mundy & Sigman, 1989; Paul et al., 2004).

Developmental testing can help the examiner distinguish between ASD and other developmental disorders; through a careful cognitive assessment, it is possible to determine whether the child's behavior is consistent with generally impaired functioning or whether the child shows specific social and communication deficits that go beyond level of functioning. For example, a 4-year-old child who does not participate in a pretend birthday party in a standard diagnostic assessment would not necessarily raise a "red flag" for autism if the child appeared to be generally functioning at a 12-month-old level; however, the same behavior in 4-year-old who was assessed on cognitive tasks as functioning closer to age level would evoke some concern about autism.

This issue is made more significant by the fact that the alternative diagnoses that are ruled out when autism is considered differ across ages and developmental levels. The most common alternative diagnoses made in toddlers are language delay and unspecified developmental delay. More specific disorders, such as learning disabilities, generalized anxiety disorder, and reactive attachment disorder, can be more confidently identified as an alternative in later preschool years, and attention-deficit/hyperactivity disorder is the most common alternative in the early school years (Bishop & Lord, 2006; Lord et al., 1999, 2000; Rutter & Lord, 1987; Schopler & Mesibov, 1988; Watson & Marcus, 1988). Many clinics have also reported a new cadre of referrals in later school age that consist of children with increasingly obvious social difficulties, particularly at school, who have had numerous diagnoses in the past and are being referred for Asperger syndrome or high-functioning autism.

For preschool-age children, the primary diagnostic distinction *within* the autism spectrum is usually between a narrow diagnosis of autism and a broader diagnosis of "almost autism," referred to as atypical autism, pervasive developmental disorder not otherwise specified (PDDNOS), or autism spectrum disorder (which would include all of the preceding). There is little information concerning the reliability over time or across raters within or across sites, even though these distinctions are included in formal diagnostic manuals. For a diagnosis of PDDNOS, DSM-IV-TR (American Psychiatric Association, 2000) requires that a child must have social deficits and additional difficulties either in communication or repetitive behaviors (or both, but falling subthreshold on at least one) or must fail to meet onset criteria.

In reality, if these criteria were interpreted literally, most children with any kind of behavior disorder would probably be labeled PDDNOS. For instance, children with ADHD often have trouble with peers and may not carry on conversations well, both of which are possible criteria for a diagnosis of PDDNOS (Barkley, 1998). Buitelaar, Van de Gaag, Klin, and Volkmar (1999) found that several ICD-10/DSM-IV items discriminated significantly between PDDNOS and nonspectrum disorders, including eye gaze, lack of reciprocity, repetitive use of language, and selective social interaction before the age of 3. Such findings, however, are not reflected in the current diagnostic criteria for PDDNOS. There is an assumption in the DSM-IV and ICD-10, it seems, that there is an as yet undefined qualitative difference between children within the spectrum and without. There is much argument about whether this undefined qualitative dimension is important and merits further investigation, is clinically useful but difficult to establish empirically, or is part of a shared clinician–researcher–parent myth that reflects more art than science.

Aside from the three terms that are used generally and often interchangeably to mean "almost autism," there is Asperger syndrome. According to the diagnostic manuals, Asperger syndrome should be diagnosed only when a child does not meet criteria for autism and has not had a language or cognitive delay (American Psychiatric Association, 1994; World Health Organization, 1992). Because most children referred at very young ages have language or other delays, even though they may eventually be remediated, diagnosing Asperger syndrome in young children is quite controversial. Adding to the controversy, many clinicians and some researchers use the term *Asperger syndrome* to describe combinations of symptoms quite specific to their own groups, such as children with autism who are clumsy but bright, children with severe social deficits who have strong verbal but poor nonverbal problem-solving skills, and children who have social deficits that are milder than those of children with autism (see Ozonoff, South, & Miller, 2000; Volkmar et al., 1996; Wing, 1981).

Childhood disintegrative disorder and Rett syndrome are the other pervasive developmental disorders within the DSM-IV system. These conditions are both quite rare. Their diagnoses are, in part, based on their different trajectories of development, as well as on a particular genetic profile, in the case of Rett syndrome (Kerr, 2002).

DEVELOPMENTAL TRAJECTORIES

The majority of children diagnosed with ASD show signs of atypical development starting in infancy. However, somewhere between one-quarter and one-third of parents of children with ASD report that their children initially appeared to be developing normally or near normally and then experienced a regression, most often between 13 and 24 months of age (Davidovitch, Glick, Holtzman, Tirosh, & Safir, 2000; Goldberg et al., 2003). This phenomenon seems to be relatively specific to autism, although it has been reported anecdotally to occur in disorders defined by anatomical abnormalities, such as agenesis of the corpus callosum, as well as in Landau–Kleffner syndrome, a neurological disorder, also called acquired epileptic aphasia (Mouridsen, 1995; Shinnar et al., 2001). Rett syndrome and childhood disintegrative disorder, both considered pervasive developmental disorders, are also partly defined by the presence of a regression.

On the basis of detailed retrospective accounts and access to early videotapes, researchers have found that children with ASD who experience a regression tend to have more early social and communicative skills than do children who do not lose skills (see Goldberg et al., 2003; Luyster et al., 2005). Table 2.1 compares the early social-communication skills of children with ASD who later experienced a regression (either in language or in other social communication skills) with those of children with ASD and no regression. A modified version of the Communicative Development Inventory (CDI; Fenson, 1989), a parent-report measure, was used to assess children's early social-communicative skills.

Although this sounds obvious (in that one would have to have the skills in order to lose them), when the preloss skills of children who later have regressions are compared with those of typically developing children, the former are described as having fewer skills than the latter (Richler et al., in press). Thus children with ASD and regression have more early social-communication skills than children with ASD and no regression but fewer early skills than typical children. There is also some evidence that, at least in the short term, children with ASD and regression have poorer social and communicative outcomes than children with ASD and no regression (Brown & Prelock, 1995; Kobayashi & Murata, 1998; Kurita, 1996). However, findings on long-term outcomes for children with ASD and regression remain unclear (Lord, Shulman, & DiLavore, 2004).

Although theoretical papers and some empirical studies have suggested relationships between regression and various phenomena, including seizures, at this point there is relatively little data showing such connections to various biological phenomena once recruitment effects are controlled for (Shinnar et al., 2001; Tuchman & Rapin, 1997). Although some researchers, several years ago, argued for an association between ASD and the measles–mumps–rubella vaccine, several population studies have found no evidence for such a connection (Dales, Hammer, & Smith, 2001; Fombonne & Chakrabarti, 2001; Kaye, del Mar Melero-Montes, & Jick, 2001; Madsen et al., 2002; Taylor et al., 2002). There have, however, been some findings suggesting that regression in ASD may be associated with parental reports of immune disorders within the family (Molloy et al., in press), as well as

TABLE 2.1. Reported Skill Mastery at 24 Months by Loss Group

Mean number of behaviors at 24 months by modified CDI section	NR (n = 188)	NWL-R (n = 38)	WL (n = 125)
Prespeech behaviors	5.21[a, b] (2.61)	7.13 (1.68)	7.07 (2.16)
Games and routines	3.32[a, b] (2.05)	4.39 (1.70)	4.50 (1.98)
Actions with objects	5.11[a] (3.08)	6.11 (3.22)	6.30 (2.62)
First communicative gestures	3.79[a, b] (2.76)	6.03 (2.73)	5.62 (2.83)
Phrase comprehension	9.79[a, b] (6.98)	13.00 (5.95)	13.94 (5.54)
Words understood only	5.92 (5.24)	6.18 (5.11)	6.94 (4.87)
Words understood and said	7.20[a] (6.81)	8.79 (6.61)	9.26 (5.62)

Note. NR, no regression; NWL-R, children who did not meet criteria for word loss but lost other social communication skills; WL, word loss. From Luyster et al. (2005). Copyright 2005 by Lawrence Erlbaum Associates, Inc. Reprinted by permission.

[a]Lower than WL group, $p < .006$.

[b]Lower than NWL-R group, $p < .006$.

parent reports of the children having histories of gastrointestinal problems (Richler et al., in press). It is important to note, however, that parent reports in these studies have not been corroborated by official medical records or biological assays; such studies are under way.

At this point, there is not a well-defined biological phenotype of regression, even though the phenomenon of regression itself seems to be occurring in quite similar ways across children. Further research, particularly in the form of prospective studies, will attempt to focus on individual trajectories among children with ASD and regression in order to assess heterogeneity in this group and to look for further associations with biological phenomena.

As discussed earlier, identifying trajectories of development may be quite helpful in making diagnoses. In general, research comparing diagnoses made by experienced clinicians for children at 2 years of age with diagnoses made by the same clinicians several years later and/or with diagnoses made by standardized measures such as the ADI-R (Le Couteur et al., 2003) and the ADOS (Lord et al., 2000) suggest that classifications of autism at age 2 are quite stable. On the other hand, much less stability has been described for diagnoses of atypical autism or PDDNOS (see Cox et al., 1999; Eaves & Ho,

2004; Lord, 1995; Stone et al., 1999, 2000). In a recent longitudinal study, we found that about half of the children in our sample who were identified as having PDDNOS or autism under age 3, when there were high levels of uncertainty on the part of the clinicians, had diagnoses of autism by age 3 that were stable until age 9. However, the remaining children were as likely to receive nonspectrum diagnoses by age 9 as they were to maintain diagnoses of PDDNOS (Lord, 1995; Lord et al., in press-a).

It is not entirely clear which measures of development and functioning are the strongest predictors of outcome in children with ASD. There is a general myth in the field of autism that the years up until age 5 constitute a "critical period" for the development of language. In general, this phenomenon is supported primarily by studies that used language at age 5 as a predictor of later language, without considering other options (such as language at age 3 or 4 or 7; Lockyer & Rutter, 1970; Venter, Lord, & Schopler, 1992). In addition, it has been proposed that children with nonverbal IQs under 50 have little chance of independence as adults. It has recently been proposed that, in reality, the threshold for possible independence should be raised to 70 (Howlin, Goode, Hutton, & Rutter, 2004). It is unclear at what point nonverbal IQs become sufficiently stable to make such a prediction, but several studies have shown that verbal and nonverbal IQs and other standard language measures administered as young as age 2 can predict how the same children will do at age 5, specifically in the areas of adaptive functioning, independence, and comorbidity with other psychiatric disorders (Thurm, Lord, Lee, & Newschaffer, 2005; Venter et al., 1992).

In addition, early intervention, now available to at least some children at age 2 or even younger, may affect the best age for making predictions about language development. For example, a child who is 3 years of age and has been in intensive treatment for 2 years but has not learned any words may be in quite a different situation than a child who receives treatment for the first time at age 3. In other words, success of intervention depends in part on what treatment the child has previously received and how effective this treatment was. Predictions from early preschool to later school age and adulthood may not be as strong for children who begin to receive intensive intervention only when they enter formal education as they are for children who have received earlier intensive intervention.

CONCLUSION

In order for clinicians to be able to provide accurate early diagnoses of ASD, to predict possible developmental trajectories, and to make appropriate recommendations for intervention, researchers must determine how best to identify children with ASD at a young age. This means identifying the most specific and reliable early signs of ASD. In order to describe these early indicators of ASD, researchers must have a good understanding of typical development, including not only the typical ages at which developmental milestones are achieved but also the ways in which typical development can vary from child to child. They must also consider the kinds of trajectories one might expect to see both across different skill areas and over time.

In searching for these early signs of ASD, researchers must look not only at early social and communicative development but also at other ways in which, from very early on, development in children with ASD differs from typical development. One exciting new area of research, for example, is early brain development in children with ASD. A recent paper by Courchesne, Carper, and Akshoomoff (2003) reported that in the first year of life, children with ASD, on average, experienced accelerated head growth relative to typically developing children. Hopefully, as we begin to uncover and confirm or disconfirm more of these early indicators of ASD, we will not only deepen our understanding of the etiology and developmental course of the disorder but will also be able to identify "at risk" children from the earliest age, so that we can closely monitor their development and provide appropriate intervention.

REFERENCES

Aldred, C., Green, J., & Adams, C. (2004). A new social communication intervention for children with autism: Pilot randomized controlled treatment study suggesting effectiveness. *Journal of Child Psychology and Psychiatry and Allied Disciplines, 45*(8), 1420–1430.

American Psychiatric Association. (1987). *Diagnostic and statistical manual of mental disorders* (3rd ed., rev. ed.). Washington, DC: Author.

American Psychiatric Association. (1994). *Diagnostic and statistical manual of mental disorders* (4th ed.). Washington, DC: Author.

American Psychiatric Association. (2000). *Diagnostic and statistical manual of mental disorders* (4th ed., text rev.). Washington, DC: Author.

Anglin, J. (1993). Vocabulary development: A morphological analysis. *Monographs of the Society for Research in Child Development, 58*(10), 1–166.

Bailey, D. B., Hatton, D., Skinner, M., & Mesibov, G. (2001). Autistic behavior, FMR-1 protein, and developmental trajectories in young males with fragile X syndrome. *Journal of Autism and Developmental Disorders, 31*, 165–174.

Baird, G., Charman, T., Baron-Cohen, S., Cox, A., Swettenham, J., Wheelwright, S., & Drew, A. (2000). A screening instrument for autism at 18 months of age: A 6-year follow-up study. *Journal of the American Academy of Child and Adolescent Psychiatry, 39*(6), 694–702.

Barkley, R. A. (1998). *Attention-deficit/hyperactivity disorder: A handbook for diagnosis and treatment* (2nd ed.). New York: Guilford Press.

Bishop, D. V., & Norbury, C. F. (2002). Exploring the borderlands of autistic disorder and specific language impairment: A study using standardized diagnostic instruments. *Journal of Child Psychology and Psychiatry and Allied Disciplines, 43*(7), 917–929.

Bishop, S. L., & Lord, C. (2006). Assessment and diagnosis of preschoolers with autism spectrum disorders. In J. L. Luby (Ed.), *Handbook of preschool mental health*. New York: Guilford Press.

Brown, J., & Prelock, P. A. (1995). Brief report: The impact of regression on language development in autism. *Journal of Autism and Developmental Disorders, 25*(3), 305–309.

Buitelaar, J. K., Van der Gaag, R., Klin, A., & Volkmar, F. (1999). Exploring the boundaries of pervasive developmental disorder not otherwise specified: Analyses of data from the DSM-IV autistic disorder field trial. *Journal of Autism and Developmental Disorders, 29*(1), 33–43.

Charman, T., & Baird, G. (2002). Practitioner review: Diagnosis of autism spectrum disorder in 2- and 3-year-old children. *Journal of Psychology and Psychiatry and Allied Disciplines, 43*(3), 289–305.

Charman, T., Drew, A., Baird, C., & Baird, G. (2003). Measuring early language development in preschool children with autism spectrum disorder using the MacArthur Communicative Development Inventory (Infant Form). *Journal of Child Language, 30*(1), 213–236.

Charman, T., Taylor, E., Drew, A., Cockerill, H., Brown, J.-A., & Baird, G. (2005). Outcome at 7 years of children diagnosed with autism at age 2: Predictive validity of assessments conducted at 2 and 3 years of age and pattern of symptom change over time. *Journal of Child Psychology and Psychiatry, 46*(5), 500–513.

Constantino, J. N. (2002). *The Social Responsiveness Scale*. Los Angeles: Western Psychological Services.

Constantino, J. N., Gruber, C. P., Davis, S., Hayes, S., Passanante, N., & Przybeck, T. (2004). The factor structure of autistic traits. *Journal of Child Psychology and Psychiatry, 45*(4), 719.

Courchesne, E., Carper, R., & Akshoomoff, N. A. (2003). Evidence of brain overgrowth in the first year of life in autism. *Journal of the American Medical Association, 290*(3), 337–344.

Cox, A., Klein, K., Charman, T., Baird, G., Baron-Cohen, S., Swettenham, J., et al. (1999). Autism spectrum disorders at 20 and 42 months of age: Stability of clinical and ADI-R diagnosis. *Journal of Child Psychology and Psychiatry and Allied Disciplines, 40*(5), 719–732.

Cuccaro, M. L., Shao, Y., Grubber, J., Slifer, M., Wolpert, C. M., Donnelly, S. L., et al. (2003). Factor analysis of restricted and repetitive behaviors in autism using the Autism Diagnostic Interview—R. *Child Psychiatry and Human Development, 34*(1), 3–17.

Dales, L., Hammer, S. J., & Smith, N. J. (2001). Time trends in autism and in MMR immunization coverage in California. *Journal of the American Medical Association, 285*(9), 1183–1185.

Davidovitch, M., Glick, L., Holtzman, G., Tirosh, E., & Safir, M. P. (2000). Developmental regression in autism: Maternal perception. *Journal of Autism and Developmental Disorders, 30*(2), 113–119.

De Giacomo, A., & Fombonne, E. (1998). Parental recognition of developmental abnormalities in autism. *European Child and Adolescent Psychiatry, 7*(3), 131–136.

Eaves, L. C., & Ho, H. H. (2004). The very early identification of autism: Outcome to age 4½–5. *Journal of Autism and Developmental Disorders, 34*(4), 367–378.

Eikeseth, S., Smith, T., Jahr, E., & Eldevik, S. (2002). Intensive behavioral treatment at school for 4- to 7-year-old children with autism: A 1-year comparison controlled study. *Behavior Modification, 26*(1), 49–68.

Fenson, L. (1989). *The MacArthur Communicative Development Inventory: Infant and Toddler Versions*. San Diego: San Diego State University.

Fenson, L., Dale, P. S., Reznick, J. S., Bates, E., Thal, D., & Pethick, S. (1994). Variability in early communicative development. *Monographs of the Society for Research in Child Development, 59*(5), 1–173.

Fombonne, E., & Chakrabarti, S. (2001). No evidence for a new variant of measles–mumps–rubella–induced autism. *Pediatrics, 108*, e58.

Goldberg, W. A., Osann, K., Filipek, P. A., Laulhere, T., Jarvis, K., Modahl, C., Flodman, P., & Spence, M. A. (2003). Language and other regression: Assessment and timing. *Journal of Autism and Developmental Disorders, 33*(6), 607–616.

Gotham, K., Risi, S., Pickles, A., & Lord, C. (2005). *The Autism Diagnostic Observation Schedule (ADOS): Revised algorithms for improved diagnostic validity*. Manuscript submitted for publication.

Hartup, W. W. (1983). Peer relations. In E. M Hetherington & P. H. Mussen (Eds.), *Handbook of child psychology, Vol. 4: Socialization, personality and social development* (4th ed., pp. 103–196). New York: Wiley.

Howlin, P., Goode, S., Hutton, J., & Rutter, M. (2004). Adult outcome for children with autism. *Journal of Child Psychology and Psychiatry, 45*, 212–229

Howlin, P., Mawhood, L., & Rutter, M. (2000). Autism and developmental receptive language disorder: A follow-up comparison in early adult life: II. Social, behavioral, and psychiatric outcomes. *Journal of Child Psychology and Psychiatry and Allied Disciplines, 41*(5), 561–578.

Kasari, C. (2002). Assessing change in early intervention programs for children with autism. *Journal of Autism and Developmental Disorders, 32*(5), 447–461.

Kaye, J. A., del Mar Melero-Montes, M., & Jick, H. (2001). Mumps, measles, and rubella vaccine and the incidence of autism recorded by general practitioners: A time trend analysis. *British Medical Journal, 322*(7284), 460–463.

Kerr, A. (2002). Annotation: Rett Syndrome: Recent progress and implications for research and clinical practice. *Journal of Child Psychology and Psychiatry, 43*(3), 277–287.

Kobayashi, R., & Murata, T. (1998). Setback phenomenon in autism and long-term prognosis. *Acta Psychiatrica Scandinavica, 98*(4), 296–303.

Kurita, H. (1996). Specificity and developmental consequences of speech loss in children with pervasive developmental disorders. *Psychiatry and Clinical Neurosciences, 50*(4), 181–184.

Le Couteur, A., Lord, C., & Rutter, M. (2003). *The Autism Diagnostic Interview—Revised*. Los Angeles: Western Psychological Services.

Lockyer, L., & Rutter, M. (1970). A five- to fifteen-year follow-up study of infantile psychosis: IV. Patterns of cognitive ability. *British Journal of Social and Clinical Psychology, 9*(2), 152–163.

Lord, C. (1991). Methods and measures of behavior in the diagnosis of autism and related disorders. *Psychiatric Clinics of North America, 14*(1), 69–80.

Lord, C. (1995). Follow-up of two-year-olds referred for possible autism. *Journal of Child Psychology and Psychiatry and Allied Disciplines, 36*(8), 1365–1382.

Lord, C., Leventhal, B. L., & Cook, E. H., Jr. (2001). Quantifying the phenotype in autism spectrum disorders. *American Journal of Medical Genetics, 105*(1), 36–38.

Lord, C., & Pickles, A. (1996). Language level and nonverbal social-communicative behaviors in autistic and language-delayed children. *Journal of the American Academy of Child and Adolescent Psychiatry, 35*(11), 1542–1550.

Lord, C., Risi, S., DiLavore, P., Shulman, C., Thurm, A., & Pickles, A. (in press-a). Autism from two to nine. *Archives of General Psychiatry*.

Lord, C., Risi, S., Lambrecht, L., Cook, E. H., Leventhal, B. L., DiLavore, P. C., et al. (2000). The Autism Diagnostic Observation Schedule—Generic: A standard measure of social and communication deficits associated with the spectrum of autism. *Journal of Autism and Developmental Disorders, 30*(3), 205–223.

Lord, C., Rutter, M., DiLavore, P., & Risi, S. (1999). *Autism Diagnostic Observation Schedule—WPS*. Los Angeles, CA: Western Psychological Services.

Lord, C., Shulman, C., & DiLavore, P. (2004). Regression and word loss in autistic spectrum disorders. *Journal of Child Psychology and Psychiatry and Allied Disciplines, 45*(5), 936–955.

Lord, C., Storoschuk, S., Rutter, M., & Pickles, A. (1993). Using the ADI-R to diagnose autism in preschool children. *Infant Mental Health Journal, 14*(3), 234–252.

Lord, C., Wagner, A., Rogers, S., Szatmari, P., Aman, M., Charman, T., et al. (in press-b). Challenges in evaluating psychosocial interventions for autistic spectrum disorders. *Journal of Autism and Developmental Disorders*.

Luyster, R., Richler, J., Risi, S., Hsu, W. L., Dawson, G., Bernier, R., et al. (2005). Early regression in social communication in autistic spectrum disorders: A CPEA study. *Developmental Neuropsychology, 27*(3), 311–336.

Madsen, K. M., Hviid, A., Vestergaard, M., Schendel, D., Wohlfahrt, J., Thorsen, P., et al. (2002). A population-based study of measles, mumps, and rubella vaccination and autism. *New England Journal of Medicine, 347*(19), 1477–1482.

Mirrett, P. L., Bailey, D. B., Roberts, J. E., & Hatton, D. D. (2004). Developmental screening and detection of developmental delays in infants and toddlers with fragile X syndrome. *Journal of Developmental and Behavioral Pediatrics, 25*(1), 21–27.

Molloy, C. A., Dawson, G., Dunn, M., Hyman, S. L., McMahon, W. M., Minshew, N., et al. (in press). Familial autoimmune thyroid disease as a risk factor for regression in children with autism spectrum disorder: A CPEA study. *Journal of Autism and Developmental Disorders*.

Moore, V., & Goodson, S. (2003). How well does early diagnosis of autism stand the test of time?: Follow-up study of children assessed for autism at age 2 and development of an early diagnostic service. *Autism, 7*(1), 47–63.

Mouridsen, S. E. (1995). The Landau–Kleffner Syndrome: A review. *European Child and Adolescent Psychiatry, 4*(4), 223–228.

Mundy, P., Hogan, A., & Doehring, P. (1996). *Early Social Communication Scales.* Coral Gables, FL: University of Miami.

Mundy, P., & Sigman, M. (1989). The theoretical implications of joint-attention deficits in autism. *Development and Psychopathology, 1*(3), 173–183.

National Research Council, Committee on Educational Interventions for Children with Autism. (2001). *Educating children with autism.* Washington, DC: National Academies Press.

Ozonoff, S., Goodlin-Jones, B. L., & Solomon, M. (2005). Evidence-based assessment of autism spectrum disorders in children and adolescents. *Journal of Clinical Child and Adolescent Psychology, 34*, 523–540.

Ozonoff, S., South, M., & Miller, J. N. (2000). DSM-IV–defined Asperger syndrome: Cognitive, behavioral and early history differentiation from high-functioning autism. *Autism, 4*(1), 29–46.

Paul, R., Miles, S., Cicchetti, D. V., Sparrow, S. S., Klin, A., Volkmar, F., et al. (2004). Adaptive behavior in autism and pervasive developmental disorder—not otherwise specified: Microanalysis of scores on the Vineland Adaptive Behavior Scales. *Journal of Autism and Developmental Disorders, 34*(2), 223–228.

Philofsky, A., Hepburn, S. L., Hayes, A., Hagerman, R., & Rogers, S. (2004). Linguistic and cognitive functioning and autism symptoms in young children with fragile X syndrome. *American Journal on Mental Retardation, 109*(3), 208–218.

Rice, M. L., Wexler, K., & Cleave, P. L. (1995). Specific language impairment as a period of extended optional infinitive. *Journal of Speech and Hearing Research, 38*(4), 850–863.

Richler, J., Luyster, R., Risi, S., Hsu, W. L., Dawson, G., Bernier, R., et al. (in press). Is there a regressive "phenotype" of autism spectrum disorder associated with the measles–mumps–rubella vaccine?: A CPEA study. *Journal of Autism and Developmental Disorders.*

Robins, D. L., Fein, D., Barton, M. L., & Green, J. A. (2001). The Modified Checklist for Autism in Toddlers: An initial study investigating the early detection of autism and pervasive developmental disorders. *Journal of Autism and Developmental Disorders, 31*(2), 131–144.

Rogers, S., Herbison, J., Lewis, C., Pantone, J., & Reis, K. (1986). An approach for enhancing the symbolic, communicative, and interpersonal functioning of young children with autism or severe emotional handicaps. *Journal of the Division of Early Childhood, 10*, 135–148.

Rogers, S., Wehner, E. A., & Hagerman, R. (2001). The behavioral phenotype in fragile X: Symptoms of autism in very young children with fragile X syndrome, idiopathic autism, and other developmental disorders. *Journal of Developmental and Behavioral Pediatrics, 22*, 409–417.

Rosenthal, R., & Jacobson, L. F. (1968). Teacher expectations for the disadvantaged. *Scientific American, 218*(4), 19–23.

Rutter, M., Bailey, A., Lord, C., & Berument, S. K. (2003). *Social Communication Questionnaire.* Los Angeles: Western Psychological Services.

Rutter, M., & Lord, C. (1987). Language impairment associated with psychiatric disorder. In W. Yule, M. Rutter, & M. Bax (Eds.), *Language development and disorders* (pp. 206–233). London: SIMP/Blackwell Scientific and Lippincott.

Schopler, E., & Mesibov, G. B. (1988). Introduction to diagnosis and assessment of autism. In E. Schopler & G. B. Mesibov (Eds.), *Diagnosis and assessment in autism* (pp. 3–14). New York: Plenum Press.

Schopler, E., Reichler, R. J., & Renner, B. R. (1988). *The Childhood Autism Rating Scale (CARS)*. Los Angeles: Western Psychological Services.

Shao, Y. J., Raiford, K. L., Wolpert, C. M., Cope, H. A., Ravan, S. A., Ashley-Koch, A. A., et al. (2002). Phenotypic homogeneity provides increased support for linkage on chromosome 2 in autistic disorder. *American Journal of Human Genetics, 70*(4), 1058–1061.

Shinnar, S., Rapin, I., Arnold, S., Tuchman, R. F., Shulman, L., Ballaban-Gil, K., et al. (2001). Language regression in childhood. *Pediatric Neurology, 24*(3), 183–189.

Siegel, B., Pliner, C., Eschler, J., & Elliott, G. R. (1988). How children with autism are diagnosed: Difficulties in identification of children with multiple developmental delays. *Journal of Developmental and Behavioral Pediatrics, 9*(4), 199–204.

Silverman, J. M., Smith, C. J., Schmeidler, J., Hollander, E., Lawlor, B. A., Fitzgerald, M., et al. (2002). Symptom domains in autism and related conditions: Evidence for familiality. *American Journal of Medical Genetics, 114,* 64–73.

Sparrow, S. S., Balla, D. A., & Cicchetti, D. V. (1984). *Vineland Adaptive Behavior Scales*. Circle Pines, MN: American Guidance Service.

Sparrow, S. S., Cicchetti, D. V., & Balla, D. A. (2005). *Vineland Adaptive Behavior Scales* (2nd ed.). Circle Pines, MN: American Guidance Service.

Spiker, D., Lotspeich, L., Kraemer, H. C., Hallmayer, J., McMahon, W., Peterson, B., et al. (1994). Genetics of autism: Characteristics of affected and unaffected children from 37 multiplex families. *American Journal of Medical Genetics, 54*(1), 27–35.

Stone, W. L., Coonrod, E. E., & Ousley, O. Y. (2000). Screening Tool for Autism in Two-Year-Olds (STAT): Development and preliminary data. *Journal of Autism and Developmental Disorders, 30*(6), 607–612.

Stone, W. L., Coonrod, E. E., Turner, L. M., & Pozdol, S. L. (2004). Psychometric properties of the STAT for early autism screening. *Journal of Autism and Developmental Disorders, 34,* 691–701.

Stone, W. L., Lee, E. B., Ashford, L., Brissie, J., Hepburn, S. L., Coonrod, E. E., et al. (1999). Can autism be diagnosed accurately in children under 3 years? *Journal of Child Psychology and Psychiatry and Allied Disciplines, 40*(2), 219–226.

Tager-Flusberg, H., Folstein, S., Kjelgaard, J., Roberts, J., Condouris, K., & Smith, J. (2001, November). *Evidence for an important language subtype in autism: Overlap between autism and specific language impairment.* Paper presented at the International Meeting for Autism Research, San Diego, CA.

Tager-Flusberg, H., & Joseph, R. M. (2003). Identifying neurocognitive phenotypes in autism. *Philosophical Transactions of the Royal Society of London: Series B. Biological Sciences, 358*(1430), 303–314.

Tager-Flusberg, H., Paul, R., & Lord, C. (2005). Language and communication in autism. In F. Volkmar, R. Paul, & A. Klin (Eds.), *Handbook of autism and pervasive developmental disorders* (3rd ed., Vol. 1, pp. 335–364). Hoboken, NJ: Wiley.

Taylor, B., Miller, E., Lingam, R., Andrews, N., Simmons, A., & Stowe, J. (2002). Measles, mumps, and rubella vaccination and bowel problems or developmental regression in children with autism: Population study [Insert]. *British Medical Journal, 324*(7333).

Thurm, A., Lord, C., Lee, L. C., & Newschaffer, C. (2005). *Predictors of language acquisition in preschool children with autism spectrum disorders.* Manuscript submitted for publication.

Trivette, C., Dunst, C., & Hamby, D. (2004). Sources of variation in consequences of everyday activity settings on child and parent functioning. *Perspectives in Education, 22*(2), 17–35.

Tuchman, R. F., & Rapin, I. (1997). Regression in pervasive developmental disorders: Seizures and epileptiform electroencephalogram correlates. *Pediatrics, 99*(4), 560–566.

Venter, A., Lord, C., & Schopler, E. (1992). A follow-up study of high-functioning autistic children. *Journal of Child Psychology and Psychiatry and Allied Disciplines, 33*(3), 489–507.

Volkmar, F., Klin, A., Schultz, R., Bronen, R., Marans, W., Sparrow, S. S., & Cohen, D. (1996). Asperger's syndrome. *Journal of the American Academy of Child and Adolescent Psychiatry, 35*, 118–123.

Watson, L., & Marcus, L. M. (1988). Diagnosis and assessment of pre-school children. In E. Schopler & G. B. Mesibov (Eds.), *Diagnosis and assessment in autism* (pp. 271–301). New York: Plenum Press.

Wetherby, A. M., & Prizant, B. M. (1998). *Communication and Symbolic Behavior Scales, Developmental profile—research edition.* Baltimore: Brookes.

Wetherby, A. M., & Prizant, B. M. (2003). *The Communication and Symbolic Behavior Scales.* Baltimore: Brookes.

Wing, L. (1981). Asperger's syndrome: A clinical account. *Psychological Medicine, 11*(1), 115–129.

World Health Organization. (1992). *The ICD 10 classification of mental and behavioral disorders: Clinical descriptions and diagnostic guidelines.* Geneva, Switzerland: Author.

PART II

Screening
and Surveillance

This section summarizes findings from the first and second wave of studies that have applied autism screens in the general population and in referred samples or clinic settings. The focus of many of these screens is the identification of impairments in early social-communicative behaviors. The importance of early detection is highlighted, and the utility and limitations of using these screens in clinical practice are outlined.

Charman and Baron-Cohen (Chapter 3) describe the state of the art of population-based autism screening, presenting perspectives from over 10 years of research. The chapter outlines research challenges, as well as successes. The critical parameters of screening instruments that have been used in general population samples are systematically reviewed. Research over the past 15 years has shown that it is possible to identify at least some cases of ASD prospectively using such screens, but each research study completed to date has also had significant limitations. The different types of screening instruments for ASD that have been empirically tested are compared, and several emerging lines of investigation are explored. The question What is the best we can expect from population-based screens? is considered. The role that screens can play in the early identification and ongoing diagnostic process is outlined.

Zwaigenbaum and Stone (Chapter 4) discuss the use of autism-specific screens in clinical practice settings. Tools that can be used by different service providers in a variety of settings are described—ranging from pediatricians in primary care settings who encounter parents with concerns about autism to practitioners in developmental clinics who use screening to triage referrals to child-find personnel who need to decide where to refer children for assessment or intervention. Available screening measures, as well as promising new approaches, are described. The authors highlight the value of ongoing studies of "high risk" infant siblings of children with autism in identifying very early behavioral manifestations of autism. Approaches to interpreting and discussing screening results with parents are also discussed.

3

Screening for Autism Spectrum Disorders in Populations

Progress, Challenges, and Questions for Future Research and Practice

TONY CHARMAN
SIMON BARON-COHEN

THE CONTEXT FOR SCREENING

The motivations for early identification of children with autism spectrum disorders (ASD) are many and pressing. One important impetus for early identification is the increasing evidence that appropriately targeted intervention improves outcome in children with ASD (see National Research Council, 2001, for a review). Direct empirical evidence that early rather than later intervention has a specific positive benefit is not yet available (Lord et al., in press). Many autism experts have asserted that this is likely to be the case for sound developmental and neurodevelopmental principles (Dawson, Ashman & Carver, 2000; Mundy & Neal, 2001; Rogers, 2001). Furthermore, there is now wide agreement that, along with a predictable and structured environment and an emphasis on developing communication skills, children with ASD should be enrolled into programs as early as possible (Dawson & Osterling, 1997; Koegel, 2000; Lord, 2000; National

Research Council, 2001; Rogers, 1998). Early identification is also important in helping parents recognize and understand their child's difficulties and needs. When early identification is coupled with advice and appropriate support, it is likely that parents will adjust better to the challenges of raising a child with ASD, bringing benefit to the child, the parents, and their wider family.

The first attempts to develop and test screening tools that might prospectively identify children with ASD began in the early 1990s (Baron-Cohen, Allen, & Gillberg, 1992; Baron-Cohen et al., 1996). This gives us an opportunity to look back on the progress that has been made in the past 10 years. Without anticipating the outcome of this review, it is clear that we have moved forward in our knowledge and that findings from research studies have usefully informed clinical practice (Baird et al., 2001; Charman & Baird, 2002; Charman, 2003; Filipek et al., 1999, 2000). However, we have not yet arrived at what might constitute an ideal end point—a screen that prospectively identifies the majority of children with ASD before their difficulties become apparent to parents and professionals (and a screen that has few "false positives"—see the next section for a definition). Note that this is an ambitious goal and might not be achievable. Despite this, we have made progress in clarifying some of the questions and challenges for research and practice in working toward this end point.

Three distinct phases of the ongoing development of screening tools for children with ASD can be identified, framed around the following questions:

1. Is it *possible* to prospectively identify cases of ASD?
2. Is it possible to prospectively identify cases of ASD *from the general population*?
3. *How best* can we prospectively identify cases of ASD from the general population?

Prospective screening in general populations is sometimes called "Level I screening" and is contrasted to "Level II" screening, in which instruments or tests are applied to children in cases in which parents or professionals or both have raised concerns about the child's development (see Siegel, 2004). The Level II use of screening tools in referred populations is covered in the chapter by Zwaigenbaum and Stone (Chapter 4, this volume).

In addressing these questions, one issue relevant to the conceptual framework of this volume is: How critical might measuring impairments and abnormalities in emerging early social-communication behaviors be for developing effective screening tools? Given that the characteristic profile seen in children with ASD also includes "positive" symptoms that mark out a child's development as atypical (e.g., sensory abnormalities; motor stereotypies), what role should identification of such symptoms play alongside characterizing developmental delays and abnormal profiles in core social and communication skills? From completed and ongoing studies, some initial conclusions can be reached on this issue and some partial answers provided to the three questions outlined here. We also outline ideas regarding novel research studies that are required in order to further develop useful screens and expedite their implementation and use in clinical services.

DEFINING SCREENING AND SURVEILLANCE

Screening and surveillance are different but related activities that involve the detection of impairments with a view to prevention or amelioration of consequent disability and handicap. Screening is the prospective identification of unrecognized disorders by the application of specific tests or examinations. Surveillance refers to the ongoing and systematic collection of data relevant to the identification of a disorder over time by an integrated health system.

Several parameters of screening instruments are important in assessing their efficacy and utility:

1. *Sensitivity* refers to the proportion of children with a disorder identified by the screen.
2. *Specificity* refers to the proportion of children without the disorder whom the screen identified as normal.
3. *Positive predictive value* refers to the proportion of children with a positive screen result who have the disorder.

Stringent criteria exist for screens to detect discrete medical conditions (Cochrane & Holland, 1969; Wilson & Jungner, 1968). Sensitivity is required to be high so that the screen misses few cases of the disorder (avoiding falsely reassuring parents). Cases of the disorder that do not meet the threshold on a particular screening instrument—that is, they are not "screen positive"—are called "false negatives." Specificity is required to be high so that few cases without the disorder are screen positive (avoiding falsely alarming parents and possible precipitous, incorrect diagnosis and costly referral for potentially inappropriate intervention, advice, or onward referral). Non-cases that do meet the threshold on a particular screening instrument—that is, they are "screen positive"—are called "false positives." Low sensitivity and specificity also have implications for health economics because the introduction and use of a screen affects the cost and efficacy of current surveillance services. Furthermore—and relevant to screening for ASD—when the sensitivity and specificity of a screen remain constant, the positive predictive value is lower the rarer a disorder is within the population (Clark & Harrington, 1999). Hall (1996) concluded that most screening tests that set out to identify neurodevelopmental disorders do not meet these stringent criteria. Glascoe (1996) has estimated that acceptable sensitivity and specificity for developmental screening tests are 70–80%, reflecting the nature and complexity of measuring the continuous process of child development (American Academy of Pediatrics, 2001).

Surveillance involves a parent–professional partnership that takes a broader look at developmental and behavioral skills and progress over time. It combines the observations of parents with the developmental knowledge of the professional and the deployment of specific tests. There is evidence that the use of screening instruments, in combination with asking parents about their concerns, improves the efficiency of an instrument (Glascoe, 1997a, 1999). An important clinical point is that the early recognition of developmental delays requires in-depth knowledge of the precursors to a particular skill (e.g., joint-attention behaviors as a precursor to spoken language), as well as clinical judgment. In this context, the use of specific screens when there is some concern on the part of the parent or professional can be a useful adjunct to clinical judgment. Despite the challenges of screening for neurodevelopmental disorders, there is professional and public agreement that early identification of child health problems is desirable. Notably, this includes identification of developmental disabilities, as well as medical diseases (American Academy of Pediatrics, 1994, 1999; Robinson, 1998). Further, over the past decade the emphasis has shifted from screening in the preschool years to screening infants from birth to 2 years of age (American Academy of Pediatrics, 1994, 1999).

These developments chime with developments within the ASD field, in which one significant change over the past 10 to 15 years in many countries has been the increasing number of children who are referred and identified in the third, and sometimes even the second, year of life (Charman & Baird, 2002). This contrasts to the picture in the 1980s and early 1990s, when many children were not diagnosed before 4 or 5 years of age or even later (Howlin & Asgharian, 1999). This shift to earlier referral and diagnosis in many services is due to several factors, including better training of health professionals and wider public recognition of ASD. These changes, in turn, have been informed by a number of strands of research that have focused on very early signs of ASD, including studying early videotapes of later-diagnosed children (e.g., Adrien et al., 1993; Baranek, 1999; Osterling, Dawson, & Munson, 2002; see Charman, 2000, for a review) and the studies testing screening tools for ASD reviewed in this chapter.

IS IT POSSIBLE TO PROSPECTIVELY IDENTIFY CASES OF ASD?

Many general developmental screening instruments exist, and some have been shown to have robust psychometric properties and norms (e.g., Ages and Stages Questionnaire [Squires, Bricker, & Potter, 1997]; Child Development Inventories [Ireton, 1992]; Denver Developmental Screening Test—Revised [Frankenburg, Dodds, Archer, Shapiro, & Bresnik, 1992]; Parents' Evaluation of Developmental Status [Glascoe, 1997b]). However, these were designed to identify the considerable proportion of children in the general population who have developmental delays in the motor, language, and cognitive domains, and not specifically children with ASD.

A number of rating scales that measure severity of autistic symptoms also exist (e.g., Autism Behavior Checklist [ABC; Krug, Arick, & Almond, 1980]; Childhood Autism Rating Scale [CARS; Schopler, Reichler, DeVellis, & Daly, 1980]). However, these have primarily been used to assess clinically referred, school-age and adult service user samples, and data on their psychometric properties are not informative to the question of how well they would work as potential screening tools for ASD in very young children. Other instruments that measure autism symptoms—such as the Autism Diagnostic Interview—Revised (ADI-R; Lord, Rutter, & Le Couteur, 1994), the Autism Diagnostic Observation Schedule—Generic (ADOS-G; Lord et al., 2000), and the Diagnostic Interview for Social and Communication Disorders (DISCO; Wing, Leekam, Libby, Gould, & Larcombe, 2002)—are detailed interview and observation schedules that are useful clinically and in research, but they are time-consuming and require rigorous training in their administration and hence are inappropriate to consider as potential screening tools.

At the beginning of the 1990s, Baron-Cohen and colleagues set out to develop a specific screening tool that aimed to prospectively identify autism in infancy. Among the wide range of autism symptoms that could have been targeted, a decision was made on empirical and theoretical grounds to focus on early social-communication impairments. Empirically, a series of experimental studies in the 1980s had shown that preschool and young school-age children with ASD were impaired relative to children with general developmental delay (or "mental retardation") in social-communication abilities such as joint attention (e.g., protodeclarative pointing, or "pointing to indicate interest"), gaze monitoring, and pretend play (Baron-Cohen, 1987, 1989; Mundy, Sigman, Ungerer, & Sherman, 1986; Sigman, Ungerer, Mundy, & Sherman, 1986). Theoretically, it seemed to make most sense to focus on what we understood as the core impairments in autism: social and communication impairments. A new instrument was developed to prospectively identify autism at 18 months of age: the CHAT (CHecklist for Autism in Toddlers). This age was chosen as an appropriate screen "window" (Aylward, 1997) because joint attention and pretend play typically emerge at this time in normal development (Carpenter, Nagell, & Tomasello, 1998). The CHAT assesses simple pretend play (appropriate use of a tea set, doll play, object substitution) and joint-attention behaviors (pointing for interest, in combination with eye contact, and following gaze) using parental report and health practitioner observation through direct testing.

The first study tested the effectiveness of the CHAT as a screening instrument in a genetic high-risk sample of forty-one 18-month-old siblings of children already diagnosed with autism (Baron-Cohen et al., 1992). Whereas none of 50 unselected 18-month-olds failed all five key items, 4 of the children in the high-risk group did so. A year later, when the children were 30 months old, a follow-up was carried out. None of the unselected children had been diagnosed with ASD. The 4 children in the high-risk group who had failed the five key items were the only children who received a diagnosis of autism at this follow-up assessment. This confirmed the prediction that absence of joint attention and pretend play in combination at 18 months of age is a marker that a child is highly likely to go on to receive a diagnosis of autism. Thus this first experiment provided us with an answer to the first question: Yes, it is possible to prospectively identify cases of ASD.

IS IT POSSIBLE TO PROSPECTIVELY IDENTIFY CASES OF ASD FROM THE GENERAL POPULATION?

Following the demonstration that it was possible to prospectively identify cases of autism at 18 months of age using the CHAT, we set about testing how well the instrument would work in identifying cases of ASD from a general population. One issue was whether there was something different about how the instrument would work in the high-risk, genetically loaded families compared with the broader group of the heterogeneous ASD population (who may have different, rather than less, genetic loading). To test the effectiveness of the CHAT in a large general population, health visitors (community nurses) and general practitioners (community doctors) in the South Thames region of the United Kingdom used the questionnaire with 18-month-olds as part of routine health surveillance (Baird et al., 2000; Baron-Cohen et al., 1996, 2000). The fact that such a surveillance "contact" between health professionals and infants already existed at this age made this in some ways a design of convenience but also coincided with the "developmental window" we had identified in terms of the typical development of joint attention and play skills. Of the total population of 40,818 eighteen-month-olds eligible for screening, 16,235 (39.8%) were screened using the CHAT. This proportion reflected the fact that only children who had a health check approximately 2 months before or after 18 months of age were included in the study and that participation in the health surveillance 18-month check was not 100%. In addition, some children with profound developmental delays, including those with severe sensory and motor impairments, were excluded, as the health practitioners decided not to impose additional assessment on parents of children with preidentified severe developmental problems. We did not receive systematic information on such exclusions.

We predicted that those children who at 18 months failed all five key items would be at the greatest risk for ASD. We called this the "high risk for autism" group. Children who failed both items that measured proto-declarative pointing (pointing for interest) but who were not in the high risk for autism group were predicted to be in the "medium risk for autism" group. Children who did not fit either of these profiles were predicted to be in the "low risk for autism" group. In order to minimize false positives, a two-stage screening procedure was adopted. Children who were initially (CHAT-1) screen positive (at the high- or medium-risk threshold) received a second administration (CHAT-2) of the screen one month later via a telephone follow-up.

Data on the parameters of the CHAT screen were estimated after a follow-up of the population at age 7 years (Baird et al., 2000; Baron-Cohen et al., 2000). Used in this two-stage way, the positive predictive value of the screening instrument was high (83% for ASD using the high-risk threshold). However, sensitivity was poor (18%), indicating that four-fifths of the children subsequently identified as having childhood autism in the study population were missed on screening. If a one-stage screening procedure only had been adopted, the proportion of children with autism identified would have increased to 38%, although in clinical use this would have entailed the assessment of more screen false positives. However, some children with language delay and intellectual disability were also identified at the high-risk threshold, and the one-stage positive predictive value for identification of *all* developmental problems was 48% (see Baird et al., 2000, for full details). The CHAT population study demonstrated that failing a combination of joint-attention and pretend-play items (using both parental report and health practitioner observation and on both administrations of the screen) indicated a significant risk for developing autism or a related pervasive developmental disorder (PDD). Interestingly, although 9% of the screened population were reported as not producing simple pretend play at age 18 months, and 4.5% were reported as not pointing for interest, failing a *combination* of joint-attention and pretend-play items (using both parental report and health practitioner observation) was very much rarer (0.23%). Thus the study demonstrated that failing the combination of joint-attention and pretend-play items indicated a significant risk for developing autism, and this was especially true when a child failed on both administrations of the screen (CHAT-1 and CHAT-2). However, although the CHAT screen had a high positive predictive value, its sensitivity was moderate at best, and the findings cannot support a recommendation for total population screening at a single time point (Baird et al., 2000).

One aspect of the study that has not been emphasized in previous publications is that we took the opportunity to compare how the CHAT worked when administered by professionals who asked questions directly of parents and who then combined this information with direct observations of the child with how the CHAT worked in the form of a questionnaire completed by parents with no professional involvement (see Charman et al., 2001). In the CHAT study, we used a version of the questionnaire mailed to 2,541 parents out of 16,235 in the population. This version of the screen included the nine parental-report items in section A of the CHAT and a parent version of item Bii, which asked whether their child followed gaze (Baird et al., 2000, p. 695). At the high-risk cutoff it did not appear that the sensitivity for detection of autism at the first screen (CHAT-1) was different for the two versions: parent + professional (failing all 5 key items) = 36.6% versus parent-only (failing the 3 key items administered) = 44.4%. Potentially this parent-only method reduces the burden on primary health care workers and is therefore a cost-effective method of screening large populations. Considerations regarding the mode of administration or delivery of screens and how these affect the balance between screen "accuracy" and costs and burden to services and professionals are considered in a later section of this chapter.

However, there are differences between the use of a screen in our research study (in which the criterion set for risk and onward referral was applied without clinical decision making) and the use of a screen in routine health surveillance (in which clinical decision making about possible developmental problems is used in combination with the risk criteria to determine referral). Fortunately, there is some evidence that skilled clinical opinion can also enhance detection. This is good surveillance, but not screening. Subsequent to our initial attempt to screen a population sample, we have used the CHAT to identify children with autism at age 24 months for inclusion in an early-intervention study (Drew et al., 2002). Only the key screening items (across both the parent-report and practitioner-observation sections) that measure joint attention and play behaviors were included in a shortened version of the screen, again administered at 18 months. In order to minimize screen false positives, health practitioners were asked to refer children who not only failed all the key items but also about whom they had concerns about possible ASD.

The children identified as failing all pointing and pretense items by parent report, confirmed by professional observation, were given a repeat CHAT (CHAT-2) by telephone within 2 weeks. Of 51 children referred to the study, 5 "passed" (i.e., fell below the high-risk threshold) on retest by telephone (compared with 26 of 38 who passed on retest in the original population study; Baird et al., 2000). Of the remaining 46, following a diagnostic assessment, 31 had autism; 5, PDD; 6, a receptive–expressive language disorder; 2, global developmental delay; and 1, ADHD. Only 1 child had no developmental problem identified at assessment. Thus, when the score on the CHAT screen was combined with clinical judgment or concern about possible autism, the positive predictive value was very high even for a one-stage (CHAT-1 only) administration (71% for all ASDs and 88% for all developmental disorders). This result concurs with studies that have used the CHAT screen in referred samples (Robins, Fein, Barton, & Green, 2001; Scambler, Rogers, & Wehner, 2001; see also Zwaigenbaum & Stone, Chapter 4, this volume, for details). A recent follow-up of this sample at age 7 years has demonstrated that in all but one case the ASD diagnosis was still considered to be clinically appropriate at this older age, when it is possible to be more confident of diagnostic decisions and differential diagnosis (Charman et al., 2005).

This second study suggests that the positive predictive value of the CHAT may be further increased in the one-stage administration when combined with a professional clinical judgment of concern regarding the child's development. Another difference between this study and the CHAT population study was that both the research team and the practitioners knew that a child who failed the key items across two administrations was highly likely to have autism, on the basis of our initial population study. However, sensitivity cannot be estimated from this study, as the screen was not used on a total population that was then followed up to identify screen false negatives. We are currently undertaking a study to test the sensitivity and specificity of two screening instruments—the Modified CHAT (M-CHAT; Robins et al., 2001) and the Social Communication Questionnaire (SCQ; Berument, Rutter, Lord, Pickles, & Bailey, 1999)—when used by community pediatricians and speech and language pathologists at the point of referral for developmental concerns, and we hope to be able to answer the question of whether improved positive predictive value, when employed as Level II screens in referred populations, comes at the cost of reduced sensitivity for these screens.

MORE RECENT ATTEMPTS TO TEST SCREENS FOR ASD IN THE GENERAL POPULATION

A full evaluation of prospective population screens is a long-term research enterprise. In the CHAT population study, we reassessed the cohort to identify all known cases of ASDs at the age of 7 years, an age at which we considered most cases of ASD would have been identified, some 6 years after the initial screening. Several other studies are under way to test the properties of other screening instruments in general populations, and although none have yet completed such a long-term follow-up, we will review the results that are emerging.

Siegel (2004) in the 1990s developed a screening test designed to be of use in several levels of health surveillance, from primary care physicians (Stage 1) to child development clinics (Stage 2) to specialist autism assessment services (Stage 3): This is the Pervasive Developmental Disorders Screening Test—II (PDDST-II; Siegel, 2004). Siegel (2004) reports strong instrument properties in samples of referred children with ASD and other developmental delays, as well as in comparison with an alternative "high risk" clinical sample of children with very low birthweight. However, the utility of the PDDST as a general population screen for ASDs has not been evaluated.

Robins et al. (2001) developed a modified version of the CHAT (the M-CHAT). They included all nine parental-report items from the original instrument (Baron-Cohen et al., 1992). Note that this included the "key" items that were used in the original CHAT study to identify our prospective risk groups (joint attention and pretend play), other early social-communication items (e.g., "bring to show," [or show-and-tell]) and items that were considered "filler items" measuring nonsocial-communication development that we expected all children to pass (e.g., "Does your child like climbing on things, such as up stairs?"; Charman et al., 2001). Robins et al. (2001) added additional items measuring other aspects of early social-communication impairments that are characteristic of autism (e.g., response to name, imitation), as well as repetitive behaviors (e.g., unusual finger mannerisms) and sensory abnormalities (e.g., oversensitivity to noise). The M-CHAT is a parent-report instrument; the health practitioner does no direct testing. The initial M-CHAT report is covered in detail by Zwaigenbaum and Stone (Chapter 4, this volume). In brief, in their initial report Robins et al. (2001) had tested 1,122 unselected children (initially at 18 months but subsequently at 24 months of age) and 171 children referred for early-intervention services. Robins et al. (2001) reported that the M-CHAT's instrument parameters were strong (i.e., it had high sensitivity, high specificity, and high positive predictive value) in this largely referred sample. Follow-up studies will allow us to estimate the instrument's parameters with an unselected or general population in order to compare them directly to those of the CHAT. In particular, we do not yet know the sensitivity of the M-CHAT in detecting cases of ASD in children about whom there have been no previous developmental concerns. It is notable for this chapter that items that best discriminated between children with ASD and children with other developmental problems were those that measured joint-attention behaviors (pointing and following a point, bringing things for show), social relatedness (interest in other children, imitation), and communication (response to name).

A group from Hong Kong has recently published data from older, already diagnosed children with ASD that examine the utility of a two-stage surveillance procedure that combines the use of the M-CHAT as a parental questionnaire and a follow-up stage employing clinician observation of behavior using items of the original CHAT screen (CHAT-23; Wong et al., 2004). The most sensitive item in this study was another form of early social communication: "Does your child imitate you?" Again, the properties of this second modified version of the CHAT have not yet been tested as a general population screen.

Buitelaar and colleagues in the Netherlands have developed a screening instrument (Early Screening of Autistic Traits; ESAT) to identify ASD in 14-month-old children (Dietz, Willemson-Swinkels, van Daalen, van Egeland, & Buitelaar, in press; Willemsen-Swinkels et al., in press). Health practitioners at a well-baby clinic appointment administered an initial screen of four items. If a child failed one or more of the four items (measuring varied play with toys, readability of emotional expression, and sensory abnormalities), the parent was offered a follow-up home visit. The choice of these items was based on comparison of frequency of endorsement of items in an unselected sample of 8- to 20-month-olds and retrospective parental reports of how their children *would have* scored on items at 14 months of age in two older, already diagnosed samples of children with ASD and children with ADHD (Willemsen-Swinkels et al., in press). At this visit a longer version of the ESAT (14 items that included many social-communication items such as eye contact, response to name, etc.) was administered, along with other developmental assessments. Children who failed 3 or more items of the 14-item ESAT were invited for a diagnostic evaluation. The Utrecht group (Dietz et al., in press; Willemsen-Swinkels et al., in press) has completed screening of 31,724 children at 14 months of age. The ESAT identified children with ASD (*n* = 18) and also children with language disorder (*n* = 18) and mental retardation (*n* = 13). Once again, establishing the instrument properties of the ESAT will require longer term follow-up of the entire population sample in order to identify missed cases. Similarly to the M-CHAT analysis conducted by Robins et al. (2001), the items that discriminated best between children with and without ASD were items assessing early social-communication impairments, including "shows interest in people," "smiles directly," and "reacts when spoken to."

One notable feature of this study, in comparison with the CHAT population study, was that the rate of refusal of diagnostic appointments was considerably higher (no parents refused to attend in the CHAT study). This may indicate that parents of children age 14 months were more reluctant to accept that their children might have developmental problems than parents of children age 18 months in the CHAT study. The issues of screen accuracy (both in terms of positive predictive value and sensitivity) and parental acceptance and recognition are important considerations when considering the "best" time to employ a general population screen for ASD (see Charman et al., 2001, 2002; Robins et al., 2001; Willemsen-Swinkels, Buitelaar, & van Engeland, 2001, for further discussion of these issues).

A group from Yokohama, Japan, has also used a novel screening tool (YACHT; Young Autism and other developmental disorders CHeckup Tool; Honda & Shimizu, 2002) in combination with an integrated surveillance system of health checks at age 18 and 36 months to identify children with ASD. The YACHT has two versions for use at 18-month (YACHT-18) and 36-month (YACHT-36) checkups and consists of social, language, motor, and hearing items. Although in the initial report no cutoff for the YACHT-18 was described, the authors calculated that, in combination with clinical decision making regarding likely problems, the initial sensitivity of the instrument was 74% (Honda & Shimizu, 2002), considerably above that of the CHAT. Once again, longer term follow-up of the whole population is needed in order to establish definitive instrument properties.

Returning to the questions that provide the framework for this chapter, how well can we answer the question, Is it possible to prospectively identify cases of ASD from the general population? Clearly, prospective identification of ASD that was unsuspected by parents and health professionals is possible, and this has now been confirmed in several studies using several different instruments (CHAT, M-CHAT, ESAT) and at several different ages, from 14 to 24 months. However, the only study that has yet conducted the long-term follow-up that is necessary to establish sensitivity, specificity, and positive predictive value of the screen in a general population is the CHAT study. Although the specificity and positive predictive value were acceptable, the sensitivity of the CHAT was too low to recommend universal screening. All these instruments are likely to be useful as part of surveillance by health professionals in combination with their clinical judgments and parents' expressions of concerns. However, the answer regarding whether any of the screens should be recommended as general population screens will await the follow-up of the ongoing studies.

HOW BEST CAN WE PROSPECTIVELY IDENTIFY CASES OF ASD FROM THE GENERAL POPULATION?

As summarized, the evidence base is not yet available to make confident recommendations as to how *best* to prospectively identify cases. In this section we review what hints are emerging from the research studies conducted to date, highlight the issues that need to be considered in further screen development, and mention several new studies that may provide clues to the best content, mode, and age for screening for ASD.

Content

There is some consensus in the studies conducted to date that delays in early social communication—the hallmark symptoms of ASD—are the most discriminating items on the screens that have been tested. In the CHAT study, impairments in joint attention and pretend play were a priori targeted as key items because these abilities are present in typical development in most cases by 18 months of age and also because research had shown them to discriminate between preschool children with ASD and children with mental retardation (Baron-Cohen et al., 1992, 1996). Post hoc analysis of items from screens that have subsequently been developed has also found that items that assess early social-communication impairment were most discriminating. In the M-CHAT study, these included joint-attention behaviors ("pointing and following a point," "bringing things to show"), social relatedness ("interest in other children," "imitation") and communication ("response to name"; Robins et al., 2001). In the ESAT study, the most discriminating of the 14 items were "shows interest in people," "smiles directly," and "reacts when spoken to" (Dietz et al., in press) and in the CHAT-23 study, the most discriminating item was "Does your child imitate you?" (Wong et al., 2004).

Although both the M-CHAT (e.g., "oversensitivity to noise"; "stares at nothing") and the ESAT (e.g., "reacts to sensory stimuli"; "shows stereotyped movements") included sensory and repetitive behaviors, these were not discriminating. Examination of the data from these studies shows that the reason was *not* that they were rarely endorsed by parents of children with ASD but that they were *also* frequently endorsed by parents of children without ASD (typically children with mental retardation). Although characteristic impairments and abnormalities are required in all three domains of behavior (social, communication, and repetitive and sensory behaviors) for a diagnosis of autism, impairments in the former two areas appear more specific to ASD, at least at this early age. It appears that even children with mental retardation are showing some of these early social-communicative competencies by their second birthdays or before. This may also reflect the fact that "third axis" repetitive, stereotyped, and sensory behaviors are more prominent at the ages of 3 to 5 years of age than they are at age 2, as has been found in several prospective studies of children first identified in toddlerhood (Charman et al., 2005; Cox et al., 1999; Stone et al., 1999). This relates to the issue of when to screen for ASD—the age of screening and the content of the screen (in terms of which items are most discriminating) are likely to be interdependent.

One final point concerns what should be assessed for each skill inquired about. The CHAT screen asks parents "Does your child *ever* . . . ?" One possibility is that the low sensitivity reflected the fact that even very rare or fleeting examples of such behaviors (more akin to "*Has* your child *ever* . . . ?") were positively endorsed by parents of children with ASD who "passed" the screen (Baird et al., 2000). Both the ESAT and the M-CHAT, by contrast, phrase questions more in the continuing present sense ("Does your child . . . ?" and "Is your child . . . ?"). This slight difference in wording might indicate to parents a more enduring and common substantiation of the behavior the item is inquiring about.

Baron-Cohen and colleagues (Baron-Cohen, Charman, Wheelwright, & Richler, 2002) have directly addressed this issue in a completely revised screening questionnaire that has recently been piloted. They developed a *quantitative* version of the CHAT (called the Q-CHAT) in order to pick up not just those children who have never produced the behavior but also those who are simply showing a reduced rate. This approach is in line with seeing autism as a *continuum* or *spectrum* disorder. The Q-CHAT retains the key items from the CHAT but "dimensionalizes" them (using a 5-point scale of frequency) so that each item scores from 1 (no symptoms) to 5 (maximal symptoms). In common with the ESAT and M-CHAT, the Q-CHAT also increased the number of key items by adding items from all three domains of the "triad" of impairments that characterize ASD; that is, items that inquire about language development, social communication, and repetitive or restricted behaviors. The Q-CHAT is still very brief (Q- stands for both "quantitative" and "quick") but now has 25 items instead of 9. So the range of the instrument is 25 (minimum) to 125 (maximum), with each item scored so that positive autism symptoms score more highly.

In a pilot study, the Q-CHAT was completed by parents of typically developing 18- and 24-month-old children and of older, already diagnosed preschool children with ASD and with mental retardation (Baron-Cohen et al., 2002). As expected, the group with ASD scored significantly higher than the other three groups. In terms of setting a threshold to detect ASD cases, 70% of the group with ASD scored at or above 68 on the Q-CHAT, compared with only 0.9% of the unselected 18-month-olds, 0.7% of the 24-month-olds, and 35.5% of the group with mental retardation. This preliminary study indicated that the revised instrument had good sensitivity in detecting children with ASD. Confirmation of the Q-CHAT's properties will require a general population screening study and appropriate follow-up. It may be that a screen that asks about frequency as opposed to presence or absence of early indicators of autism will be more sensitive, but conclusions will await the outcome of future studies and will require the use of sophisticated signal-detection analysis methods.

Creating the most accurate and reliable screens may require more than rephrasing questions to make them transparent. As an alternative to the questionnaire format, one could use photographs or videotape to present behaviors to parents and ask, "Does your child do this?" (e.g., protodeclarative pointing). Such a screen might allow more accurate reporting of behaviors that are not always transparent in the written word to parents (as well as allowing a "language free" measure).[1]

Looking much further into the future, screens for ASD might not rely on parents or professionals reporting on children's behavior and development. One day it might be possible to use biological markers, for example, head circumference (Courchesne, Carper & Akshoomoff, 2003) or neuropeptides (Nelson et al., 2001), as the basis for screens for ASD. However, more biological approaches might never be good candidate screens for the following reasons. The behavioral phenotype of ASD might be arrived at by a number of different pathogenic routes, and thus the autistic spectrum includes individuals with different ultimate etiologies. Even when biological or genetic markers are found, they may not be present in all individuals with the phenotype. Thus both case definition and methods of early identification for the whole spectrum of disorders may continue to be reliant on the behavioral and developmental picture alone.

Mode

Both parent questionnaire (CHAT; ESAT; M-CHAT) and combined parental questionnaire and health-professional administration (CHAT; CHAT-23; ESAT) modes of administration have been shown to be able to prospectively identify cases of autism. In part, the decision to use parent-only compared with parent-and-professional administration will be based on economics and considerations regarding service burden and acceptability. However, we do have some data from screening studies to address the issue of how much parents and professionals agree. As reported earlier, in the CHAT study there was no difference in the overall sensitivity between parent-only and parent-and-professional administered CHAT screens (Charman et al., 2001). However, for at least a proportion of the screen false negatives (children with ASD who were not above threshold), parents reported that children could point for interest or pretend play, but these behaviors were not observed by the health practitioner during administration of section B of

---

[1] I am grateful to Peter Mundy for this suggestion (see Delgado, Venezia, & Mundy, 2004).

the screen. The pattern was striking in that the reverse was rarely the case. For example, for the 41 cases of childhood autism in which CHAT-1 was administered by a health practitioner, 17 were discrepant for point for interest; and in 16 of these cases, the parents reported that their children did point for interest, but this behavior was not elicited by the health practitioner, with one case only showing the opposite profile. For pretend play, 11 disagreements appeared—10 cases in which the parent-only reported that the child pretended compared with one case in which the practitioner-only did (Charman et al., 2001). In the ESAT study (Dietz et al., in press) there was reasonable overall agreement between the parent-completed and researcher-rated versions of the 14-item ESAT administered at the home visit (Dietz et al., in press). However, for children without ASD (but with language delay and mental retardation), parents tended to rate their children as more impaired than the researcher did. By contrast, for the children with ASD, the reverse was the case, with the researcher rating children as more impaired than parents did. It may be that the subtle impairments shown by toddlers with autism are more difficult for parents to recognize than the broader range of signs of developmental delay recognized by parents of children with mental retardation.

Other modes of administration will also need to be explored. For example, Raymaekers and Roeyers (2003) are undertaking a study in which the SCQ is being completed by nursery staff to identify ASD in 3-year-old children attending kindergarten classes in Belgium. There is some evidence that with older school-age children, screens can identify cases of ASD not identified at younger ages (Childhood Asperger Syndrome Test [CAST]; Williams et al., 2005), although the focus of this chapter and much of the research currently under way in the field is on screening in toddlerhood or preschool.

Age

The age of application of a screen for autism is a critical issue in terms of its screening properties. In part, this reflects the nature of autism as a developmental disorder, as well as the rapid development of early social-communication skills in the second year of life in the typically developing population. One important finding from the CHAT study was that although the two-stage administration increased the positive predictive value (from 26% to 75% for childhood autism at the high-risk threshold), it reduced sensitivity (from 38% to 18% for childhood autism at the high-risk threshold; compare Baird et al., 2000, Table 1 and Table 2). Although development might account for some of the children who fell out of "risk status" between the first (CHAT-1) and second (CHAT-2) administrations of the CHAT, thus reducing its sensitivity, several other factors might also account for this finding. Parents may become sensitized to behaviors previously demonstrated by their children that previously they had not noticed or construed in the terms inquired about on the screen. Alternatively, the second administration was done by the research team, not community practitioners, and the researchers likely had a clearer sense of the behaviors about which the screen inquired (see Baird et al., 2000; Charman et al., 2001, 2002; Willemsen-Swinkels et al., 2001, for discussion).

Considerations of the "best" age at which to screen might differ for different types of screen items. With "negative" items that index delays and deficits in social-communication abilities, some children may fail these items and be identified by a screen at an earlier age due to developmental delays (rather than autism), and they might develop these skills (at least to a level to pass the screen item) by a later age. Consistent with this account, true-positive children with autism had lower IQs than the false-negative children with autism in the CHAT study (Baird et al., 2000). In contrast, in terms of severity of autistic symptoms as measured by the ADI-R, there were no differences between the autism true positives and false negatives. Thus relying on developmental items specific to an age inevitably misses the more able child and reduces the screen's sensitivity. These considerations will also, however, affect the screen's specificity and positive predictive value. When screened at an earlier age, more children without ASD will fall above the screen threshold due to general developmental delay. Although a direct comparison is not possible, there is a suggestion of such a pattern when comparing the proportions of ASD versus other developmental delays identified in the CHAT (Baird et al., 2000) and ESAT (Dietz et al., in press) studies. Screening using the CHAT at 18 months of age identified proportionally more children with ASD than with other developmental delays (Baird et al., 2000, Figs. 1 and 2). By contrast, in the ESAT study screening at 14 months of age, proportionally more children with non-ASD developmental delays were identified than children with ASD (Dietz et al., in press, Fig. 2). As discussed earlier, in terms of "positive" symptoms of ASD, such as repetitive, rigid, and sensory behaviors, the developmental story may be different, as these behaviors might have more clearly emerged and might be more specific to autism at an older age.

CLINICAL ISSUES IN SCREENING AND SURVEILLANCE

The prospective identification of children with ASD—in particular, in cases in which parents and professionals had not previously had concerns about a child's development—presents new challenges to clinical practice. These include the utility of standardized assessment instruments with young preschoolers, the reliability of early diagnosis and how the diagnosis is put to parents, and the ability to indicate prognosis (Charman & Baird, 2002).

A number of studies have examined the stability and accuracy of diagnosis, both in samples of children referred for assessment at an early age and from the CHAT screening study (Charman et al., 2005; Cox et al., 1999; Gillberg et al., 1990; Lord, 1995; Stone et al., 1999). The consensus from these studies is that diagnosis of childhood autism is stable in the third and even the second year of life and that experienced clinical judgment, taking information from a variety of sources, is more reliable than the use of standard assessment instruments (Charman & Baird, 2002). Diagnosis of the broader range of ASD may be less accurate, as has been found for older samples. In particular, less severe ASD presentations may be misdiagnosed as developmental or language delay in very young children. Furthermore, the particular pattern of symptoms that presents in a 2-year-old with ASD may differ from that seen at the more prototypic age of 4 or 5 years. In particular, overt repetitive and stereotyped behaviors may be less notable, although where these are seen alongside the social and communicative impairments, they are highly indicative of ASD (Charman et al., 2005; Charman & Baird, 2002; Rogers, 2001; Stone et al., 1999). One question is how well these research findings would translate into everyday clinical practice, especially when the mix of developmental problems seen in a particular clinic is wide. However, a recent clinic-based study has also found good stability of diagnosis from the second to third years of life (Moore & Goodson, 2003).

Providing a prompt service in addressing parental concern is, of course, very different from finding a problem that a parent does not suspect. Parents will inevitably notice ASD at some stage. However, one consequence of screening for undetected cases of ASD is that for some parents their first recognition that something might be wrong will follow "failure" of a screen and consequent discussion about their child's development with the professional involved in the screening process. These different views need to be borne in mind by health professionals. The difficulties of recognition, belief, and acceptance are far from easy when the professional is giving completely unexpected information. The negotiation of realization of a possible problem is one of the skills of effective surveillance. For a parent to make use of information about his or her child, it first has to make sense, and he or she has to be ready to agree with it. Conversely, with older children about whom parents may already have significant concerns and for whom they are keen to seek access to limited service resources, parents may put pressure on professionals to arrive at a definitive diagnosis in order to "qualify" for such services before the clinical picture and diagnostic certainty have fully emerged.

Clinical work is often concerned with those children who do not clearly meet full criteria for childhood autism but who have apparently milder social problems or mixed developmental difficulties. Clinical experience also suggests that some children who show definite features of autism earlier make remarkable developmental progress. Therefore, caution must be used, especially under 3 years, for those children with features of the broader autistic spectrum. It is our clinical experience that parents understand the difficulties of certainty in developmental assessment. Most appreciate honesty on the professional's part about the difficulty of reaching a precise prognosis on a very young child and can understand a frank discussion about the possible outcomes if accompanied by appropriate advice and help for intervention. Understanding why one's child behaves as he or she does is halfway to doing something about it.

One additional clinical factor to consider is the discussion of "risk status" with parents and what it means when a particular child fails a screen. Instrument statistics refer to whole samples rather than to one individual child. Thus there is a difference in scientific terms between a screen positive predictive value of 90% (that indicates that 9 out of 10 children from a previous sample who met this risk threshold went on to receive a diagnosis of the disorder being screened for) and the everyday notion that a child has "a 9 in 10 chance" of having the disorder (which is strictly incorrect due to sampling issues). In practice, even when tests have very high positive predictive value, the initial screening process should be seen as the beginning of an ongoing process of referral, further assessment, and reassessment at a later date. In short, being screen positive does not constitute a diagnosis, but it should be the beginning of a dialogue between the parent and professional about the child's development, with additional assessments being couched as helpful checks to make sure things are going all right. This situation is not without anxiety, both for the parents and for the professional. A straightforward, honest, and informed approach to the screening process and any possible consequences of being screen positive (couched in terms of further checks as much as in terms of likelihood of having a particular disorder) are required.

CONCLUSIONS

Overall, there is some evidence that screening for ASD in referred children in cases in which a concern about development has already been identified may result in better sensitivity than screening for ASD in an unselected, general population (Drew et al., 2002; Robins et al., 2001; Scambler et al., 2001; Siegel, 2004; Stone, Coonrod, Ousley, 2000; Stone, Coonrod, Turner, & Pozdol, 2004). This is relevant to the question of what criteria should be set for acceptable sensitivity, specificity, and positive predictive value for screens for ASD. It is very likely that sensitivity will always be lower for unselected than for referred samples. One important question is whether the ultimate goal of research should be the development of a universal population screen to identify undetected cases of ASD or the development of instruments that can be used, in combination with parental and professional expressions of concern regarding a child's development, in ongoing health surveillance. Another consideration is whether screens should target ASD specifically or whether they should also attempt to identify children with language and general developmental delays (mental retardation) or other neurodevelopmental conditions. As the compass of "caseness" is broadened, some of the false positives (e.g., children with significant language delay identified by an ASD screen) become true positives. However, broadening the range of disorders to include, for example, children with language delay in addition to ASD will not necessarily make the task of developing screens with acceptable instrument parameters any easier. Two recent systematic reviews on screening for speech and language delays concluded that limitations in the sensitivity and specificity of available screening instruments, as well as difficulties in identifying the boundaries of "caseness" in relation to demonstrated treatment efficacy and need, meant that universal population screening could not be recommended (Law, Boyle, Harris, Harkness, & Nye, 2000; Pickstone, Hannon, & Fox, 2002). Only further research will reveal whether a screen for ASD (and possibly other language and developmental disabilities) will have robust enough instrument parameters to recommend it for universal screening or whether the instruments are more suited to improve decision making as part of ongoing health surveillance and training. However, in the past decade considerable progress has been made in the field, and we await the findings from many ongoing studies internationally with keen anticipation.

ACKNOWLEDGMENTS

We are grateful to our research collaborators on the CHAT project for many discussions over the years that have helped develop and inform our views on this topic: Gillian Baird, Antony Cox, Auriol Drew, John Swettenham, and Sally Wheelwright. Our work on screening has been funded by the Medical Research Council and the Health Foundation in the United Kingdom.

REFERENCES

Adrien, J. L., Lenoir, P., Martineau, J., Perrot, A., Hameury, L., Larmande, C., et al. (1993). Blind ratings of early symptoms of autism based upon family home movies. *Journal of the American Academy of Child and Adolescent Psychiatry, 32*, 617–626.

American Academy of Pediatrics, Committee on Children with Disabilities. (1994). Screening infants and young children for developmental disabilities. *Pediatrics, 93*, 863–865.

American Academy of Pediatrics, Committee on Children with Disabilities. (1999). The pediatrician's role in the development and implementation of an Individual Education Plan (IEP) and/or an Individual Family Service Plan (IFSP). *Pediatrics, 104*, 124–127.

American Academy of Pediatrics, Committee on Children with Disabilities. (2001). Developmental surveillance and screening of infants and young children. *Pediatrics, 108*, 192–196.

Aylward, G. P. (1997). Conceptual issues in developmental screening and assessment. *Journal of Developmental and Behavioral Pediatrics, 18*, 240–249.

Baird, G., Charman, T., Baron-Cohen, S., Cox, A., Swettenham, J., Wheelwright, S., et al. (2000). A screening instrument for autism at 18 months of age: A six-year follow-up study. *Journal of the American Academy of Child and Adolescent Psychiatry, 39*, 694–702.

Baird, G., Charman, T., Cox, A., Baron-Cohen, S., Swettenham, J., Wheelwright, S., et al. (2001). Screening and surveillance for autism and pervasive developmental disorders. *Archives of Diseases in Childhood, 84*, 468–475.

Baranek, G. T. (1999). Autism during infancy: A retrospective video analysis of sensory-motor and social behaviors at 9–12 months of age. *Journal of Autism and Developmental Disorders, 29*, 213–224.

Baron-Cohen, S. (1987). Autism and symbolic play. *British Journal of Developmental Psychology, 5*, 139–148.

Baron-Cohen, S. (1989). Perceptual role-taking and protodeclarative pointing in autism. *British Journal of Developmental Psychology, 7*, 113–127.

Baron-Cohen, S., Allen, J., & Gillberg, C. (1992). Can autism be detected at 18 months? The needle, the haystack and the CHAT. *British Journal of Psychiatry, 138*, 839–843.

Baron-Cohen, S., Charman, T., Wheelwright, S., & Richler, J. (2002, May). *Development of a new screening instrument for autism spectrum disorders: The Q-CHAT*. Paper presented at the International Meeting for Autism Research, Orlando, FL.

Baron-Cohen, S., Cox, A., Baird, G., Swettenham, J., Nightingale, N., Morgan, K., et al. (1996) Screening for autism in a large population at 18 months of age: An investigation of the CHAT (CHecklist for Autism in Toddlers). *British Journal of Psychiatry, 168*, 158–163.

Baron-Cohen, S., Wheelwright, S., Cox, A., Baird, G., Charman, T., Swettenham, J., et al. (2000). The early identification of autism: The Checklist for Autism in Toddlers (CHAT). *Journal of the Royal Society of Medicine, 93*, 521–525.

Berument, S. K., Rutter, M., Lord, C., Pickles, A., & Bailey A. (1999). Autism screening questionnaire: Diagnostic validity. *British Journal of Psychiatry, 175*, 444–451.

Carpenter, M., Nagell, K., & Tomasello, M. (1998). Social cognition, joint attention and communicative competence from 9 to 15 months of age. *Monographs of the Society for Research in Child Development, 63*, 1–143.

Charman, T. (2000). Theory of mind and the early diagnosis of autism. In S. Baron-Cohen, H. Tager-Flusberg, & D. Cohen (Eds.), *Understanding other minds: Perspectives from autism and developmental cognitive neuroscience* (2nd ed., pp. 422–441). Oxford, UK: Oxford University Press.

Charman, T. (2003). Screening and surveillance for autism spectrum disorder in research and practice. *Early Child Development and Care, 173,* 363–374.

Charman, T., & Baird, G. (2002). Practitioner review: Diagnosis of autism spectrum disorder in 2– and 3–year-old children. *Journal of Child Psychology and Psychiatry, 43,* 289–305.

Charman, T., Baron-Cohen, S., Baird, G., Cox, A., Wheelwright, S., Swettenham, J., et al. (2001). Response to Robins, Fein, Barton, & Green, "The Modified CHecklist for Autism in Toddlers: An initial study investigating the early detection of autism and pervasive developmental disorders." *Journal of Autism and Developmental Disorders, 31,* 145–148.

Charman, T., Baron-Cohen, S., Baird, G., Cox, A., Wheelwright, S., Swettenham, J., et al. (2002). Response to Willemsen-Swinkels, Buitelaar, & van Engeland, "Is 18 months too early for the CHAT?" *Journal of the American Academy of Child and Adolescent Psychiatry, 41,* 235–236.

Charman, T., Taylor, E., Drew, A., Cockerill, H., Brown, J. A., & Baird, G. (2005). Outcome at 7 years of children diagnosed with autism at age 2: Predictive validity of assessments conducted at 2 and 3 years of age and pattern of symptom change over time. *Journal of Child Psychology and Psychiatry, 46,* 500–513.

Clark, A., & Harrington, R. (1999). On diagnosing rare disorders rarely: Appropriate use of screening instruments. *Journal of Child Psychology and Psychiatry, 40,* 287–290.

Cochrane, A., & Holland, W. (1969).Validation of screening procedures. *British Medical Bulletin, 27,* 3–8.

Courchesne, E., Carper, R., & Akshoomoff, N. (2003). Evidence of brain overgrowth in the first year of life in autism. *Journal of the American Medical Association, 290,* 337–344.

Cox, A., Klein, K., Charman, T., Baird, G., Baron-Cohen, S., Swettenham, J., et al. (1999). Autism spectrum disorders at 20 and 42 months of age: Stability of clinical and ADI-R diagnosis. *Journal of Child Psychology and Psychiatry, 40,* 719–732.

Dawson, G., Ashman, S. B., & Carver, L. J. (2000). The role of early experience in shaping behavioral and brain development and its implications for social policy. *Development and Psychopathology, 12,* 695–712.

Dawson, G., & Osterling, J. (1997). Early intervention in autism. In M. Guralnick (Ed.), *The effectiveness of early intervention* (pp. 307–326). Baltimore: Brookes.

Delgado, C. E. F., Venezia, M., & Mundy, P. (2004, May). *The Pictorial Infant Communication Scale.* Poster presented at the International Conference on Infant Studies, Chicago, IL.

Dietz, C., Willemsen-Swinkels, S. H. N., van Daalen, E., van Engeland, H., & Buitelaar, J. K. (in press). Screening for Autistic Spectrum Disorder in children aged 14 to 15 months: II. Population screening with the Early Screening of Autistic Traits (ESAT): Design and general findings. *Journal of Autism and Developmental Disorders.*

Drew, A., Baird, G., Baron-Cohen, S., Cox, A., Slonims, V., Wheelwright, S., et al. (2002). A pilot randomised control trial of a parent training intervention for preschool children with autism. *European Child and Adolescent Psychiatry, 11*, 266–272.

Filipek, P. A., Accardo, P. L., Ashwal, S., Baranek, G. T., Cook, E. H., Dawson, G., et al. (2000). Practice parameters: Screening and diagnosis of autism. *Neurology, 55*, 468–479.

Filipek, P. A., Accardo, P. L., Baranek, G. T., Cook, E. H., Dawson, G., Gordon, B., et al. (1999). The screening and diagnosis of autistic spectrum disorders. *Journal of Autism and Developmental Disorders, 29*, 439–484.

Frankenburg, W. K., Dodds, J., Archer, P., Shapiro, H., & Bresnik B. (1992). The Denver II: A major revision and restandardization of the Denver Developmental Screening Test. *Pediatrics, 89*, 91–97.

Gillberg, C., Ehlers, S., Schaumann, H., Jakobsson, G., Dahlgren, S. O., Lindblom, R., et al. (1990). Autism under age 3 years: A clinical study of 28 cases referred for autistic symptoms in infancy. *Journal of Child Psychology and Psychiatry, 31*, 921–934.

Glascoe, F. P. (1996). Developmental screening. In M. Wolraich (Ed.), *Disorders of development and learning: A practical guide to assessment and management* (2nd ed.). St. Louis, MO: Mosby.

Glascoe, F. P. (1997a). Parents' concerns about children's development: Prescreening technique or screening test? *Pediatrics, 99*, 522–528.

Glascoe, F. P. (1997b). *Parents' evaluations of developmental status.* Nashville, TN: Ellsworth & Vandermeer Press.

Glascoe, F. P. (1999). The value of parents' concerns to detect and address developmental and behavioral problems. *Journal of Paediatrics and Child Health, 35*, 1–8.

Hall, D. M. B. (1996). *Health for all children: The report of the Joint Working Party on Child Health Surveillance* (3rd ed.). Oxford, UK: Oxford University Press.

Honda, H., & Shimizu, Y. (2002). Early intervention system for preschool children with autism in the community. *Autism: The International Journal of Research and Practice, 6*, 239–257.

Howlin, P., & Asgharian, A. (1999). The diagnosis of autism and Asperger syndrome: Findings from a systematic survey. *Developmental Medicine and Child Neurology, 41*, 834–839.

Ireton, H. (1992). *Child Development Inventories.* Minneapolis, MN: Behavioral Science Systems.

Koegel, L. K. (2000). Interventions to facilitate communication in autism. *Journal of Autism and Developmental Disorders, 30*, 383–391.

Krug, D. A., Arick, J., & Almond, P. (1980). Behavior checklist for identifying severely handicapped individuals with high levels of autistic behavior. *Journal of Child Psychology and Psychiatry, 21*, 221–229.

Law, J., Boyle, J., Harris, F., Harkness, A., & Nye, C. (2000). The feasibility of universal screening for primary language delay: Findings from a systematic review. *Developmental Medicine and Child Neurology, 42*, 190–200.

Lord, C. (1995). Follow-up of two-year-olds referred for possible autism. *Journal of Child Psychology and Psychiatry, 36*, 1365–1382.

Lord, C. (2000). Commentary: Achievements and future directions for intervention in communication and autism spectrum disorders. *Journal of Autism and Developmental Disorders, 30,* 393–398.

Lord, C., Risi, S., Lambrecht, L., Cook, E. H., Leventhal, B. L., DiLavore, P. C., et al. (2000). The Autism Diagnostic Observation Schedule—Generic: A standard measure of social and communication deficits associated with the spectrum of autism. *Journal of Autism and Developmental Disorders, 30,* 205–223.

Lord, C., Rutter, M., & Le Couteur, A. (1994). Autism Diagnostic Interview—Revised. *Journal of Autism and Developmental Disorders, 24,* 659–686.

Lord, C., Wagner, A., Rogers, S., Szatmari, P., Aman, M., Charman, T., et al. (in press). Challenges in evaluating psychosocial interventions for autistic spectrum disorders. *Journal of Autism and Developmental Disorders.*

Moore, V., & Goodson, S. (2003). How well does early diagnosis of autism stand the test of time?: Follow-up study of children assessed for autism at age 2 and development of an early diagnostic service. *Autism, 7,* 47–63.

Mundy, P., & Neal, R. (2001). Neural plasticity, joint attention and autistic developmental pathology. *International Review of Research in Mental Retardation, 23,* 139–168.

Mundy, P., Sigman, M., Ungerer, J., & Sherman, T. (1986). Defining the social deficits of autism: The contribution of non-verbal communication measures. *Journal of Child Psychology and Psychiatry, 27,* 657–669.

National Research Council, Committee on Educational Interventions for Children with Autism. (2001). *Educating children with autism.* Washington, DC: National Academies Press.

Nelson, K. B., Grether, J. K., Croen, L. A., Dambrosia, J. M., Dickens, B. F., Jelliffe, L. L., et al. (2001). Neuropeptides and neurotrophins in neonatal blood of children with autism or mental retardation. *Annals of Neurology, 49,* 597–606.

Osterling, J. A., Dawson, G., & Munson, J. A. (2002). Early recognition of 1-year-old infants with autism spectrum disorder versus mental retardation. *Development and Psychopathology, 14,* 239–251.

Pickstone, C., Hannon, P., & Fox, L. (2002). Surveying and screening preschool language development in community-focused intervention programmes: A review of instruments. *Child, Care, Health and Development, 28,* 251–264.

Raymaekers, R., & Roeyers, H. (2003, November). *Identification of autism in preschoolers.* Paper presented at the International Congress on Autism—Europe, Lisbon, Portugal.

Robins, D. L., Fein, D., Barton, M. L., & Green, J. A. (2001). The Modified CHecklist for Autism in Toddlers: An initial study investigating the early detection of autism and pervasive developmental disorders. *Journal of Autism and Developmental Disorders, 31,* 131–144.

Robinson, R. (1998). Effective screening in child health. *British Medical Journal, 316,* 1–2.

Rogers, S. J. (1998). Empirically supported comprehensive treatments for young children with autism. *Journal of Clinical Child Psychology, 27,* 167–178.

Rogers, S. (2001). Diagnosis of autism before the age of 3. *International Review of Mental Retardation, 23,* 1–31.

Scambler, D., Rogers, S. J., & Wehner, E. A. (2001). Can the checklist for autism in toddlers differentiate young children with autism from those with developmental delays? *Journal of the American Academy of Child and Adolescent Psychiatry, 40,* 1457–1463.

Schopler, E., Reichler, R. J., DeVellis, R., & Daly K. (1980). Towards objective classification of childhood autism: Childhood Autism Rating Scale (CARS). *Journal of Autism and Developmental Disorders, 10,* 91–103.

Siegel, B. (2004). *Pervasive Developmental Disorders Screening Test—II (PDDST-II).* San Antonio, TX: Harcourt.

Sigman, M., Mundy, P., Sherman, T., & Ungerer, J. (1986). Social interactions of autistic, mentally retarded and normal children and their caregivers. *Journal of Child Psychology and Psychiatry, 27,* 647–655.

Squires, J., Bricker, D., & Potter, L. (1997). Revision of a parent-completed development screening tool: Ages and Stages Questionnaires. *Journal of Pediatric Psychology, 22,* 313–328.

Stone, W. L., Coonrod, E. E., & Ousley, O. Y. (2000). Brief report: Screening Tool for Autism in Two-Year-Olds (STAT): Development and preliminary data. *Journal of Autism and Developmental Disorders, 30,* 607–612.

Stone, W. L., Coonrod, E. E., Turner, L. M., & Pozdol, S. L. (2004). Psychometric properties of the STAT for early autism screening. *Journal of Autism and Developmental Disorders, 34,* 691–701.

Stone, W. L., Lee, E. B., Ashford, L., Brissie, J., Hepburn, S. L., Coonrod, E. E., et al. (1999). Can autism be diagnosed accurately in children under three years? *Journal of Child Psychology and Psychiatry, 40,* 219–226.

Willemsen-Swinkels, S. H., Buitelaar, J. K., & van Engeland, H. (2001). Is 18 months too early for the CHAT? *Journal of the American Academy of Child and Adolescent Psychiatry, 40,* 737–738.

Willemsen-Swinkels, S. H. N., Dietz, C., van Daalen, E., Kerkhof, I. H. G. M., van Engeland, H., & Buitelaar, J. K. (in press). Screening for Autistic Spectrum Disorders in children aged 14 to 15 months: I. The development of the Early Screening of Autistic Traits (ESAT) Questionnaire. *Journal of Autism and Developmental Disorders.*

Williams, J., Scott, F., Stott, C., Allison, C., Bolton, P., Baron-Cohen, S., et al. (2005). The CAST (Childhood Asperger Syndrome Test). Test accuracy. *Autism, 9,* 45–68.

Wilson, J., & Jungner, G. (1968). *Principles and practice of screening for disease* (Public Health Papers No. 34). Geneva, Switzerland: World Health Organization.

Wing, L., Leekam, S. R., Libby, S. J., Gould, J., & Larcombe, M. (2002). The Diagnostic Interview for Social and Communication Disorders: Background, interrater reliability and clinical use. *Journal of Child Psychology and Psychiatry, 43,* 307–325.

Wong, V., Hui, L. H., Lee, W. C., Leung, L. S., Ho, P. K., Lau, W. L., et al. (2004). A modified screening tool for autism (Checklist for Autism in Toddlers [CHAT-23]) for Chinese children. *Pediatrics, 114,* e166–e176.

4

Early Screening for Autism
Spectrum Disorders in
Clinical Practice Settings

LONNIE ZWAIGENBAUM
WENDY STONE

The early identification of children with autism spectrum disorders (ASD) (Wing, 1996) is an essential public health need. Recent population-based studies indicate that approximately 2–3 in 1,000 children have autism and that perhaps 5–6 in 1,000 have some form of ASD (Bertrand et al., 2001; Chakrabarti & Fombonne, 2001; Scott, Baron-Cohen, Bolton, & Brayne, 2002; Yeargin-Allsopp et al., 2003). The demand for clinical services for children with ASD in some regions has increased by as much as 400–600% over the past 10 years. Several authors (Bryson, 1996; Fombonne, 1999, 2003; Gillberg & Wing, 1999) have suggested that this increase may be due to broadening of diagnostic criteria, inclusion of a wider range of children, and greater awareness among health professionals. Although recent service registry (Croen, Grether, Hoogstrate, & Selvin, 2002) and population-based (Yeargin-Alsopp et al., 2003) data suggest that children are being diagnosed earlier than in the past, the diagnosis is still often not

88

made until years after parents initially identify concerns (Howlin & Moore, 1997; Siegel, Pliner, Eschler, & Elliott, 1988; Stone & Rosenbaum, 1988).

Concerted efforts directed at earlier detection and diagnosis of ASD are well justified. Earlier diagnosis of ASD provides greater opportunities for children to benefit fully from intensive autism-specific intervention. All available evidence points to much better outcomes with early intervention (Dawson & Osterling, 1997; Rogers, 1996, 1998; Smith, Groen, & Wynn, 2000). Although there have been no studies that have systematically examined the relative benefits of beginning intervention at one age versus another, one report by Harris and Handleman (2000) suggests that children who enter treatment at an earlier age may show greater gains in IQ and are more likely to achieve full integration on school entry. In addition to reducing the burden of suffering and enhancing quality of life for affected children and their families, early intervention may reduce the considerable lifetime costs associated with providing care to an individual with autism (Jacobson & Mulick, 2000; Jarbrink & Knapp, 2001). Also, most parents of children with autism begin to identify concerns (Coonrod & Stone, 2004; De Giacomo & Fombonne, 1998; Ohta, Nagai, Hara, & Sasaki, 1987; Rogers & DiLalla, 1990) and seek assistance (Howlin & Moore, 1997; Siegel et al., 1988) by the time their children are 2 years old. Reducing the interval between the time children are first seen for clinical assessment and the time they receive a definitive diagnosis would reduce the frustration and despair that many parents experience with long delays. Earlier diagnosis also allows parents to be better informed at an earlier stage in their family planning about recurrence risk to later-born children (Simonoff, 1998), as well as better able to monitor these children for early signs of autism (Zwaigenbaum et al., 2005) and other related developmental concerns (Bailey, Palferman, Heavey, & Le Couteur, 1998; Dawson et al., 2002).

Although universal, community-wide screening for ASD may be the ideal and continues to be an important goal, efforts thus far (as outlined by Charman & Baron-Cohen, Chapter 3, this volume) have met with only modest success, in part due to the relatively low detection rates of available tools. Notably, parents of children with ASD often seek assistance from a community professional (typically their family physician) because of developmental concerns when the child is around the age of 18–24 months. Typically, parents recall that there was limited inquiry into their concerns, which were generally minimized or dismissed regardless of the circumstances (Howlin & Asgharian, 1999; Howlin & Moore, 1997). Referrals ultimately followed as developmental impairments became more apparent, but often the children were seen by a series of consultants, whose assessments resulted in further delays and misinformation. This experience may be shared by other parents with developmental concerns and is not necessarily unique to autism. However, each of these clinical encounters, from the initial contact with the family physician to subsequent appointments with early-intervention service coordination agencies, community-based professionals (who may not have specific expertise in autism), or the local developmental center, represents an opportunity to identify children with clear signs of autism and to move quickly to a specialized assessment that is more likely to result in a definitive diagnosis. Similarly, children with ASD may initially present with developmental delays or language delays that lead to involvement with generic early-identification and intervention programs, speech and language services, and therapeutic day-care or preschool services. If there were a way to systematically and efficiently identify, out of the diverse population attending such programs, which children are most likely to have an ASD, this would be another opportunity for a timely referral to a specialized diagnostic assessment so that intervention could be tailored appropriately. Hence, whereas universal (or "first level") screening may reach a broader segment of the community, an alternative and complementary approach is to conduct targeted screening in clinical practice settings. "Second level" screening of children already identified as having developmental concerns may prove to be an efficient approach to identifying children with ASD because many initially come to attention due to language delays or other developmental concerns.

Notably, consensus panels comprising several professional groups, including the American Academy of Neurology (Filipek et al., 2000), the American Academy of Child and Adolescent Psychiatry (Volkmar, Cook, Pomeroy, Realmuto, & Tanguay, 1999), and the American Academy of Pediatrics (AAP Committee on Children with Disabilities, 2001), among others, have issued practice parameters endorsing screening in clinical practice settings. The recommended assessment model involves a combination of surveillance (a continuous process by which decisions regarding the need for further evaluation are made based on best clinical judgment and often multiple sources of data; Dworkin, 1989) and screening (by which decisions are made based on a cutoff point on a specific instrument). The consensus panel representing these professional groups recommended that health care providers use surveillance approaches to identify children at risk, including developmental screening questionnaires and clinical acumen to detect delays in speech or overall development, and to detect specific behavioral "red flags" for autism (Filipek et al., 1999, 2000). Specific indicators of speech delay that warrant immediate further evaluation were listed as: (1) no babbling by 12 months, (2) no gesturing by 12 months, (3) no single words by 16 months, and (4) no 2-word phrases (excluding rote or echolalic phrases) by 24 months. Additional red flags for autism listed by Filipek et al. (2000) for the clinician to consider include any loss of language or social skills at any age, diminished social-communicative behaviors (including eye contact, orienting to faces, social smiling, pointing, showing, and other attempts to get parents' attention) and social responsiveness (including lack of response to child's name being called or to parent's efforts to play and interact and lack of interest in and/or avoidance of other children), and atypical play and/or sensory-oriented behaviors (lack of imitative play, lack of interest in toys or interests limited to repetitive activities such as spinning wheels of toy car, odd or repetitive ways of moving hands and fingers, etc.) The consensus panel recommended that when children are identified with delays or other specific behavioral red flags, they be given an autism screening tool to determine which children should be referred for a more comprehensive and autism-specific diagnostic assessment.

With increasing availability of screening tools designed for use in clinical practice settings, we will begin to see the impact of this approach to early detection of autism on diagnostic patterns, utilization of health and intervention services, and, ultimately, on the function and well-being of children with ASD. Although these potential effects are still on the horizon, we have preliminary data from several second-level screens to help guide initial clinical decisions regarding the use of these tools. This chapter describes screening tools for autism that have been used to assess referred populations in clinical practice settings, the potential applications of these tools, and other issues related to the potential effects of second-level screening for targeted children and for the health system in general.

To set the stage for a detailed discussion of currently available tools, we briefly review terms used to evaluate the psychometric properties of screening instruments. *Sensitivity* refers to the proportion of children with ASD who are correctly identified by the screen (a child with the disorder who is not identified by the screen is considered to be a "false negative"). *Specificity* refers to the proportion of children who do not have ASD who are correctly classified by the screen (a child who does not have autism yet fails the screen is considered to be a "false positive"). *Positive predictive value* (PPV) is the likelihood of having the diagnosis, given a positive screen. *Negative predictive value* (NPV) is the likelihood of not having the diagnosis, given a negative screen (Sackett, Haynes, Guyatt, & Tugwell, 1991). Sensitivity and specificity are properties of the screening test, whereas PPV and NPV are related to the specificity and sensitivity of the test, respectively, as well as to the base rate of ASD in the group being screened. As noted earlier, when cases of ASD are identified in the general community (as in universal screening), this is considered first-stage screening, whereas second-stage screening (the focus of this chapter) implies that the target population has been selected based on developmental concerns or other risk indicators.

AUTISM SCREENING TOOLS USED IN SECOND-STAGE SCREENING

CHecklist for Autism in Toddlers

The CHecklist for Autism in Toddlers (CHAT) was described in detail in Chapter 3, this volume. Although it was developed and has been mainly used for screening in the general community (Baron-Cohen, Allen, & Gillberg, 1992; Baron-Cohen et al., 1996), there is one published study that assesses the sensitivity and specificity of the CHAT in a clinical sample. Scambler, Rogers, and Wehner (2001) evaluated the CHAT with 26 children with established diagnoses of autism, based on at least three of the following: the DSM-IV checklist (American Psychiatric Association, 1994), the Autism Diagnostic Interview—Revised (ADI-R), the Autism Diagnostic Observation Scale (ADOS), and a best-estimate review. Also, 18 children with other developmental delays were evaluated, including 6 with Down syndrome. These children ranged in age from 2 to 3 years, with a mean age of roughly 33 months. The developmental-delay group had somewhat higher verbal and overall adaptive skills than the autism group. The CHAT (high-risk criteria: child must fail protodeclarative pointing, gaze monitoring, and pretend play on a single administration) correctly identified 12 of 26 children in the autism group (sensitivity = 46%). The medium-risk criteria suggested by Baird et al. (2000; i.e., the child must fail protodeclarative pointing, but gaze monitoring and/or pretend play can be present) identified an additional 5 of 26 children in the autism group (overall sensitivity = 65%). Scambler et al.'s (2001) further modification to these medium-risk criteria—notably, that the child must fail protodeclarative pointing *or* pretend play but may pass the other key items—identified an additional 5 children in the autism group (overall sensitivity = 85%). No child with a diagnosis of developmental delay failed the CHAT, regardless of the criteria used (specificity = 100%).

Although these data are encouraging, there are several reasons for a cautious interpretation. First, previous CHAT research suggests that estimates of screening sensitivity may be inflated in the absence of prospective follow-up (Baird et al., 2000). Assessing agreement between screening and diagnostic measures in a cross-sectional study is very different from using a screening tool to predict future diagnoses in a longitudinal study. Second, the modified criteria were generated post hoc to maximize sensitivity and specificity in the current data set. These criteria need to be replicated in an independent sample to confirm better differentiation of autism from developmental delay than the original CHAT cutoffs. Third, it is important to note that Scambler et al. (2001) studied a convenience sample of children with established diagnoses whose parents had volunteered to participate in a longitudinal study of developmental problems. This was not a consecutive series of children referred for diagnostic assessment. Hence it is unclear whether estimates of sensitivity and specificity would generalize to any real-life clinical setting; in particular, there may have been a selection bias toward children with more obvious diagnostic presentations. Nevertheless, Scambler et al.'s (2001) findings suggest that using broader thresholds and targeting children who are 2 years (rather than 18 months) old for screening may yield higher sensitivity while retaining very high specificity. Notably, a modification of the CHAT has been developed with these goals in mind.

Modified CHecklist for Autism in Toddlers

The Modified CHecklist for Autism in Toddlers (M-CHAT; Robins, Fein, Barton, & Green, 2001) differs from the CHAT in two main ways: (1) the M-CHAT includes several additional items, covering a broader range of developmental domains than the CHAT, including sensory and motor abnormalities, imitation, and response to name; and (2) the M-CHAT is a parent-completed questionnaire, with no observational component. Two questions are included that cover critical CHAT items (pointing to show and pretending, but not gaze monitoring), as are the other seven items from the questionnaire portion of the CHAT, not all of which were intended to be specific to autism (Charman et al., 2001). Also, the M-CHAT is administered at 24 months rather than 18 months.

Robins et al. (2001) report an initial evaluation of the M-CHAT in toddlers being seen for routine checkups with their community pediatrician or family doctor (N = 1,122 from 98 selected practices) and in toddlers referred to early-intervention programs due to language delays or other nonspecific developmental concerns (N = 171). Initially, screening was conducted at 18 months using a 30-item questionnaire. Subsequently, based on analysis involving the first 600 participants, the M-CHAT was shortened to 22 items, and the timing of administration was changed from 18 months to 24 months. In addition, a 23rd item (social referencing) was added, and the cutoff criteria that identified children for further evaluation were changed. Parents were contacted by phone if (1) the child failed 3 of 23 items (that is, at least 3 of 23 behavioral markers were endorsed), (2) the child failed 2 of 8 items selected based on a discriminant function analysis (DFA) of the first 600 participants (shortened to 6 items when the overall scale was shortened to 23), or (3) the referral source noted concerns. Out of the total sample, parents of 132 out of 1,293 children were contacted. The purpose of the phone interview was to confirm parents' responses on the M-CHAT, not to collect new information. Positive screens were confirmed in 58 of 132 toddlers, who were then seen by the investigators for further evaluation.

Assessment of these 58 toddlers included standardized measures of cognitive, adaptive, and communication skills and best clinical judgment using a semistructured diagnostic interview based on DSM-IV criteria and the Childhood Autism Rating Scale (CARS). Based on this assessment, 39 children were diagnosed with ASD at a mean age of 27.6 months. This number included 3 of 1,122 who were referred at well-child visits and 36 of 171 referred by early-intervention services. Children who did not meet M-CHAT criteria or who were "OK on phone interview" (Robins et al., 2001, p. 139) did not receive further assessment. Sensitivity and specificity of the M-CHAT for a clinical diagnosis of ASD, with 3 of 23 items as the screening cutoff, were estimated to be 97% and 95%, respectively. With a cutoff of 2 of the 6 items loading most strongly on the DFA (pointing to indicate interest, responding to name, showing interest in other children, bringing objects to show, looking where someone points, imitating), sensitivity and specificity were 95% and 98%, respectively. It is important to note that *these calculations assume that there were no cases of autism among the group of children who were not seen for clinical assessment.* This group consisted of 1,235 of the 1,293 children originally screened, including 74 children who failed the original screen (as a parent-completed questionnaire) but whose risk status was not confirmed during the phone interview. Sensitivity and specificity for a cutoff on the entire set of nine CHAT items was also calculated and compared with estimates for the M-CHAT. Notably, this is not how the CHAT is actually scored, so it does not give an equal comparison of the two measures (Charman et al., 2001).

The M-CHAT holds considerable promise in terms of both potential sensitivity and relative ease of administration. There has been considerable interest in using the M-CHAT in clinical settings, and a Chinese-language translation has been described (Wong et al., 2004). However, there are important methodological concerns with the design and interpretation of the data from its initial investigation. First, the sensitivity and specificity of the M-CHAT *cannot* truly be estimated based on initial data in Robins et al. (2001), because children below the screening cutoff received no further evaluation. Calculating sensitivity as the proportion of children diagnosed with ASD who exceeded the cutoff simply provides a check that the authors followed their stated procedures in determining which children would receive a clinical assessment. One child received a diagnosis but had only two positive items; presumably this child was assessed prior to the change in cutoff criteria (i.e., one of the first 600 participants) or else had two of the six items chosen by the initial DFA.

Second, by conducting assessments on only those children who failed the questionnaire and phone interview, the authors may have introduced a significant expectation bias into their diagnostic assessments. This is particularly relevant given that: (1) the diagnostic measures used in this study

(DSM-IV and CARS) involve a high degree of clinical judgment and (2) a remarkably high proportion (36 of 171; 21%) of the group referred from early-intervention services received a diagnosis of ASD. This is a group that the authors described as unselected for ASD other than having a language delay or nonspecific developmental concern. Admittedly, there is a paucity of data on the distribution of diagnoses among children in generic early-intervention programs (Britain, Holmes, & Hassanein, 1995). However, the rate of ASD in Robin et al.'s (2001) referral sample is similar to the rate observed in children with delays who were seen in neurology and developmental clinics at a tertiary care center, where one might expect children to be more severely impaired than in a community intervention sample (Shevell, Majnemer, Rosenbaum, & Abrahamowicz, 2001). Findings from the CHAT follow-up (Baird et al., 2000; Cox et al., 1999) suggest that some children identified with developmental delays near age 2, particularly those who score subthreshold on autism screening, may be diagnosed with ASD at a later age. This finding suggests that even more than 21% of Robins et al.'s (2001) referral group will ultimately receive a diagnosis of ASD. Additional follow-up, preferably blind to initial M-CHAT status and including a sample of screen-negative participants, will be needed to resolve this issue. Robins and colleagues have subsequently presented findings involving 657 children from their original sample who were rescreened at 4 years, but again, only those children who screened positive on the questionnaire and phone interview were seen for diagnostic assessment (Robins et al., 2002). Follow-up assessment of the M-CHAT screening samples is still under way.

Screening Tool for Autism in Two-Year-Olds

The Screening Tool for Autism in Two-Year-Olds (STAT) was developed by Stone and Ousley (1997) for second-stage screening; that is, to help differentiate children with autism from children with other disorders once developmental concerns are identified. Scoring is based on behaviors observed during structured tasks. The STAT was designed for use in children between 24 and 35 months of age, and its items cover (item counts in parentheses) motor imitation (4), play skills (2), requesting (2), and directing attention (4). The two items covering requesting were included to facilitate interaction but were not scored in the initial STAT evaluation by Stone, Coonrod, and Ousley (2000). Cutoff criteria were initially established based on a "development sample" of 7 children with autism and 33 children with other developmental disorders and then were evaluated in a "validation sample" of 12 children with autism and 21 children with other disorders. The development and validation samples were recruited from consecutive referrals to a university-based developmental evaluation center, and the entire group ranged in age from 24 to 35 months. Diagnosis was based on clinical assessment using DSM-IV criteria, scores on the CARS, and standard measures of cognitive development (procedures similar to those used by Robins et al., 2001, to evaluate the M-CHAT). Screening with the STAT and diagnostic assessment were completed independently at the same clinic visit (i.e., a concurrent design). Cutoff criteria were established based on findings in the development sample. To pass each of the three domains (imitation, play, and directing attention), the child must receive credit on at least two items within that domain (i.e., half the imitation items, both play items, half the directing-attention items). Because all 7 children with autism failed at least two domains compared with 3 of 33 in the nonautism group, this was used as the overall criterion for failing the STAT. Results for the validation sample are reported separately, providing an independent assessment of this criterion: 10 of 12 children with autism failed at least two domains (sensitivity = 83%), compared with 3 of 21 in the nonautism group (specificity = 86%).

The scoring system of the STAT was revised more recently, based on signal-detection analyses in a sample of 26 children with autism (AUT) and 26 children with language impairment or other developmental delays (DD/LI); children with pervasive developmental disorder not otherwise specified (PDDNOS) were not included (Stone, Coonrod, Turner, & Pozdol, 2004). Participants were recruited from a regional diagnostic center, and the two groups were matched on chronological age (CA) and mental age (MA). As in the previous study (Stone et al., 2000), the sample was divided equally into a development sample and a validation sample. The STAT was scored somewhat differently than before, with the four domains (including requesting) weighted equally (i.e., individual items were weighted inversely to the number items in the domain to which they belong), generating a total score of 0–4. Receiver Operating Curves determined that a cutoff of 2 for "high risk" in the developmental sample was associated with maximal sensitivity (100%) and very good specificity (roughly 80%). This cutoff was associated with a sensitivity of 92% and specificity of 85% in the validation sample. The STAT, using this cutoff, was further evaluated in a sample of 50 children with autism, 39 with DD/LI, and 15 with PDDNOS. The main findings were: (1) excellent interobserver and test–retest reliability for the STAT classification of high risk versus low risk (kappas = 1.0 and .90, respectively); (2) excellent agreement between the STAT and ADOS (autism cutoff) when the sample was restricted to children with autism and DD/LI (only 2 of 52 children scoring in the STAT high-risk range failed to exceed the ADOS threshold for autism); and (3) children with a clinical diagnosis of PDDNOS were roughly equally divided into the high-risk and low-risk categories by the STAT (Stone et al., 2004).

Overall, the STAT has a number of strengths as a second-level screen.

It can discriminate children with autism from those with DD/LI with a high degree of sensitivity and specificity, and there is excellent agreement between the STAT high-risk category and an ADOS classification of autism. Its interactive format also allows for greater standardization and assessment of qualitative differences between autism and DD/LI that may be difficult to ascertain in a questionnaire format, and it generates rich observational data that can help guide initial intervention planning. The potential limitations of the STAT are that it is not designed to detect children with PDDNOS and that it requires more training and expertise than parent questionnaires. The STAT is certainly not the only screening tool to show reduced sensitivity for cases of PDDNOS; for example, the CHAT had extremely low sensitivity for PDDNOS (Baird et al., 2000). Moreover, this problem with identification of PDDNOS is not limited to screening measures; diagnostic agreement and diagnostic stability have been found to be lower for the diagnosis of PDDNOS than for the diagnosis of autism (Eaves & Ho, 2004; Stone et al., 1999). Nevertheless, in many districts, intervention services may not discriminate by diagnostic subtype within the autism spectrum. Children with PDDNOS show substantial benefit with early intensive intervention (Smith et al., 2000), and they make up 40–75% of the total number of children on the spectrum in recent epidemiological studies (Bertrand et al., 2002; Chakrabarti & Fombonne, 2001). These figures raise questions about the utility of a screening tool that has a sensitivity of 90% only for the children at the severe half of the autism spectrum; however, this issue may not be easily resolved given the sometimes subtle and heterogeneous manifestations of PDDNOS. The second issue is that the STAT is more resource-intensive than a parent questionnaire such as the M-CHAT, but it may also generate richer, more clinically meaningful data. This is a trade-off that needs to be considered by clinicians and other service providers. Regardless, the STAT is clearly a strong candidate for second-stage screening and has been implemented in a number of clinical settings in Canada and the United States. Additional research is being conducted on identifying screening cutoffs for PDDNOS, as well as for children older than 36 months and younger than 24 months.

Pervasive Developmental Disorders Screening Test–II

The Pervasive Developmental Disorders Screening Test–II (PDDST-II) is a parent-report questionnaire developed by Siegel and colleagues (Siegel, 2004), and includes components designed for first-stage and second-stage screening. Its psychometric properties have been presented at professional meetings (Siegel, 2001) and are now described in a published manual (Siegel, 2004). There are three components (stages) of the PDDST-II, the first two of which involve screening for ASD in clinical practice settings (Stage 3, which is not discussed further, discriminates autism from PDDNOS).

The PDDST-II, Stage 1, was designed to be used in primary care settings and includes 23 items based on behaviors emerging between 12 and 24 months. The standardization sample included 656 preschool children who had been referred due to suspected autism (not all actually had an ASD, but all had at least a few autistic symptoms) (Siegel, 2004) and 256 ex-preterm infants who were expected to show a high rate of early atypical development (but not autism). Sensitivity and specificity estimates are based on agreement between item and group classification. For example, a true positive is recorded when a child in the suspected-autism group scores positive on a PDDST-II item. Hence, although this instrument is intended to be used as a first-stage screen, its evaluation is based on classification into groups defined by clinical suspicion (rather than by individual diagnoses) and does not include a community-based cohort of children unselected for developmental concerns. Further evaluation of the PDDST-II, Stage 1, in a community setting will be needed to evaluate its utility as a first-stage screen.

The PDDST-II, Stage 2, was designed for use in developmental clinics in which children are often first assessed for possible developmental disorders. The index population included patients with diagnoses of autistic disorder or PDDNOS (N = 318). The comparison group consisted of patients clinically referred for autism evaluation but who eventually received nonautistic spectrum disorder diagnoses, such as mental retardation or developmental language disorders (N = 62). Estimates of sensitivity and specificity for the PDDST-II for this sample are not yet available. Note that the usual role of a second-stage screen is to identify those children most likely to have ASD out of a larger group referred due to a broad range of developmental concerns. In contrast, the evaluation data for the PDDST-II, Stage 2, addresses the question Which children referred due to clinical suspicion of *autism* are most likely to have the diagnosis? There is also the limitation of a very high base rate of autism/ASD in the test sample, which increases estimates of positive predictive value of the instrument to beyond that which could be expected in an unselected group of children with developmental concerns of a more general nature.

Eaves and Ho (2004) recently reported their clinical experience using the PDDST, Stages 1 and 2, as part of their initial diagnostic assessment of 49 children referred for suspected autism, seen initially at around 2.5 years of age (PDDST data available for 35 children). All 35 children for whom PDDST data were available scored above the screening threshold, and 30 received clinical diagnoses of autism. Although the authors did not calculate sensitivity and specificity, estimates from this small sample would be 100% for sensitivity and 0% for specificity (because all children screened positive). Notably, only 4 of 14 children without PDDST data were diagnosed with autism, suggesting that the screen may have been used selectively based on strong diagnostic suspicion. Given that the 34 children had diagnoses of autism and that an additional 9 were diagnosed with PDDNOS (i.e., ASD diagnoses in 43 of 49 children; 88%) the PDDST was not truly being used as a second-stage screen in this sample; rather, there may have been other intake procedures that triaged children with a high likelihood of diagnosis to this specialty clinic.

PROMISING MEASURES UNDER DEVELOPMENT

Systematic Observation of Red Flags

Wetherby et al. (2004) describe a coding scheme for behavioral "red flags" that appears to discriminate between children with ASD, children with language and/or other developmental delays (DD), and children who are typically developing (TD). The Systematic Observation of Red Flags (SORF) was developed to complement assessment using the Communication and Symbolic Behavior Scales Developmental Profile (CSBS-DP; Wetherby & Prizant, 2002). The CSBS-DP consists of three main components: a 24-item parent questionnaire designed to be completed quickly by a parent in a doctor's office or other community setting (the Infant–Toddler Checklist), a more detailed four-page follow-up Caregiver Questionnaire, and an interactive, observational assessment (the behavioral sample), each of which covers communicative, social, and symbolic play behaviors. The SORF consists of 29 items that are coded from videotapes of the CSBS-DP behavioral sample.

Wetherby et al. (2004) evaluated the SORF in a sample of 3,021 children ages 12–24 months and not previously identified with developmental delays. These children were recruited from selected child-care and health care agencies serving families of young children. An additional 5 children under 24 months with known DD (including 2 children with Down syndrome) were also included in this study. A multistage assessment process was used to identify ASD, DD, and TD comparison groups. First, parents completed the Infant–Toddler Checklist of the CSBS-DP. Second, children scoring below the 10th percentile on the Checklist ($N = 377$), a random sample of children scoring above this cutoff ($N = 230$), and the 5 children with known delays were selected for further assessment using the behavioral sample of the CSBS-DP, with roughly 20% sample loss at this stage. Third, children scoring below the 10th percentile on the behavior profile, a random sample of children above this cutoff, and the 5 children with known DD were selected for cognitive and language assessment using the Mullen Scales of Early Learning at age 2–3 years. The Mullen was completed for 298 of 445 children (i.e., an additional 30% sample loss). Fourth, children with communication delays (based on the CSBS-DP at 12–24 months, not on the Mullen) were selected for further assessment, which included 71 children from the main sample and the 5 with known DD. Based on parent-reported intervention history from a related study, 10 of 71 were suspected of having ASD. These 10 children with suspected ASD, 21 other randomly selected children with "communication delay," and the 5 children with known delays formed a group of 36 children who were then evaluated for best-estimate diagnosis. This evaluation was completed by a clinical psychologist and a speech/language pathologist on the study team, based on a review of the child's Vineland Adaptive Behavior Scales, the Mullen Scales, and the ADOS at age 2–3 years (previous clinical diagnoses substituted for the ADOS for 2 children). Overall, 18 children were diagnosed with ASD (9 with autism, 9 with PDDNOS), and 18 children with DD; 18 children who completed the first three steps of the study and who had no indication of ASD or communication delay were selected as the TD comparison group.

Videotapes of the CSBS-DP behavioral sample for the ASD, DD, and TD children from the final sample were recoded using the SORF. Interrater reliability of items coded on the SORF was excellent for trained, experienced raters in the study group (mean Cohen kappa = 0.94, range 0.82–1.00). Significant group differences were found in ratings on 13 of 29 items, primarily covering joint attention (e.g., lack of warm, joyful expression with gaze; lack of pointing), vocalization (e.g., unusual prosody; lack of vocalization with consonants), and repetitive movements (e.g., repetitive movements or posturing of body, arms, hands, or fingers; repetitive movements with objects). Post hoc testing indicated significant differences between all three groups (i.e., ASD > DD > TD) for 9 items and differences between ASD and TD, but not ASD and DD, for 4 items (including lack of pointing, vocalization with consonants, and conventional toy play). A DFA using these 13 items correctly predicted group membership for all children with ASD and TD and for 15 of 18 children with DD (3 classified as TD).

Wetherby and colleagues (2004) also assessed the CSBS-DP Infant–Toddler Checklist at 12–24 months to screen for communication impairment (i.e., the combined ASD and DD group vs. TD, and ASD vs. TD, excluding the DD group). Estimates of sensitivity and specificity were very high (89% and 89%, respectively, for the former comparison and 94% and 89%, respectively, for the latter). However, both the screen (the Infant–Toddler Checklist) and the communication delay classification (i.e., lower 10th percentile on the behavioral profile) are components of the CSBS-DP at 12–24 months, so these estimates are not easily interpreted. Assessment of ASD was also not fully independent of the screen: Possible diagnoses were ascertained from intervention history, which was determined only in the communication-delay group. Notably, the CSBS-DP has shown excellent sensitivity and specificity for independently determined communication delays in other studies (Wetherby, Goldstein, Cleary, Allen, & Kublin, 2003).

The SORF has a number of strengths. Initial data presented by Wetherby et al. (2004) suggest that the SORF is sensitive to both autism and PDDNOS at 2–3 years. The SORF covers a wide breadth of social and communicative functions that are recognized as core deficits of autism in preschoolers, and there are nine items that discriminate between children with ASD and DD. Also, the CSBS-DP behavioral profile (which generates the videotaped behaviors from which the SORF is coded) is a rich, interactive assessment that could identify targets for subsequent intervention and that could conceivably be integrated into a preschool developmental assessment (or speech and language) program to identify children needing diagnostic assessment for ASD.

However, the data presented by Wetherby et al. (2004) are preliminary. The SORF is coded retrospectively from the videotaped behavioral profile, rather than being used prospectively during an interactive assessment. Also, by selecting only the 13 of 29 items that differentiated between ASD, DD, and TD at the $p < .002$ level, it is not surprising that the discriminant function analysis separated the three groups so distinctly. As Wetherby et al. (2004) note, validation of these findings in an independent sample is necessary before conclusions about the SORF 13-item algorithm and estimates of sensitivity and specificity can be made with confidence. The diagnostic groups being compared are a mix of children taken from a heterogeneous community sample screened with the CSBS-DP and a small number of children referred with developmental delay (3 of whom were among the 18 children with ASD in the final sample), and the diagnosis of ASD was heavily reliant on the ADOS in the absence of a standardized diagnostic interview. Further studies are warranted that assess the CSBS-DP behavior profile and the SORF as second-level screens for ASD.

Social Communication Questionnaire

The Social Communication Questionnaire (SCQ), originally named the Autism Screening Questionnaire (ASQ; Berument, Rutter, Lord, Pickles, & Bailey, 1999), is a 40-item parent questionnaire designed for use with individuals age 4 and older. Items were derived from the Autism Diagnostic Interview—Revised (ADI-R; Lord, Rutter, & LeCouteur, 1994). Preliminary data from 2- to 4-year-olds indicate more modest estimates of sensitivity and specificity than in the original test sample of older individuals (Corsello, Cook, & Leventhal, 2003). The SCQ has also been used to identify children with ASD from among samples of children with specific genetic disorders (for example, Cohen syndrome; Howlin & Karpf, 2004) and to compare 6- to 9-year-old children with ASD and pragmatic language impairment (Bishop & Norbury, 2002). Additional research on the utility of the SCQ as a second-level screening with younger samples is warranted.

Autism Observation Scale for Infants

There is growing interest in prospective studies of infants at high risk for ASD as a potential means to identify novel behavioral (and biological) markers. Infant siblings of children with ASD are particularly well suited for prospective studies, as recurrence risk may be as high as 8–9% (Ritvo et al., 1989) and risk status is known from birth and is independent of any hypothesized markers. Although there are a number of methodological and practical challenges related to this research design (Zwaigenbaum et al., in press), several studies are under way, and initial data suggests that early behavioral markers for autism may be detected as early as 12 months of age, raising the possibility of earlier screening. These studies also provide context for the development and evaluation of new measures of ASD-related behaviors that could be modified and evaluated as possible screening tools that might be administered in clinical practice settings at an earlier age than are currently available measures. For example, the Autism Observational Scale for Infants (AOSI; Bryson, Brian, McDermott, Rombough, & Zwaigenbaum, in press) was developed to aid systematic data collection in an infant-siblings sample on early abnormalities in several developmental domains relevant to autism, including visual attention, early play behaviors including imitation, affective responses, early social-communicative behaviors (such as eye gaze, social referencing, and reciprocal smiling), behavioral reactivity, and sensory–motor development. Infants are engaged in semistructured play and systematic presses are designed to assess various target behaviors, which are rated on a scale from 0 to 3, on which 0 implies normal function and higher values represent increasing deviation. For example, "social babbling" is rated 0 if there are clear four-step sequences of back-and-forth vocalizations with the examiner (two turns each), 1 if there are only two-step sequences (i.e., the infant vocalizes in response to something the examiner says but does not respond a second time in sequence), 2 if the infant's vocalizations are unrelated to the examiner's vocalizations, and 3 if the infant rarely or never vocalizes.

Reliability analyses indicate that absolute agreement between trained raters on the AOSI is > 90% on each item, and measures of interrater agreement on the total score using intraclass correlations (ICCs) at 6, 12, and 18 months are 0.71, 0.90, and 0.92, respectively, each on a sample of 26–34 infants. Test–retest reliability (at 12 months) is also good (ICC = 0.63; Bryson et al., in press). Also, preliminary data indicate that the AOSI can distinguish between siblings with and without autism as early as 12 months of age (Zwaigenbaum et al., 2005). The presence of seven or more risk markers (that is, items scored 1 or above) at 12 months prospectively identified 6 of 7 children diagnosed with autism at 24 months, compared with 2 of 58 nonautistic siblings and 0 of 23 controls. As such, the sensitivity and specificity of the AOSI for autism in this initial sample of siblings, using a cutoff point of seven markers, are 84% and 98%, respectively. Individual 12-month AOSI risk markers that predict autism at 24 months include atypical eye contact, visual tracking, disengagement of visual attention, orienting to name, imitation, social smiling, reactivity, social interest, and sensory-oriented behavior (Zwaigenbaum et al., 2005). Clearly, these findings must be replicated in other high-risk samples, as well as nonsibling samples, that might be assessed in community settings (e.g., infants referred to early-intervention programs) before the AOSI can be applied in clinical practice. However, these data illustrate how prospective studies of high-risk infants may lead to the development of new measures that might be used for earlier screening.

IMPLICATIONS FOR CLINICAL PRACTICE

Although most of the screening instruments described in this chapter are still at an early stage in the transition from research to community settings, there are good reasons to believe that ASD screening tools can address important clinical needs in a number of practice environments. In many situations, health and child-care professions currently rely on best clinical judgment to make decisions about which children to refer to specialized clinics for diagnostic assessment. The accuracy of informal impressions regarding which children are likely to have autism has not been studied systematically. Presumably, the sensitivity of informal assessment by community physicians, for example, to the early risk markers of ASD has been poor given that, until recently, a relatively small proportion of affected children were referred for diagnostic assessment before 3 years of age (Howlin & Moore, 1997).

Matching the Screening to the Setting

One of the important distinctions between types of second-stage screening measures is how information is gathered: from parent questionnaires (e.g., M-CHAT) or from direct interaction with the child (e.g., STAT). Clearly, each source of information has advantages, as well as limitations. Parent questionnaires are convenient to use in that they are quick and easy to score and require minimal training. However, two critical assumptions underlying the use and interpretation of parent questionnaires are that: (1) parents are able to read and comprehend the screening questions and that (2) parents interpret the questions in the manner intended by the author. Literacy requirements, different frames of reference, and potential for reporter bias can thus affect the utility of this type of screening. In contrast, interactive measures have the advantage of enabling the service provider to elicit behaviors directly, through structured interactions with the child. By focusing on behaviors that represent core features of autism (e.g., social interactions, communication, imitation, and play), interactive measures can yield information relevant not only to determining autism risk status but also to identifying specific goals for intervention programming. Thus the ability to provide targeted intervention may be facilitated through the use of interactive screening tools. However, these tools often require training and involve more professional time than do parent questionnaires and thus are not feasible for use in all clinical settings.

Several considerations can guide the choice of which type of screening to use in different clinical or community settings: the type of service provided, the time allotted for each visit, and the background and training of the clinician. Table 4.1 illustrates the implications of these different factors for the use of parental report versus interactive screening measures. As illustrated in the table, interactive measures are less useful in settings involving brief visits or professionals who have limited experience with autism.

A simple parent questionnaire with clear criteria for establishing risk status, such as the M-CHAT, may be invaluable to the community physician who lacks experience with developmental and behavioral assessment and may lead to earlier and more consistent referrals. Similarly, a brief interactive assessment such as the STAT may be an essential tool in a second-level assessment by a community pediatrician or psychiatrist who may not be experienced in ASD diagnosis but who can make more evidence-based decisions regarding which children should be referred immediately for a specialized assessment. In fact, there is strong evidence that the availability of an early identification tool and involvement in a screening program can increase community physicians' awareness of early signs and lead to earlier detection and referral, independent of the screening properties of the particular tool (Charman & Baird, 2002). Also, recent epidemiological studies have indicated that trained health personnel, by simply observing children in their homes and asking parents about their concerns, identified four out of five children with autism, generally prior to the age of 2–2½ years (Chakrabarti & Fombonne, 2001, 2005). In fact, the average age of diagnosis (roughly 3½ years) in recent epidemiological studies (Bertrand et al., 2001; Chakrabarti & Fombonne, 2001) is considerably younger than that reported by parents of children born 10–20 years ago (Howlin & Moore, 1997). Screening tools ultimately assist physicians by providing a standard-

TABLE 4.1. Matching the Characteristics of Early Screening Tools to Clinical Settings

Feature of setting	Type of Stage 2 screening	
	Parent report	Interactive
Time allotted per child visit		
Under half-hour	Y	N
Over half-hour	Y	Y
Type of service provided		
Diagnostic assessment	Y	Y
Developmental/skill assessment		
(e.g., speech–language, occupational therapy)	Y	Y
Early intervention (e.g., specialized preschool,		
speech–language therapy)	Y	Y
Clinical training and experience		
No autism experience	Y	N
Autism experience—below age 5	Y	Y
Autism experience—age 5 or older	Y	N

Note. Y's indicate suitable matches between the features of the setting and the type of screening. N's indicate less compatibility between the setting and the screening type.

ized method of collecting information about early signs, much as questionnaires that cover parental concerns can be used as part of general developmental surveillance to detect children with other developmental problems (Glascoe, 2003).

Similarly, a second-stage ASD screening tool could increase the efficiency of intake and triage processes at developmental evaluation clinics. Children referred due to developmental or language delay could be directed to general assessment clinics or diagnostic clinics specialized to ASD, depending on parental questionnaires and/or brief observations using one of the second-level screens described in this chapter. In fact, regional assessment clinics often use standardized intake tools to identify likely diagnoses based on parental questionnaires or interviews. For example, the Brief Child and Family Telephone Interview (Cunningham, Pettingill, & Boyle, 2000), derived from a DSM-based symptom checklist used in a general population study of pediatric mental health (Boyle et al., 1993), is widely used in Canada to determine initial service plans for children referred to regional centers. However, currently very little data exist on the use of ASD screening tools in such settings (Eaves & Ho, 2004), and it would certainly be worthwhile to assess the accuracy and cost-efficiency of such a practice relative to current intake procedures, which in some centers are highly resource intensive and poorly evaluated.

Early-intervention, day-care/preschool, and speech and language services are the introduction to developmental services for many families of children with ASD. Providers in these settings are often the first to observe the at-risk child's development in sufficient depth to identify early markers of autism. The use of a standardized ASD screen may help ensure that children with ASD are detected earlier and more consistently, so that children can be referred for a specialized diagnostic assessment in a timely manner. For example, experience with the M-CHAT shows that a brief questionnaire can sensitively detect children with ASD as early as 18–24 months of age from early-identification/intervention settings. An interactive assessment such as the STAT could be used as part of intake to speech and language services. Further research assessing the utility of ASD screening tools in a wide range of community-based therapeutic settings is warranted.

Understanding and Explaining Screening Results

Although early identification and intervention for children with ASD have been advocated by several medical panels, including the American Academy of Pediatrics and the American Academy of Neurology, several obstacles to using screening measures in clinical practice settings may include reluctance to "label" a young child and/or discomfort conveying difficult information to parents. The issue of labeling young children has many facets, including the fear of imparting a "life sentence," the limited availability of (or knowledge about) intervention services for young children with ASD, and the possibility that one's screening results will not be confirmed by subsequent diagnostic evaluation (i.e., false positives). These concerns may be placed in proper perspective by considering the fact that the process of screening is much different from that of conducting a diagnostic evaluation. The purpose of autism screening, especially in referral populations, is to identify the need for further specialized evaluation that can rule in or rule out the diagnosis. Screening is a means to obtaining autism-specialized services, not an end in itself. Screening will inevitably result in some false positives, as well as some false negatives.

Because one of the goals of a screening program is to identify as many children with ASD as possible at an early age, it is important to consider the potential impact of a positive screen in a child who does not have ASD. Early identification through autism screening may be of benefit to children with other (non-ASD) developmental problems, such as language delay; however, the benefits for children who are typically developing are less obvious. It must be clearly communicated to families that a positive screen simply suggests the need for further assessment and does not imply a diagnosis. Hence timely access to a more comprehensive developmental assessment is essential not only to confirm the diagnosis of autism but also to clarify the clinical status of the broader group of toddlers who screen positive. The evaluation of autism screening programs should take into account the impact on all children and families who are targeted.

In many cases, the process of screening can serve as a focal point for communication with parents about important areas of the child's development. Screening questionnaires can be reviewed with parents so that specific endorsements can be clarified. Discrepancies between parental reports and clinician observations can be discussed, so that differences in perspective can be explained and understood. Likewise, interactive measures can serve as a rich format for discussion about children's observed strengths and weaknesses and can provide live exemplars for behaviors that warrant monitoring or perhaps intervention. Explaining the results of screening becomes less daunting for the service provider and less threatening for the parent when conducted within a conversational context that is based on shared observations and in which parental input and feedback are solicited and respected.

Availability of Follow-Up Services

As indicated earlier, screening is just the first step in securing appropriately specialized services for young children with ASD. Following a positive screen, it is essential to obtain a more comprehensive diagnostic assessment and evaluation of service needs so that an individually tailored intervention plan can be developed and implemented. Although service systems and pathways may vary across districts and service regions, there are certain unfortunate similarities that transcend geography: long waiting lists for diagnostic evaluations and a paucity of evidence-based interventions for children under 3 years old.

The availability of diagnostic evaluation centers and autism-specialized personnel is limited by economic constraints, as well as staffing issues. Diagnostic evaluations for children with ASD can be both time- and personnel-intensive, and clinical settings in which these services are offered are often in high demand. It is not uncommon for parents of a 24-month-old child to be told by an evaluation center that there is a 6-month wait—or longer—for a diagnostic evaluation. Clearly, it is not reasonable for a young child to wait that long before receiving services. One alternative route to specialized services for children in this situation is through the use of interactive screening measures. As mentioned earlier, these interactive measures can provide information not only about the child's risk for ASD but also about specific strengths and needs in core areas such as socialization, communication, and play. A positive screen can thus be used to develop goals so that specialized services may be started in the interim period between the initial referral and the diagnostic evaluation.

The need to tie early screening and diagnosis to timely access to effective ASD-specific interventions was discussed in detail in Chapter 3, this volume. It is reasonable to hypothesize that earlier initiation of treatment for autism may take advantage of ongoing brain development and plasticity, although we are still learning to what extent this will translate to better functional outcomes. Although effective interventions exist for autism, there are currently no evidence-based intervention programs specifically designed to treat autism in children under the age of 2, and none of the more generic treatment strategies for other at-risk children have been studied in this population. Existing programs may need to be modified to be more developmentally appropriate and targeted to the unique needs of this age group, taking into account factors such as attention span, differences in engagement, difficulties self-regulating, and potential for sensory overload.

The potential benefits of early identification and screening programs depend on whether health and other service systems are prepared to accommodate the increased numbers of children who will require expert diagnostic assessment and to offer intervention services in a timely manner to those children who receive a diagnosis. Ultimately, if an investment of resources is made to ensure earlier initiation of treatment and if this leads to improved outcomes, early screening may prove to be a cost-effective, as well as ethically responsible, strategy through reduction in long-term disability. However, without the allocation of additional resources to diagnostic and treatment services supporting the implementation of a screening program, the end result may simply be longer wait lists and added frustration for families. Screening programs will also require clinicians with the expertise to make relevant differential diagnoses in children referred for assessment, as children with other disorders who are identified through the process of screening will have service needs as well.

CONCLUSIONS

There are a growing number of ASD screening tools designed for use in clinical practice settings. "Second-level" screening for ASD can both extend and complement general population screening, providing opportunities to detect children with early signs at many points of entry into the health and developmental service systems. Further development of screening measures that can identify the full range of autism (i.e., including PDDNOS) is necessary, as is evaluation of the sensitivity and specificity of ASD screening tools in a broader range of community settings. In addition, service planning will be essential to ensure timely access to specialized diagnostic and intervention programs for all children identified through the process of screening.

REFERENCES

AAP Committee on Children with Disabilities. (2001). Technical report: The pediatrician's role in the diagnosis and management of autistic spectrum disorder in children. *Pediatrics, 107,* E85.

American Psychiatric Association. (1994). *Diagnostic and statistical manual of mental disorders* (4th ed.). Washington, DC: American Psychiatric Association.

Bailey, A., Palferman, S., Heavey, L., & Le Couteur, A. (1998). Autism: The phenotype in relatives. *Journal of Autism and Developmental Disorders, 28,* 369–392.

Baird, G., Charman, T., Baron-Cohen, S., Cox, A., Swettenham, J., Wheelwright, S., et al. (2000). A screening instrument for autism at 18 months of age: A 6-year follow-up study. *Journal of the American Academy of Child and Adolescent Psychiatry, 39,* 694–702.

Baron-Cohen, S., Allen, J., & Gillberg, C. (1992). Can autism be detected at 18 months? The needle, the haystack, and the CHAT. *British Journal of Psychiatry, 161,* 839–843.

Baron-Cohen, S., Cox, A., Baird, G., Swettenham, J., Nightingale, N., Morgan, K., et al. (1996). Psychological markers in the detection of autism in infancy in a large population. *British Journal of Psychiatry, 168,* 158–163.

Bertrand, J., Mars, A., Boyle, C., Bove, F., Yeargin-Allsopp, M., & Decoufle, P. (2001). Prevalence of autism in a United States population: The Brick Township, New Jersey, investigation. *Pediatrics, 108,* 1155–1161.

Berument, S. K., Rutter, M., Lord, C., Pickles, A., & Bailey, A. (1999). Autism screening questionnaire: Diagnostic validity. *British Journal of Psychiatry, 175,* 444–451.

Bishop, D. V., & Norbury, C. F. (2002). Exploring the borderlands of autistic disorder and specific language impairment: A study using standardised diagnostic instruments. *Journal of Child Psychology and Psychiatry, 43,* 917–929.

Boyle, M. H., Offord, D. R., Racine, Y., Fleming, J. E., Szatmari, P., & Sanford, M. (1993). Evaluation of the revised Ontario Child Health Study scales. *Journal of Child Psychology and Psychiatry, 34,* 189–213.

Britain, L. A., Holmes, G. E., & Hassanein, R. S. (1995). High-risk children referred to an early-intervention developmental program. *Clinical Pediatrics, 34,* 635–641.

Bryson, S. E. (1996). Brief report: Epidemiology of autism. *Journal of Autism and Developmental Disorders, 26,* 165–167.

Bryson, S. E., Brian, J., McDermott, C., Rombough, V., & Zwaigenbaum, L. (in press). The Autism Observational Scale for Infants: Scale development and assessment of reliability. *Journal of Autism and Developmental Disabilities.*

Chakrabarti, S., & Fombonne, E. (2001). Pervasive developmental disorders in preschool children. *Journal of the American Medical Association, 285,* 3141–3142.

Chakrabarti, S., & Fombonne, E. (2005). Pervasive developmental disorders in preschool children: Confirmation of high prevalence. *American Journal of Psychiatry, 162,* 1133–1141.

Charman, T., & Baird, G. (2002). Practitioner review: Diagnosis of autism spectrum disorder in 2- and 3-year-old children. *Journal of Child Psychology and Psychiatry*, *43*, 289–305.

Charman, T., Baron-Cohen, S., Baird, G., Cox, A., Wheelwright, S., Swettenham, J., et al. (2001). The Modified Checklist for Autism in Toddlers [Commentary]. *Journal of Autism and Developmental Disorders*, *31*, 145–148.

Coonrod, E. E., & Stone, W. L. (2004). Early concerns of parents of children with autistic and nonautistic disorders. *Infants and Young Children*, *17*, 258–268.

Corsello, C. M., Cook, E., Jr., & Leventhal, B. L. (2003, April). *A screening instrument for autism spectrum disorders*. Paper presented at the meeting of the Society for Research in Child Development, Tampa, FL.

Cox, A., Klein, K., Charman, T., Baird, G., Baron-Cohen, S., Swettenham, J., et al. (1999). Autism spectrum disorders at 20 and 42 months of age: Stability of clinical and ADI-R diagnosis. *Journal of Child Psychology and Psychiatry*, *40*, 719–732

Croen, L. A., Grether, J. K., Hoogstrate, J., & Selvin, S. (2002). The changing prevalence of autism in California. *Journal of Autism and Developmental Disorders*, *32*, 207–215.

Cunningham, C. E., Pettingill, P., & Boyle, M. (2000). *The Brief Child and Family Phone Interview (BCFPI)*. Hamilton, Ontario: Canadian Centre for the Study of Children at Risk, Hamilton Health Sciences Corporation, McMaster University.

Dawson, G., & Osterling, J. (1997). Early intervention in autism: Effectiveness and common elements of current approaches. In M. J. Guralnick (Ed.), *The effectiveness of early intervention* (pp. 307–326). Baltimore: Brookes.

Dawson, G., Webb, S., Schellenberg, G. D., Dager, S., Friedman, S., Aylward, E., et al. (2002). Defining the broader phenotype of autism: Genetic, brain, and behavioral perspectives. *Developmental Psychopathology*, *14*, 581–611.

De Giacomo, A., & Fombonne, E. (1998). Parental recognition of developmental abnormalities in autism. *European Journal of Child and Adolescent Psychiatry*, *7*, 131–136.

Dworkin, P. H. (1989). British and American recommendations for developmental monitoring: The role of surveillance. *Pediatrics*, *84*, 1000–1010.

Eaves, L. C., & Ho, H. H. (2004). The very early identification of autism: Outcome to age 4½–5. *Journal of Autism and Developmental Disorders*, *34*, 367–378.

Filipek, P. A., Accardo, P. J., Ashwal, S., Baranek, G. T., Cook, E. H., Jr., Dawson, G., et al. (2000). Practice parameter: Screening and diagnosis of autism: Report of the Quality Standards Subcommittee of the American Academy of Neurology and the Child Neurology Society. *Neurology*, *55*, 468–479.

Filipek, P. A., Accardo, P. J., Baranek, G. T., Cook, E. H., Jr., Dawson, G., Gordon, B., et al. (1999). The screening and diagnosis of autistic spectrum disorders. *Journal of Autism and Developmental Disorders*, *29*, 439–484.

Fombonne, E. (1999). The epidemiology of autism: A review. *Psychological Medicine*, *29*, 769–786.

Fombonne, E. (2003). Epidemiological surveys of autism and other pervasive developmental disorders: An update. *Journal of Autism and Developmental Disorders*, *33*, 365–382.

Gillberg, C., & Wing, L. (1999). Autism: Not an extremely rare disorder. *Acta Psychiatrica Scandinavica, 99,* 399–406.

Glascoe, F. P. (2003). Parents' evaluation of developmental status: How well do parents' concerns identify children with behavioral and emotional problems? *Clinical Pediatrics, 42,* 133–138.

Harris, S. L., & Handleman, J. S. (2000). Age and IQ at intake as predictors of placement for young children with autism: A four- to six-year follow-up. *Journal of Autism and Developmental Disorders, 30,* 137–142.

Howlin, P., & Asgharian, A. (1999). The diagnosis of autism and Asperger syndrome: Findings from a survey of 770 families. *Developmental Medicine and Child Neurology, 41,* 834–839.

Howlin, P., & Karpf, J. (2004). Using the Social Communication Questionnaire to identify "autistic spectrum" disorders associated with other genetic conditions: Findings from a study of individuals with Cohen syndrome. *Autism, 8,* 175–182.

Howlin, P., & Moore, A. (1997). Diagnosis in autism: A survey of over 1200 patients in the UK. *Autism, 1,* 135–162.

Jacobson, J. W., & Mulick, J. A. (2000). System and cost research issues in treatments for people with autistic disorders. *Journal of Autism and Developmental Disorders, 30,* 585–593.

Jarbrink, K., & Knapp, M. (2001). The economic impact of autism in Britain. *Autism, 5,* 7–22.

Lord, C., Rutter, M., & Le Couteur, A. J. (1994). Autism Diagnostic Interview—Revised: A revised version of a diagnostic interview for caregivers of individuals with possible pervasive developmental disorders. *Journal of Autism and Developmental Disorders, 24,* 659–685.

Ohta, M., Nagai, Y., Hara, H., & Sasaki, M. (1987). Parental perception of behavioral symptoms in Japanese autistic children. *Journal of Autism and Developmental Disorders, 17,* 549–563.

Ritvo, E. R., Jorde, L. B., Mason-Brothers, A., Freeman, B. J., Pingree, C., Jones, M. B., et al. (1989). The UCLA–University of Utah epidemiologic survey of autism: Recurrence risk estimates and genetic counseling. *American Journal of Psychiatry, 146,* 1032–1036.

Robins, D. L., Fein, D., Barton, M. L., & Green, J. A. (2001). The Modified CHecklist for Autism in Toddlers: An initial study investigating the early detection of autism and pervasive developmental disorders. *Journal of Autism and Developmental Disorders, 31,* 131–144.

Robins, D., Fein, D., Barton, M., Green, J., Dixon, P., Kleinman, J., et al. (2002, November). *The Modified CHecklist for Autism in Toddlers (M-CHAT): Autism is detected at 2 years old.* Paper presented at the International Meeting for Autism Research, Orlando, FL.

Rogers, S. J. (1996). Brief report: Early intervention in autism. *Journal of Autism and Developmental Disorders, 26,* 243–246.

Rogers, S. J. (1998). Empirically supported comprehensive treatments for young children with autism. *Journal of Clinical Child Psychology, 27,* 168–179.

Rogers, S. J., & DiLalla, D. L. (1990). Age of symptom onset in young children with pervasive developmental disorders. *Journal of the American Academy of Child and Adolescent Psychiatry, 29,* 863–872.

Sackett, D. L., Haynes, R. B., Guyatt, G. H., & Tugwell, P. (1991). Helping patients follow the treatments you prescribe. In D. L. Sackett, R. B. Haynes, G. H. Guyatt, & P. Tugwell (Eds.), *Clinical epidemiology: A basic science for clinical medicine* (pp. 249–281). Toronto, Ontario, Canada: Little, Brown.

Scambler, D., Rogers, S. J., & Wehner, E. A. (2001). Can the CHecklist for Autism in Toddlers differentiate young children with autism from those with developmental delays? *Journal of the American Academy of Child and Adolescent Psychiatry, 40,* 1457–1463.

Scott, F. J., Baron-Cohen, S., Bolton, P., & Brayne, C. (2002). Brief report: Prevalence of autism spectrum conditions in children aged 5–11 years in Cambridgeshire, UK. *Autism, 6,* 231–237.

Shevell, M. I., Majnemer, A., Rosenbaum, P., & Abrahamowicz, M. (2001). Etiologic yield of autistic spectrum disorders: A prospective study. *Journal of Child Neurology, 16,* 509–512.

Siegel, B. (2001, April). *Early screening and diagnosis in autism spectrum disorders: The Pervasive Developmental Disorders Screening Test (PDDST).* Paper presented at the meeting of the Society for Research in Child Development.

Siegel, B. (2004). *The Pervasive Developmental Disorders Screening Test–II (PDDST-II).* San Antonio, TX: Psychological Corporation.

Siegel, B., Pliner, C., Eschler, J., & Elliott, G. R. (1988). How children with autism are diagnosed: Difficulties in identification of children with multiple developmental delays. *Journal of Developmental and Behavioral Pediatrics, 9,* 199–204.

Simonoff, E. (1998). Genetic counseling in autism and pervasive developmental disorders. *Journal of Autism and Developmental Disorders, 28,* 447–456.

Smith, T., Groen, A. D., & Wynn, J. W. (2000). Randomized trial of intensive intervention for children with pervasive developmental disorder. *American Journal of Mental Retardation, 105,* 269–285.

Stone, W. L., Coonrod, E. E., & Ousley, O. Y. (2000). Brief report: Screening Tool for Autism in Two-Year-Olds (STAT): Development and preliminary data. *Journal of Autism and Developmental Disorders, 30,* 607–612.

Stone, W. L., Coonrod, E. E., Turner, L. M., & Pozdol, S. L. (2004). Psychometric properties of the STAT for early autism screening. *Journal of Autism and Developmental Disorders, 34,* 691–701.

Stone, W. L., Lee, E. B., Ashford, L., Brissie, J., Hepburn, S. L., Coonrod, E. E., et al. (1999). Can autism be diagnosed accurately in children under 3 years? *Journal of Child Psychology and Psychiatry, 40,* 219–226.

Stone, W. L., & Ousley, O. Y. (1997). *STAT Manual: Screening Tool for Autism in Two-Year-Olds.* Unpublished manuscript, Vanderbilt University.

Stone, W. L., & Rosenbaum, J. L. (1988). A comparison of teacher and parent views of autism. *Journal of Autism and Developmental Disorders, 18,* 403–414.

Volkmar, F., Cook, E. H., Jr., Pomeroy, J., Realmuto, G., & Tanguay, P. (1999). Practice parameters for the assessment and treatment of children, adolescents, and adults with autism and other pervasive developmental disorders. *Journal of the American Academy of Child and Adolescent Psychiatry, 38*(Suppl. 12), 32S–54S.

Wetherby, A., Goldstein, H., Cleary, J., Allen, L., & Kublin, K. (2003). Early identification of children with communication disorders: Concurrent and predictive validity of the CSBS Developmental Profile. *Infants and Young Children, 16,* 161–174.

Wetherby, A., & Prizant, B. (2002). *Communication and Symbolic Behavior Scales Developmental Profile—First normed edition.* Baltimore: Brookes.

Wetherby, A. M., Woods, J., Allen, L., Cleary, J., Dickinson, H., & Lord, C. (2004). Early indicators of autism spectrum disorders in the second year of life. *Journal of Autism and Developmental Disorders, 34,* 473–493.

Wing, L. (1996). Autistic spectrum disorders. *British Medical Journal, 312,* 327–328.

Wong, V., Hui, L. H., Lee, W. C., Leung, L. S., Ho, P. K., Lau, W. L., et al. (2004). A modified screening tool for autism (Checklist for Autism in Toddlers [CHAT-23]) for Chinese children. *Pediatrics, 114,* e166–e176.

Yeargin-Allsopp, M., Rice, C., Karapurkar, T., Doernberg, N., Boyle, C., & Murphy, C. (2003). Prevalence of autism in a U.S. metropolitan area. *Journal of the American Medical Association, 289,* 49–55.

Zwaigenbaum, L., Bryson, S., Rogers, T., Roberts, W., Brian, J., & Szatmari, P. (2005). Behavioral markers of autism in the first year of life. *International Journal of Developmental Neurosciences, 23,* 143–152.

Zwaigenbaum, L., Thurm, A., Stone, W., Baranek, G., Bryson, S., Iverson, J., et al. (in press). Studying the emergence of autism spectrum disorders in high risk infants: Methodological and practical issues. *Journal of Autism and Developmental Disorders.*

PART III

Evidence-Based Interventions

This section presents a discussion of different treatment approaches that specifically target early social-communicative development in young children with ASD. Chapters focus on interventions that address the core social-communicative deficit areas seen in toddlers and preschool children with autism: joint attention, communication and language, play, and imitation. Attention to theoretical, as well as evidence-based, support for the specific intervention approaches is provided.

Yoder and McDuffie (Chapter 5) summarize a range of intervention approaches that focus on the development of joint-attention skills in young children with ASD and other developmental disorders. They provide theoretical and empirical evidence for the contributions of initiating joint attention and responding to joint attention to subsequent language development. Interventions for improving joint attention are described along a continuum that ranges from discrete trials to naturalistic approaches, and the strengths and limitations of each are described. The authors outline an agenda for future research that includes an increased focus on randomized group experiments, assessment of generalization and maintenance of treatment effects, and identification of predictors of responsiveness to treatment. Implications for current clinical practice are also discussed.

Rogers (Chapter 6) adopts a historical perspective in describing and evaluating intervention approaches that focus on the development of language. Behavioral, pragmatic, naturalistic, and developmental approaches to developing language competence are compared, and the relative strengths and weakness of each approach for young children with ASD are outlined. The different mechanisms that might underlie improved language in different intervention programs are discussed. This chapter proposes the existence of subgroups of children with ASD who have different language profiles and trajectories and discusses strategies for selecting appropriate treatments for each group.

Wolfberg and Schuler (Chapter 7) highlight the importance of social interactions with peers and describe the development of the social and symbolic components of peer play in children with typical development and children with ASD. Interventions that focus on the development of peer play skills—including adult-directed, child-centered, and peer-mediated approaches—are discussed in terms of their utility for young children with ASD. A comprehensive intervention model for promoting peer play is presented, along with a case illustration and suggestions for future research.

Nadel and Aouka (Chapter 8) conceptualize imitation as serving the important developmental functions of promoting learning and fostering communication. They summarize the many component skills underlying the development of imitation abilities (e.g., representation, motor planning), as well as the specific skills required to perform different types of imitation tasks in different types of settings. Proposed mechanisms that underlie imitation abilities in prompted versus spontaneous imitative exchanges are compared in both typically developing children and children with ASD. The authors outline a model whereby the stimulation of imitation and recognition of being imitated can be used to enhance autonomous actions and to help develop an awareness of self- and other agency.

Howlin (Chapter 9) reviews a variety of alternative and augmentative strategies for improving communication and social interaction in nonverbal children with ASD. Programs developed specifically for children with ASD (e.g., Picture Exchange Communication System), as well as more general augmentative approaches (e.g. sign language), are evaluated with respect to their theoretical basis and empirical findings. The potential for computers to play a role as augmentative communication systems for young children with ASD is outlined. Clinical recommendations about when to introduce augmentative systems, how to match specific systems to individual children, and how to increase children's motivation to communicate based on the review of the empirical literature are provided.

5

Treatment of Responding to and Initiating Joint Attention

PAUL J. YODER
ANDREA S. MCDUFFIE

This chapter reviews treatment approaches for and evidence concerning the efficacy of treatments on the development of two types of joint attention: responding to joint attention (RJA) and initiating joint attention (IJA). First, we define the term *joint attention* and provide the rationale for focusing on responding to and initiating joint attention. Second, we present two theories predicting that IJA and RJA have developmental consequences on language development. Third, we present the empirical support for the association between these types of joint attention and language. Fourth, we present the rules of evidence for judging whether a treatment affects IJA and RJA. Fifth, we present the primary treatment approaches targeting IJA and RJA. Sixth, we briefly review the extent to which internally valid studies have demonstrated treatment effects on IJA or RJA in children with disabilities, with a special interest in effects on children with autism. Seventh, we propose probable mechanisms by which treatments may affect joint attention. Eighth, we suggest areas of future research. Finally, we draw some clinical implications of our review.

DEFINITION OF JOINT ATTENTION
USED IN THIS CHAPTER

The definition of *joint attention* used in this chapter focuses on responding to and initiating joint attention. These two types of behavior actively indicate that both partner and object are included in the child's focus of attention. RJA is defined as the child's ability to follow an adult's attentional directive (Seibert, Hogan, & Mundy, 1982). IJA refers to the infants' use of eye contact, affect, gesture, vocalization, or symbolic communication to spontaneously share positive affect or interest about a referent (Mundy & Stella, 2000; Seibert et al., 1982). It is the social emphasis of RJA and IJA that makes them particularly important for diagnosing and predicting the developmental status of children with severe deficits in social cognition (e.g., children with autism).

We are aware that not all researchers will agree with our decision to focus exclusively on these two types of joint attention. After all, some researchers have used the term *joint attention* to refer to many different social-cognitive behaviors (Sigman & Kasari, 1995). The original definition of joint attention included RJA (Scaife & Bruner, 1975). Later concepts of joint attention (e.g., Adamson & Bakeman, 1984) considered joint attention to be a state of engagement rather than a particular behavior. One such state of engagement is *passive* joint attention (Bakeman & Adamson, 1984). Passive joint attention results when the mother actively manipulates or talks about an object during the time the baby is engaged in onlooking or object play (Bakeman & Adamson, 1984). There is shared object focus during passive joint attention, but the baby shows little awareness of the social partner.

Current definitions of joint attention vary widely in the research literature. Recent discussions of joint attention even include motor imitation with objects (Carpenter, Nagell, & Tomasello, 1998; Nadel, 2002) as a joint-attention behavior. The common requirement across most definitions of joint attention is that the infant demonstrate simultaneous or sequential coordinated attention between object and person (Adamson & Chance, 1998; Bakeman & Adamson, 1984). Coordinated attention is shown in RJA and is often shown in IJA, requesting, and social interaction behaviors (Bates, Camaioni, & Volterra, 1975; Mundy & Sigman, 1989; Mundy, Sigman, Ungerer, & Sherman, 1986; Wetherby & Prutting, 1984).

We do not include social interaction or requesting in this chapter. These functions are not impaired to the same extent in children with autism as are RJA and IJA (Mundy, Sigman, & Kasari, 1994; Mundy et al., 1986; Stone, Ousley, Yoder, Hogan, & Hepburn, 1997; Wetherby & Prutting, 1984). For example, Mundy et al. (1994) found no difference between children with ASD and developmentally matched typically developing children whose mental age was over 20 months. Requesting and social interaction lack the almost exclusively social motivation of IJA. In marked contrast to IJA, there is much more evidence that intentional communication with the pragmatic functions of requesting and social interaction can and have been facilitated in children with autism by a range of intervention methods. By "intentional communication," we mean the use of gestures, vocalization, gaze, and/or facial expressions that demonstrate coordinated attention to object and person or the use of conventional or symbolic means to communicate (Bates, 1979). A careful consideration of the studies in a recent review of "social communication" interventions for children with autism (Hwang & Hughes, 2000b), revealed that almost all of the outcome variables were types of requesting or social interaction (not IJA) or were superordinate categories of intentional communication that did not differentiate child communication acts by pragmatic function. The unusually large and persisting deficit in IJA and RJA in children with autism, the particularly social nature of IJA and RJA, and the paucity of information on effective interventions for this population motivate our choice to focus on RJA and IJA in this chapter.

RATIONALE FOR PREDICTING AN ASSOCIATION BETWEEN RJA AND IJA WITH LANGUAGE DEVELOPMENT

There are two broad classes of theories about why RJA and IJA are related to later language development. Organismic theories focus on RJA or IJA as behavioral manifestations of foundational skills for later language development (e.g., Tomasello, 1995). Eliciting-operations theories focus on the child's elicitation of adult facilitating input, which then bootstraps continued language development (Shatz, 1987; Yoder & Warren, 1993).

Social-pragmatic (Tomasello, 1995) and social-approach (Mundy, 1995) theories are two examples of organismic explanations for the importance of IJA and RJA. Social-pragmatic theorists suggest that the use of RJA and IJA represents the child's understanding that the partner's focus of attention may be different from her own (i.e., an example of understanding others' intentions). To enable reciprocal communication, the child must make sure that the focus of attention is mutually shared (Tomasello, 1995). RJA is used to follow the adult's current focus of attention, whereas IJA is used to direct adult attention to match the child's current focus. Establishing shared focus on objects or events increases the probability that the child will attend to and accurately process incidental linguistic input from the environment. Social-approach theory suggests that initiating joint attention represents a motivation to engage in social interaction, which results in the acquisition of socially transmitted skills such as language (Mundy, 1995). For example, children may use IJA frequently because they find social interaction especially rewarding for its own sake (Mundy, 1995). Bloom (1993) suggests that the desire to socially connect or "share the contents of mind" motivates child language acquisition.

The basic assumption of eliciting-operations theory is that language development is dependent on bidirectional, reciprocal social interaction between child and adult partner (Sameroff, 1983; Yoder & Warren, 1993). This model emphasizes the effect of RJA and IJA on the responses of communicative partners and the effect of the parent's behavior on the child's language development. IJA may be important to later language learning because it elicits adult verbal labels for the object that is the focus of shared attention (Yoder & Warren, 1993). In fact, Yoder and Warren (1999b) demonstrated that such maternal responsivity mediated the relationship between prelinguistic intentional communication and later language. Eliciting-operations theory would predict that RJA results in increased language learning because the adult often labels a referent object once the child has followed the adult's focus of attention. Both the child's eliciting behavior and the adult's facilitating response are important components of the eliciting-operations explanation.

Common to the theories that propose that IJA and RJA should be important to language acquisition is the notion that real developmental change is dependent on more than adding new responses to the child's behavioral repertoire. Instead, it is the ability or the motivation that the new forms of behavior reveal or the social consequences of their use that is most important. This presumption has critical implications for the targeting of joint-attention behaviors in treatments. That is, even if the increased behavior resembles joint attention in overt form (e.g., coordinated attention to object and person), unless such increased responding indicates increased understanding of communicative intentions or increased motivation to share the contents of mind, or unless it results in increased parental linguistic mapping, neither organismic nor eliciting-operations theories would expect subsequent effects on language development.

EMPIRICAL EVIDENCE FOR THE ASSOCIATION OF RJA AND IJA TO LANGUAGE IN CHILDREN WITH AUTISM

In children with autism, there is replicated evidence for the concurrent relationship between RJA and receptive vocabulary (Loveland & Landry, 1986; Mundy et al., 1986), even when controlling for chronological age, initial language level (Sigman & Ruskin, 1999), and initial mental age (Mundy et al., 1986). Currently, there is no empirical evidence for a predictive relationship between RJA and receptive language outcomes for children with autism. Because of a publication bias against reporting null findings, it is difficult to determine whether this association has been adequately considered. There is replicated evidence for both the concurrent (Mundy et al., 1986; Carpenter, Pennington, & Rogers, 2002) and predictive (Sigman & Ungerer, 1984) relationship between RJA and expressive vocabulary, even when controlling for chronological age, initial language level (Sigman & Ruskin, 1999), and initial mental age (Mundy et al., 1986).

As for IJA, there is replicated evidence for a concurrent relationship between IJA and receptive language (Sigman & Ruskin, 1999) in children with autism, even when controlling for mental age (Mundy et al., 1986). There is also replicated evidence for the concurrent relationship between IJA and expressive language (Mundy et al., 1986; Sigman & Ruskin, 1999). Replicated evidence exists for a predictive relationship between IJA and expressive language (Charman et al., 2003), even while controlling for chronological age and initial language status (Sigman & Ruskin, 1999). Another report (Mundy, Sigman, & Kasari, 1990) found both a significant concurrent and short-term predictive relationship between joint attention and language for children with autism. However, this study considered RJA and IJA as a single ability and did not distinguish between receptive and expressive language outcomes.

In sum, there is theoretical and empirical support for the hypothesis that RJA and IJA have developmental and diagnostic importance for children with autism. Therefore, it is surprising that so few interventions target RJA and IJA in this population.

EVIDENCE THAT THE BEHAVIOR
THAT CHANGES IS REALLY JOINT ATTENTION

Changes in responses that resemble IJA and RJA in behavioral form can occur during intervention without changing the underlying constructs of interest. Many children, especially children with autism, learn a therapy register (Johnson, 1988) or response set during intervention. In general, a therapy register is a style of interaction that is activated by the presence of the interventionist or the characteristics of the therapy setting. A therapy register for IJA might be an implicit rule such as: "When I am with this adult (in this room, playing with these toys), I'm supposed to look at the adult frequently. If I do this, I get something I like (i.e., positive reinforcement). If I do not do this, something I like is removed (i.e., time out from positive reinforcement)."

For us to be convinced that important changes in IJA and RJA have occurred, the newly learned behaviors must generalize across people, materials, and settings. Additionally, behavior change must be maintained months after the end of the treatment sessions. Newly learned behaviors can be important for development only if, when measured, their function for the child is similar to that seen in the natural environment. For example, if IJA indicates the child's motivation to engage in social-approach behavior, then behaviors representative of IJA should be self-initiated and their pragmatic function should appear to be declarative. Similarly, RJA may indicate the child's ability to shift attention and establish joint reference. RJA may increase the probability of processing adult verbal labels. Therefore, the ultimate test of whether our purported measures of IJA or RJA are construct-valid is whether increasing IJA or RJA has subsequent effects on language, a skill that both types of joint attention are thought to facilitate (Cronbach & Meehl, 1955). Admittedly, this last criterion is a tall order.

RULES OF EVIDENCE FOR INFERRING A TREATMENT EFFECT ON JOINT-ATTENTION DEVELOPMENT

John Stuart Mill (Beakley & Ludlow, 1992) stated the rules of evidence for causal attribution to be (1) an association between the proposed cause and the proposed effect, (2) the temporal occurrence of the proposed cause before the proposed effect, and (3) ruling out of alternative explanations for the aforementioned facts. The final criteria is by far the most difficult to establish. Contemporary research methods call such "alternative explanations" threats to internal validity (Cook & Campbell, 1979). The most common threats to internal validity in the intervention literature are (1) maturation, (2) history, and (3) instrumentation. Much discussion of maturation and history as alternative explanations for the covariance of treatment and change in behavior has taken place (Cook & Campbell, 1979). Suffice it to say that many children with autism can and have changed quite dramatically even on indices of degree of delay (e.g., standard scores) due to maturation and/or participation in traditional treatments available in the 1980s and 1990s (Sigman & Ruskin, 1999). Although the mean developmental quotient (DQ) did not change in Sigman and Ruskin's (1999) research, the DQs of many individual children did change, as is shown in the authors' discussion of the stability of mental retardation status. The point is that even indices of degree of delay can and do change without a particular treatment. Therefore, treatment research must demonstrate that behavioral changes attributed to interventions extend beyond changes that would have occurred due to maturation and history (e.g., participation in other treatments).

Instrumentation, another threat to internal validity, is of particular note for treatment studies of IJA that allow the measurement conditions of the dependent variable to vary between baseline and treatment phases. At least one study with children with autism (Lewy & Dawson, 1992) has shown that merely altering the interaction style of the adult examiner (e.g., child-led play vs. adult-led play) had a dramatic effect on the child's use of IJA. These findings could not be attributed to development because order of conditions was counterbalanced within subject and both conditions occurred on the same day.

Changing measurement conditions in ways that favor the treatment phase are particularly likely in two research designs. First, instrumentation effects can explain apparent treatment effects when dependent variables are measured within treatment sessions of baseline–treatment phase (AB) research designs. This occurs because the treatment usually supports the increased use of existing skills through skillful adult interaction, whereas the baseline condition usually provides less support of existing-skill use. Additionally, an apparent, but false, treatment effect can be observed when parents serve as both interventionists and examiners/informants. The treatment usually changes the parents' interactions in ways that scaffold the performance of existing IJA skills. Therefore, there is a change in conditions under which parents report or elicit IJA concurrent with the treatment. The difference between increased performance and increased independent competence is critical to determining whether important developmental changes have occurred in the child and whether these changes can be attributable to the treatment.

In sum, evidence that treatment affects IJA and RJA must meet two criteria. First, we need evidence that the changes are generalized and maintained and are measured in a way that allows us to observe the self-initiated nature and declarative function of the IJA behavior. Second, we need evidence of behavioral change in the context of a research design that rules out nontreatment (e.g., maturation, history, and instrumentation) explanations for the apparent association of treatment experience and changes in joint attention.

A CONTINUUM OF CURRENT
IJA AND RJA INTERVENTIONS

Available joint-attention treatments vary along the naturalistic–discrete-trial continuum (Prizant, Wetherby, & Rydell, 2000). By *naturalistic*, we mean treatments that are similar to naturally occurring parent–child interactions. By *discrete trial*, we mean treatments that use drill and practice methods that put a premium on high frequency of correct child responding to adult-provided antecedents per unit of time. We discuss here four general approaches to joint-attention treatment. Figure 5.1 illustrates where these four approaches fall along the naturalistic–discrete trial continuum. We close this section of the chapter with a summary of the differences in intervention approaches.

Developmental-Responsive Approaches

At the extreme naturalistic end of the continuum is a class of interventions we call developmental-responsive approaches. Two examples of this approach are responsive teaching (RT; Mahoney & MacDonald, 2003; Mahoney & Perales, 2003) and the developmental, individual-difference, relationship-based (DIR) model (Greenspan & Wieder, 2000).

The RT model is better specified in the published literature than the DIR model, so we use their materials to discuss how this class of interventions address joint-attention goals. RT uses the same intervention strategies for both types of joint attention. The authors of the RT approach indicate the following intervention strategies to address joint attention goals: (1) get into the child's world; (2) observe the child's behavior; (3) imitate the child's actions and communications; (4) accompany communication with intonation, pointing, and nonverbal gestures; (5) repeat activities the child enjoys; (6) read the child's behavior as an indicator of interest; (7) follow the child's attentional lead; and (8) be sensitive to the child's sensations. The authors provide the following rationale: (1) following the child's attentional, play, and interest leads facilitates eye contact; (2) contingent responsiveness to child communication acts facilitates increased frequency and efficiency of intentional communication; and (3) using multiple cues simultaneously results in children following adult attentional cues.

RT and other developmental-responsive approaches give the highest priority to a positive emotional relationship between the therapist and child. The explicit assumption is that a positive emotional relationship with the interventionist motivates IJA and monitoring for RJA cues. This class of approaches avoids adult prompts for specific forms of child behavior (e.g., eye contact) and avoids punishment or time-out procedures for undesired child performance. It is thought that both prompting and punishment or time-out techniques may produce negative affective reactions in children that are counterproductive to establishing and maintaining a highly positive relationship between adult and child. For example, our clinical experience indicates that some children close their eyes and turn away or fuss when intrusive prompts are used. Similarly, time-out and punishment can cause children to have tantrums. Both classes of reactions would be counterproductive to facilitating IJA, which depends on the child's desire to share positive affect with the interventionist.

The weaknesses of RT include not distinguishing the developmental or

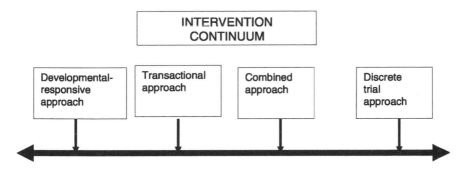

FIGURE 5.1. The relative position of the four intervention approaches along the naturalistic–discrete trial continuum.

precursor mechanisms for developing requests from those for developing IJA. Additionally, there is an implicit assumption that acquiring coordinated attention to object and person and requesting contribute to the subsequent development of RJA and IJA—an untested assumption. When applied to children with autism, it may be that adding prompts for more advanced forms of communication can improve the efficiency of treatment for IJA and RJA, above and beyond that shown for developmental-responsive approaches. The next approach uses such prompts.

Discrete Trial Training Approaches

The discrete trial training (DTT) approach is at the opposite end of the naturalistic–discrete trial continuum. The potential advantage of the DTT approaches is that new communicative forms are efficiently taught. To our knowledge, RJA has not yet been targeted using a DTT approach.

An intervention presented by Buffington, Krantz, McClannahan, and Poulson (1998) illustrates this approach to addressing IJA. The treatment follows a traditional behavioral teaching paradigm. An adult provides a discriminative stimulus that has both a verbal (e.g., "Let's talk about something on the _____") and nonverbal (e.g., presence of a pinwheel) component. The desired child response is very well defined (e.g., saying "look" while looking at and pointing to pinwheel). If the response is incorrect or incomplete, or if no response is given, the adult models the correct response. If the child still gives no response, the adult provides a physical prompt for the gestural component of the expected child response (e.g., adult physically manipulates the child's hand into the shape of a point and directs that point toward the referent) and asks the child to imitate the desired verbal response (e.g., "Say 'look' "). Reinforcement unrelated to the communication message is provided contingent on complete, correct responses (e.g., token reinforcement).

An implicit assumption of DTT approaches is that, if adults consistently and appropriately respond to trained behaviors, teaching the overt form of the behavior will eventually result in use of the behavior for the function adults assign. This assumption has not yet been tested in children with autism, who may not be reinforced by adult interest or shared positive affect.

Transactional Approaches

Transactional approaches attempt to combine the advantages of developmental-responsive and DTT approaches. They are designed to efficiently teach IJA forms by using a graduated system of prompts in a game-like, interactional framework that may enhance the reinforcement value of social interaction. These approaches have directly targeted IJA, not RJA.

Two examples of transactional approaches to intervention are the social-communication, emotional regulation, and Transactional Support (SCERTS) model (Prizant et al., 2000) and responsive education and prelinguistic milieu teaching (RPMT; Yoder & Warren, 2002). Both of these models acknowledge that primary social partners must be responsive to children's communication for the intervention methods to be effective (Prizant et al., 2000; Yoder & Warren, 2002). Similar to the developmental-responsive approaches, transactional intervention approaches select targets using the developmental literature to inform probable sequence of acquisition, follow the child's attentional and play leads, and attempt to build game-like, turn-taking routines with the child. Similar to the DTT approach, transactional approaches prompt the child to use slightly more developmentally advanced communicative behaviors.

To avoid potential negative effects of prompt use, several principles guide the use of prompts for communication. To increase the probability that children will maintain their engagement with the adult and the object of interest, prompts are used only after the child has initiated a communication act (i.e., the occasion for an incidental teaching episode) and when the motivation for continued engagement in the activity is high (e.g., deep within a turn-taking routine). To avoid prompt dependency, the level of help the prompt provides is the minimum needed at that moment to elicit the desired child behavior. For example, when the child gives the object to the teacher, to prompt for eye-gaze coordination the teacher may engage in the following sequence: (1) The teacher may delay her response if the child still does not gaze to the adult; (2) she might say "look at me" if the child still does not look at the adult; (3) the teacher may intercept the child's gaze. To avoid power plays, such repeated prompting within a given incidental teaching episode is used only when the child's motivation to communicate is high. For example, such repeated prompting might be used if the child is deep in a routine (such as asking for a ball to roll in a ball maze for the third consecutive turn). Prompts are gradually faded once the child consistently responds to a given level of prompting. Finally, transactional approaches rarely use physical prompts, again attempting to avoid coercing children to respond. IJA forms expressing positive affect (e.g., smile and pointing with attention to the message recipient) are modeled in pragmatically appropriate contexts for the declarative function (e.g., celebrating the knocking down of a tower). Transactional approaches avoid using negative consequences to respond to the child's failure to use desired behavior.

It is presumed that the child learns that moments of social connectedness are rewarding (e.g., mutual enjoyment of Jack's arrival). It is also assumed that children can elicit more of such moments by producing IJA behaviors the adult is modeling (e.g., pointing to Jack and laughing when he arrives). We do not yet have empirical support that these assumptions are true for children with autism. But there is reason to be optimistic because it has been shown that modeling IJA is related to later frequency of IJA use in children with autism (Siller & Sigman, 2002).

Combined Approaches

A final set of approaches combines elements of both transactional and DTT approaches. We call this the combined approach, because such treatments explicitly combine aspects of these two types of treatment approaches. These approaches combine the transactional and DTT approaches either by using elements of each to create a new method (e.g., Whalen & Schreibman, 2003) or by using one approach and then the other within the same treatment session (e.g., Kasari, Freeman, & Paparella, 2000). Whalen and Schreibman (2003) combined elements of pivotal response training (a transactional approach) and elements of the DTT approach. Kasari et al. (2000) used DTT followed by a method that the authors called milieu language teaching (a transactional approach). Both explicitly targeted IJA, as well as RJA.

To date, the Whalen and Schreibman (2003) treatment has been described in much greater detail than the Kasari et al. (2000) treatment. Therefore, we describe the former as an example of the combined approaches. After behavioral compliance training, children are taught to respond to attention-directing cues (i.e., RJA training). Children are taught to respond to highly redundant, proximal attention-directing cues (e.g., adult puts hand on the target object) before learning to respond to more subtle cues (e.g., adult gazes at target object). Before asking children to respond to more distal attention-directing cues (e.g., showing the target object vs. pointing to the target object), the adult provides access to preferred toys contingent on the child making eye contact with the adult. The expected child response is engagement (visual attention to or touching) with the adult's referent for at least 5 seconds. The reward for correct responding is allowing the child to play with the object (i.e., positive reinforcement). If the child does not respond as expected, all toys are removed (i.e., time-out from positive reinforcement). After two incorrect responses, the adult physically prompts the child to touch (and eventually look at) the new toy. Mastery criterion is 80% compliance to attentional directives in four out of five consecutive sessions.

IJA training occurs after mastery of the RJA training. Coordinated gaze shift and pointing for a declarative function are the targets. Child engagement with a preferred toy for more than 10 seconds is considered an opportunity for IJA. If IJA does not occur within 10 seconds of the previous instance of IJA, the preferred toy is removed (i.e., time-out from positive reinforcement). After two such instances, the child is physically prompted to move the object and look at the adult's eyes. The adult concurrently says, "show," and points to her eye as an additional prompt. As gaze shifting increases, prompts are faded. Criteria for mastery include spontaneous gaze shifts between the preferred object and the adult in at least 30% of opportunities for four out of five consecutive sessions. The 30% criterion is based on observations of typically developing children.

Summary

Table 5.1 summarizes the characteristics of the intervention approaches. The four intervention approaches differ in their tendency to (1) follow the child's momentary focus of interest, (2) directly prompt desired child behaviors, (3) consider a positive relationship between the adult and child as paramount, (4) explicitly teach the self-initiated declarative function of IJA, and (5) explicitly teach RJA. Developmental-responsive and transactional approaches follow the child's momentary attentional lead and explicitly attempt to support a positive relationship between the child and adult. Transactional, combined, and DTT approaches directly prompt the child to elicit communication behaviors. Transactional and combined approaches explicitly teach the self-initiated, declarative function of new communication forms. The developmental-responsive and combined approaches explicitly focus on RJA, as well as IJA.

REVIEW OF EFFICACY EVIDENCE FOR JOINT-ATTENTION TREATMENT APPROACHES

Although the primary focus of this chapter is on children with autism, studies on children with other disabilities were included in this review because so few internally valid studies on children with autism were found in the lit-

TABLE 5.1. Characteristics of Joint-Attention Intervention Approaches

	Developmental-responsive	Transactional	Combined	Discrete trial training
Nurturing relationship	X	X		
Contingent responsiveness	X	X	X	
Follow child's lead	X	X	X	
Developmental skill progression	X	X	X	
Routines as context for communication	X	X	X	
Incidental teaching		X		
Adult responsiveness as R+	X	X	X	
Child-selected toy as R+			X	
Tokens as R+				X
Compliance training			X	X
Verbal prompts		X	X	X
Physical prompts			X	X
Removal of toy as time-out			X	
Targets RJA	X		X	
Targets IJA	X	X	X	X

Note. R+, reward.

erature. In addition, studies that teach children to ask questions to elicit linguistic input (e.g., Taylor & Harris, 1995), although considered examples of IJA by some (Wetherby & Prizant, 1993), were excluded because not everyone would agree that question asking represents IJA (e.g., Mundy, 1995).

First, we identified the population of potentially relevant studies through the reference sections of recent existing reviews of social communication in children with autism (Goldstein, 2002; Hwang & Hughes, 2000a; Koegel, 2000; McConnell, 2002). Second, we used PsycINFO and Medline searches using descriptor terms of the synonyms for IJA and RJA, joint attention, autism, and treatment. Third, references for studies identified with the preceding methods were searched for additional articles. Thirty-seven studies were identified as potentially relevant.

For our review of efficacy of current joint-attention treatments, we eliminated studies that (1) did not distinguish their communication outcomes by pragmatic function, (2) did not examine the declarative function, (3) did not measure IJA or RJA separately from other types of joint attention, and (4) did not measure RJA or IJA apart from global measures of autism symptomatology or child development. We also eliminated studies (1) with relatively poor internal validity, (2) with only within-treatment session results (i.e., that did not measure generalization of trained responses), and (3) with results that reversed back to near baseline levels during the maintenance phase in all participants. This selection process left five studies for review (Buffington et al., 1998; Leew, 2001; Whalen & Schreibman, 2003; Yoder & Warren, 1999a, 2002). However, these criteria left us without representative tests for the developmental-responsive and DTT approaches. Thus we included two more studies that we judged to provide the best test of these two treatment approaches (Mahoney & Perales, 2003; Buffington et al., 1998, respectively).

To date, Mahoney and Perales (2003) provides the strongest test of the RT model for children with autism. Unfortunately, their dependent variables did not distinguish between joint attention and other aspects of child development. Additionally, their research design (i.e., correlation between gains in the outcome with different levels of the independent variable) does not allow us to rule out nontreatment explanations for the observed changes in the dependent variable. At present, we conclude that we do not know the extent to which the developmental-responsive approach facilitates generalized and maintained IJA and RJA.

Buffington et al. (1998) is the strongest published test of the DTT approach for what might be considered joint-attention outcomes in children with autism. These authors targeted several behaviors labeled as representative of "attention directing," "affective," and "reference" categories. Results were graphed using these aggregated categories as dependent variables. All three categories are *potential* examples of IJA. On closer examination, non-IJA examples were lumped with IJA examples for all three categories. For example, "Can I have that?" with an outstretched hand toward desired object, and "Look!" with a point, were both included under the category of "attention directing." The former example clearly has a requesting function. Additionally, the antecedents in generalization probes were extremely similar to those used in the teaching conditions, increasing the probability that a therapy register could account for the results. For example, when *teaching* the child to say "Look!," the adult said, "Let's talk about something on the pinwheel" while holding the pinwheel. When *testing* the child's "look" response, the adult said, "Find something on the globe" while holding the globe. Additionally, the structure of the generalization probe always contained a verbal antecedent to stimulate the trained behavior, thus eliminating the reader's opportunity to observe whether the trained behaviors were self-initiated by the child for the purpose of sharing interest. At present, it has not been shown that the DTT approach facilitates generalized IJA.

Of the available treatments, we know the most about the efficacy of the transactional approach to facilitating IJA. However, our knowledge is restricted to children with developmental delays. Three studies used a transactional approach to facilitate IJA in 2- to 3-year-olds with developmental delays without autism (Leew, 2001; Yoder & Warren, 1999a, 2002). In all three studies, generalized IJA was tested. Generalization was tested across person, materials, and interaction style. IJA was considered to be child-initiated communication for declarative purposes.

Yoder and Warren (1999a, 2002) used a randomized group experiment to control for threats to internal validity. Their first study showed greater generalized and maintained (6 months after treatment ended) IJA use in the prelinguistic milieu teaching (PMT) group than in the comparison group, but only in children whose parents were quite responsive to their children's communication before treatment began (Yoder & Warren, 1999a). It should be noted that staff, not parents, were the interventionists in this study. Therefore, the parents provided important background support for clinic based treatment.

Given the importance of parental responsivity, Yoder and Warren (2002) added parental responsivity education to PMT in their next study (RPMT). Using a randomized group experiment, they found that RPMT facilitated generalized and maintained (6 months after the end of treatment) IJA in children who began the treatment with relatively little IJA.

Based on the findings of Yoder and Warren (1999a), Leew (2001) restricted her sample to children of very responsive parents. Using a multiple-baseline across-subjects design, she found that abrupt changes (within 1 month of the onset of treatment) in frequency of IJA occurred in generalization sessions during the treatment phase in two out of four participants. Interestingly, her data showed that the behaviors that were eventually used for generalized IJA were first used in the requesting function. This pattern suggests the possibility that new forms of communication were first learned in an existing function, requesting, and later generalized to a new function, declaratives.

Finally, Whalen and Schreibman (2003) tested the efficacy of one variant of the combined approach. They used a multiple-baseline across-subjects design with a maintenance phase and generalization probes with 4 participants with autism. This review focuses on the generalization results from the Whalen and Schreibman study.

When changes in IJA or RJA occur several weeks or months after the onset of the treatment in some children but not in others, it weakens our confidence that the treatment caused the changes because other explanations for the changes cannot be eliminated (Kazden, 1982). Unfortunately, the graphs that illustrate the potential effects on generalized RJA in Whalen and Schreibman (2003) do not provide enough information to determine at what point after the onset of the treatment increases occurred. However, it should be noted that two out of five of the participants showed increased

RJA in generalization contexts, even at the 3-month follow-up period. Only four children in the Whalen and Schreibman (2003) study finished IJA training. Of these four children, two out of four showed generalized, maintained increases in IJA. However, this increase was not seen until the maintenance phase. In the other two children, the generalized changes in RJA or IJA reversed to near baseline levels at the maintenance check. Such reversals suggest that initial changes may have been due to therapy sets, not true joint-attention development. True development seldom reverses.

In sum, with regard to facilitating IJA or RJA, the developmental-responsive and DTT approaches have not been put to a rigorous test. In contrast, we are confident that a transactional approach has had an effect on generalized and maintained IJA increases in subgroups of children with developmental delays without autism. Although seen in only one study, it appears that these subgroups can be described as children who initially have low IJA. This bodes well for children with autism, who also have low IJA. However, the effects of such transactional approaches have not yet been tested on children with autism. Finally, we have compromised confidence that a combined approach has had an effect on generalized and maintained RJA and IJA in a subgroup of children with autism. The Whalen and Shreibman (2003) study design did not allow identification of characteristics of the subgroup of children with the best-maintained outcomes. However, anecdotal reports support the hypothesis that these children's parents were particularly attentive during treatment and seemed to actively reinforce use of trained behaviors outside of therapy (Whalen, personal communication, September 2003).

Regardless of the treatment approach used, it is highly probable that effective treatments that target generalized and maintained joint attention will need to be implemented more often and for longer periods than were used in the reviewed studies. Although it is difficult to determine the intensity of a parent-implemented treatment (e.g., RT), the amount of professional contact in the RPMT studies was about 24 hours of treatment (i.e., 20 minutes a day, 3 times a week for 6 months), and the intervention described in the Whalen and Schreibman (2003) study occurred for a maximum of 43 hours (i.e., 1.5 hours a day for up to 29 days). The required intensity of treatment to affect generalized and maintained joint attention in most children with autism is still unknown.

POTENTIAL MECHANISMS OF TREATMENT EFFECTS

If future research supports the hypothesis that treatment can affect RJA and IJA in children with autism, we will want to know the probable mechanism by which the effect occurs. The mechanisms must account for the ontogeny and maintenance of IJA and RJA in children with potentially little social interest and potentially little interest in spoken language or objects. Gains in IJA and RJA will probably not be maintained unless children are reinforced by social interaction (for IJA) and linguistic or object-knowledge information (for RJA).

For IJA, two candidate mechanisms are probable. First, studies that support the transactional approach (i.e., Leew, 2001; Yoder & Warren, 1999a, 2002) suggest that prompts and functional reinforcement can be successful in helping children learn to use new behaviors to communicate (i.e., the transfer of stimulus control hypothesis). The Leew (2001) study suggested that new communicative forms are first learned in old communicative functions, such as requests, and later generalize to the new declarative function.

Some readers will note that it is not obvious that this would occur in children who do not view social interaction as rewarding, because the motivation for declaratives is primarily to attain social attention. However, it is possible that the pairing of the functional rewards attained through requesting with social rewards obtained from adults in the context of enjoyable interactions may lead children with autism to experience social interactions as generally more rewarding (i.e., acquired reward value hypothesis). This pairing of functional and social rewards has long been hypothesized to enable many people with severe disabilities to learn to use IJA (e.g., Halle, Reichle, Drasgow, & Reinoehl, 1995). There is precedence for expression of affection acquiring reinforcing properties via paired association with primary reinforcers in children with autism (Lovaas et al., 1966). Regardless of its origin, once a child experiences social interaction as rewarding, adult models of IJA may help children to begin using newly acquired behavioral forms to attain social rewards. Siller and Sigman (2002) showed that parental modeling of IJA behavior was predictive of later IJA use in children with autism.

Transfer of stimulus control and acquired reward value hypotheses may also explain how the environment affects generalized and maintained RJA. Prompting and reinforcement may be used to teach children to monitor and follow adult attentional directives. There are some conditions and types of attentional directives to which children with autism are most likely to respond. The literature on children with Down syndrome provides evidence supporting the hypothesis that children follow attentional directives when they are unengaged (i.e., introductions) more than when they are already engaged with an object other than the adult's referent (i.e., redirections; Landry & Chapiesky, 1990; Legerstee, Varghese, & van Beek, 2002). This hypothesis has not yet been tested with children with autism. When being directed to a novel referent outside the child's current focus of attention, children with autism are more likely to follow perceptually salient adult cues than more subtle adult attentional directives (Leekam, Hunnisett, & Moore, 1998). With this in mind, it is interesting to recall that Whalen and Schreibman (2003) used an instructional sequence that progressed from more to less salient attentional cues when teaching RJA. Once the child became more fluent at deploying attention to salient attentional directives (e.g., shows), less salient attentional directives were used (e.g., gaze shifts).

Presumably, the reward for compliance with attentional directives in the natural environment is the acquisition of linguistic information or demonstration of object function or effect. If particular children are not currently using words to communicate, or if they do not look to adults for new information about objects, it is possible that linguistic and play interventions may increase the probability that such children will eventually come to experience such information as rewarding (i.e., acquired reward value hypothesis). The notion that referential language may actually precede RJA in some children with autism has cross-sectional support (Carpenter, Pennington, & Rogers, 2002). Additionally, children may become more interested in adult demonstrations of the function or effect of the referent once they repeatedly experience the utility of such exposure to expanding their object knowledge. At present, the acquired reward value hypothesis is the more tenuous of the two hypotheses.

FUTURE RESEARCH

Regardless of the mechanism of change, meaningful (i.e., generalized and maintained) changes in behaviors that can legitimately be called IJA and RJA have been shown to increase in subgroups of young children with developmental delay or autism. The data do not tell us with confidence that our treatments caused these changes in children with autism. Nor do they tell us which children with autism probably respond to joint-attention treatment. However, our consideration of the probable mechanisms of environmental influence on joint attention, the efficacy data and our clinical experience suggest that it is probable that some treatments affect the joint-attention skills of some children with autism. This subgroup of children may be those who find social interaction and linguistic and object knowledge reinforcing.

Randomized group experiments are needed to test these hypotheses. Future research must use research designs that allow confident inferences of treatment effects without requiring abrupt shifts in the dependent variable immediately following the onset of treatment. We have argued that generalization and maintenance of joint-attention outcomes are critical for differentiating therapy registers from important developmental changes in joint attention. Generalized changes in joint-attention outcomes are likely to occur many months after treatment onset in some children with autism. Only randomized group experiments are likely to afford confident inferences that the treatment caused such changes in children who are slow to generalize difficult skills such as RJA and IJA.

Past intervention literature consistently shows that some children respond to treatment and others do not, regardless of the treatment used. Therefore, it is clear that randomized group experiments must include measures of pretreatment child characteristics that are potential predictors of response to joint-attention treatment. These predictors may identify the subgroups in which the joint-attention treatments work. It is important to note that predictors of a treatment response are not the same as predictors of growth or correlates of individual differences in outcomes within a treatment group. The latter class of findings does not control for nonintervention explanations for growth in the outcomes. In fact, it is quite possible for children to show relatively fast growth on an outcome variable *and* be in the subgroup of children who are particularly ill-suited to a treatment. For example, children with relatively *high* frequency of vocal communication with consonants tend to show relatively fast expressive language growth (Yoder & Warren, 2004). In the same sample, it was children who showed relatively *low* frequency of such vocal communication whose language benefited from the prelinguistic treatment they received (Yoder & Warren, 2002). When we want to identify predictors of treatment response, we are looking for evidence that the difference between the comparison and experimental groups varies as a function of the pretreatment characteristic (i.e., statistical interactions between pretreatment variables and treatment group assignment). We call this a "moderated treatment effect."

The effect sizes of moderated treatment effects are typically between 10 and 20% of the variance after controlling for the main effects of the treatment and pretreatment predictor (Yoder & Warren, 1998, 1999a, 2001, 2002; Yoder, Kaiser, & Alpert, 1991; Yoder et al., 1995). To detect such effect sizes, relatively large samples are needed, because the relevant unit of analysis is the participant. That is, we want to know what is different about the participants who respond to the treatment versus those who do not. Because the effect sizes of these differences are likely to be moderate, there will be several exceptions to the general pattern of results. These exceptions will prevent small sample size designs from detecting the pattern with confidence. In contrast, larger sample sizes allow us to detect such effect sizes.

CLINICAL IMPLICATIONS

If the aforementioned mechanisms are accurate, then the transactional approach holds promise for facilitating IJA. The combined approach holds promise for facilitating RJA, particularly when used in combination with linguistic and/or play treatments. In both models, parents and other adults have a large role to play in encouraging the development of IJA and RJA in children with autism. We proposed that both types of joint attention are developmentally meaningful only if their typical and functional consequences maintain their use. For IJA to generalize and be maintained, parents must socially reward IJA attempts and provide the word for the referent of interest (i.e., linguistically map). For RJA to generalize and be maintained, parents must either name or demonstrate the function or effect of object referents after children shift their attention to match the adult's focus. We have argued that joint-attention treatment is likely to be less effective and more difficult to implement in children with less social interest, less interest in speech, and more restricted interest in objects.

In general, predictors of response to treatment may or may not be affected by treatment. Those that can be affected by treatment become reasonable treatment goals. We have much evidence that treatments can be successful in teaching many children with autism to talk (Koegel, 2000). There is some, but less, evidence that children with autism can be taught to expand the cognitive level of their play, thereby increasing the number of objects for which they have object schema (Lifter, 2000). We have the least amount of information about the efficacy of treatment in helping children with autism to experience social interactions as rewarding.

Although current research has not provided all of the needed answers, clinicians need to treat children with autism now. To provide guidance to clinicians in this endeavor, we offer the following considered suggestions. It is critical to distinguish among the types of joint attention when we create goals. We must select treatment approaches or use treatment elements that explicitly address the eventual function that the joint-attention ability usually has in the natural environment. Finally, measuring generalization and maintenance of newly learned joint-attention skills is critical to judging success of treatment.

Specific to treating IJA, it should be noted that the transactional approaches are most effective when children show sustained engagement with a variety of objects. It is probable that individuals with extremely short attention spans and extremely perseverative object play will need modifications of the transactional approaches (e.g., use of enticement, special positioning considerations, carefully timed introductions of new materials). It is also likely that at least 20 hours a week of transactional treatments for at least 6 months will be necessary to facilitate generalized and maintained IJA in many children.

When using the combined approaches, such as the treatment described in Whalen and Schreibman (2003), careful attention to maintenance of gains in RJA will be necessary. Maintenance may be facilitated by teaching many adults to provide opportunities for and differentially reward compliance with progressively more distal adult attentional cues. The treatment intensity Whalen and Schreibman (2003) used (about 30 hours of training) was sufficient for induction but not clearly sufficient for maintenance of new RJA skills. It is possible that further training that is targeted at altering parent–child interaction designed to support maintenance of new RJA skills would be effective, but research does not yet support this hypothesis.

Both treatments are likely to be more successful if children seek to know more about how objects are used. Extremely perseverative object use probably undermines the child's motivation to engage in RJA and introduces obstacles to IJA generalization. Treatments that attempt to expand the children's generalized use of objects (e.g., Lifter, Sulzer-Azaroff, Anderson, & Cowdery, 1993) may be a very important alteration to both transactional and combined approaches when treating children with extremely perseverative object use.

CONCLUSION

In this chapter, we provided a rationale for focusing on RJA and IJA as the most important aspects of joint attention for the diagnosis and development of children with autism. We followed with a discussion of the importance of generalization and maintenance to determining whether developmentally important changes in joint-attention skills have occurred. We also indicated the importance of controlling for threats to internal validity when determining whether measured changes in joint-attention skills occur in response to a particular treatment. We then described four intervention approaches that differ in the extent to which they prompt desired behaviors and put a premium on the positive affective relationship between adults and children. From a review of the internally valid efficacy studies, we concluded that transactional approaches hold promise for facilitating generalized IJA and that combined approaches hold promise for facilitating generalized RJA. However, the present literature does not yet support a strong claim that either treatment causes generalized and maintained changes in joint attention in children with autism.

Additionally, we noted that substantial intensity of treatment is probably necessary to observe treatment effects on generalized and maintained joint attention in many children with autism. We followed this efficacy review with a discussion of how transfer of stimulus control mechanisms could explain the ontogeny of behaviors that may eventually come to serve IJA and RJA functions. But we also discussed the caveat that gains in IJA and RJA will probably not be maintained unless the children experience social interaction (for IJA) and linguistic or object knowledge information (for RJA) as reinforcing. We suggested the possibility that object and linguistic knowledge and social interaction may acquire reinforcing properties as children experience the need for and the rewarding experiences of these types of consequences for RJA and IJA. Finally, we argued that randomized group experiments with pretreatment measures of potential predictors of response to treatment will be necessary to address the deficits in our present knowledge base about effective joint-attention treatments for children with autism. We suggested that degree of social interest, awareness or interest in language, and play level or degree of perseverative object use are potential predictors of response to joint-attention treatment in children with autism.

REFERENCES

Adamson, L. B., & Bakeman, R. (1984). Mothers' communicative acts: Changes during infancy. *Infant Behavior and Development, 7*(4), 467–478.

Adamson, L. B., & Chance, S. E. (1998). Coordinating attention to people, objects and symbols. In A. M. Wetherby, S. F. Warren, & J. Reichle (Eds.), *Transitions in prelinguistic communication* (pp. 15–37). Baltimore: Brookes.

Bakeman, R., & Adamson, L. B. (1984). Coordinating attention to people and objects in mother–infant and peer–infant interaction. *Child Development, 55*(4), 1278–1289.

Bates, E. (1979). Intentions, conventions, and symbols. In E. Bates, L. Benigni, I. Bretherton, L. Camaioni, & V. Volterra (Eds.), *The emergence of symbols: Cognition and communication in infancy* (pp. 33–68). New York: Academic Press.

Bates, E., Camaioni, L., & Volterra, V. (1975). The acquisition of performatives prior to speech. *Merrill-Palmer Quarterly, 21*, 205–226.

Beakley, B., & Ludlow, P. (1992). *The philosophy of the mind: Classical problems/contemporary issues*. Cambridge, MA: MIT Press.

Bloom, L. (1993). *The transition from infancy to language: Acquiring the power of expression*. New York: Cambridge University Press.

Buffington, D., Krantz, P., McClannahan, L., & Poulson, C. (1998). Procedures for teaching appropriate gestural communication skills to children with autism. *Journal of Autism and Developmental Disorders, 28*, 535–545.

Carpenter, M., Nagell, K., & Tomasello, M. (1998). Social cognition, joint attention and communicative competence from 9 to 15 months of age. *Monographs of the Society for Research in Child Development, 63*(4).

Carpenter, M., Pennington, B., & Rogers, S. (2002). Interrelations among social-cognitive skills in young children with autism. *Journal of Autism and Developmental Disorders, 32*, 91–106.

Charman, T., Baron-Cohen, S., Swettenham, J., Baird, G., Drew, A., & Cox, A. (2003). Predicting language outcome in infants with autism and pervasive developmental disorder. *International Journal of Language and Communication Disorders, 38*, 265–285.

Cook, T., & Campbell, D. (1979). *Quasi-experimentation: Design and analysis issues for field settings*. Boston: Houghton-Mifflin.

Cronbach, L. J., & Meehl, P. E. (1955). Construct validity in psychological tests. *Psychological Bulletin, 52,* 281–302.

Goldstein, H. (2002). Communication intervention for children with autism: A review of treatment efficacy. *Journal of Autism and Developmental Disorders, 32,* 373–396.

Greenspan, S., & Wieder, S. (2000). Developmental approach to difficulties in relating and communicating in autism spectrum disorders and related syndromes. In A. Wetherby & B. Prizant (Eds.), *Autism spectrum disorders: A transactional developmental perspective* (Vol. 9, pp. 279–303). Baltimore: Brookes.

Halle, J., Reichle, J., Drasgow, E., & Reinoehl, M. (1995). Assessment and intervention of severe language delays in children. *Journal of Behavioral Education, 5,* 173–188.

Hwang, B., & Hughes, C. (2000a). The effects of social interactive training on early social communicative skills of children with autism. *Journal of Autism and Developmental Disorders, 30,* 331–343.

Hwang, B., & Hughes, C. (2000b). Increasing social communicative skills of preverbal preschool children with autism through social interactive training. *Journal of Association of Persons with Severe Handicaps, 25,* 18–28.

Johnson, J. (1988). Generalization: The nature of change. *Language, Speech, and Hearing Services in Schools, 19,* 314–329.

Kasari, C., Freeman, S., & Paparella, T. (2000). Early intervention in autism: Joint attention and symbolic play. In L. Glidden (Ed.), *International review of research in mental retardation* (Vol. 23, pp. 207–237). San Diego, CA: Academic Press.

Kazden, A. (1982). *Single-case research designs: Methods for clinical and applied settings.* New York: Oxford University Press.

Koegel, L. K. (2000). Interventions to facilitate communication in autism. *Journal of Autism and Developmental Disorders, 30,* 383–391.

Landry, S. H., & Chapiesky, M. (1990). Joint attention of six-month-old Down syndrome and preterm infants: I. Attention to toys and mother. *American Journal on Mental Retardation, 94,* 488–498.

Leekam, S. R., Hunnisett, E., & Moore, C. (1998). Targets and cues: Gaze-following in children with autism. *Journal of Child Psychology and Psychiatry, 39*(7), 951–962.

Leew, S. V. (2001). *The relationship of prelinguistic milieu training to the increased use of communication forms associated with proto-declaratives.* Unpublished dissertation, Vanderbilt University, Nashville, TN.

Legerstee, M., Varghese, J., & van Beek, Y. (2002). Effects of maintaining and redirecting infant attention on the production of referential communication in infants with and without Down syndrome. *Journal of Child Language, 29,* 23–48.

Lewy, A., & Dawson, G. (1992). Social stimulation and joint attention in young autistic children. *Journal of Abnormal Child Psychology, 20*(6), 555–566.

Lifter, K. (2000). Linking assessment to intervention for children with developmental disabilities or at risk for developmental delay: The Developmental Play Assessment (DPA) instrument. In C. Schaefer (Ed.), *Play diagnosis and assessment* (pp. 228–261). New York: Wiley.

Lifter, K., Sulzer-Azaroff, B., Anderson, S. R., & Cowdery, G. E. (1993). Teaching play activities to preschool children with disabilities: The importance of developmental considerations. *Journal of Early Intervention, 17*(2), 139–159.

Lovaas, I., Freitag, G., Kinder, M., Rubenstein, B., Schaeffer, B., & Simmons, J. (1966). Establishment of social reinforcers in two schizophrenic children on the basis of food. *Journal of Experimental Child Psychology, 4,* 109–125.

Loveland, K. A., & Landry, S. H. (1986). Joint attention and language in autism and developmental language delay. *Journal of Autism and Developmental Disorders, 16*(3), 335–349.

Mahoney, G., & MacDonald, J. (2003). *Responsive teaching: Parent-mediated developmental intervention.* Cleveland, OH: Case Western Reserve University.

Mahoney, G., & Perales, F. (2003). Using relationship-focused intervention to enhance the social-emotional functioning of young children with autism spectrum disorders. *Topics in Early Childhood Disorders, 23,* 77–89.

McConnell, S. (2002). Interventions to facilitate social interaction for young children with autism: Review of available research and recommendations for educational intervention and future research. *Journal of Autism and Developmental Disorders, 32,* 351–372.

Mundy, P. (1995). Joint attention and social-emotional approach behavior in children with autism. *Development and Psychopathology, 7,* 63–82.

Mundy, P., & Sigman, M. (1989). Second thoughts on the nature of autism. *Development and Psychopathology, 1,* 213–217.

Mundy, P., Sigman, M., & Kasari, C. (1990). A longitudinal study of joint attention and language development in autistic children. *Journal of Autism and Developmental Disorders, 20,* 115–129.

Mundy, P., Sigman, M., & Kasari, C. (1994). Joint attention, developmental level, and symptom presentation in young children with autism. *Development and Psychopathology, 6,* 389–401.

Mundy, P., Sigman, M., Ungerer, J., & Sherman, T. (1986). Defining the social deficits in autism: The contribution of non-verbal communication measures. *Journal of Child Psychology and Psychiatry, 27,* 657–669.

Mundy, P., & Stella, J. (2000). Joint attention, social orienting, and nonverbal communication in autism. In A. Wetherby & B. Prizant (Eds.), *Autism spectrum disorders: A transactional developmental perspective* (Vol. 9, pp. 55–77). Baltimore: Brookes.

Nadel, J. (2002). Imitation and imitation recognition: Functional use in preverbal infants and nonverbal children with autism. In A. Meltzof & W. Prinz (Eds.), *The imitative mind: Development, evolution, and brain bases* (pp. 42–62). Cambridge, UK: Cambridge University Press.

Prizant, B., Wetherby, A., & Rydell, P. (2000). Communication intervention issues for children with autism spectrum disorders. In A. Wetherby & B. Prizant (Eds.), *Autism spectrum disorders: A transactional developmental perspective* (Vol. 9, pp. 193–224). Baltimore: Brookes.

Sameroff, A. (1983). Developmental systems: Contexts and evolution. In P. Mussen (Ed.), *Handbook of child psychology* (Vol. 1, pp. 237–294.). New York: Wiley.

Scaife, M., & Bruner, J. (1975). The capacity for joint visual attention in the infant. *Nature, 253,* 265–266.

Seibert, J. M., Hogan, A. E., & Mundy, P. C. (1982). Assessing interactional competencies: The Early Social-Communication Scales. *Infant Mental Health Journal, 3*(4), 244–258.

Shatz, M. (1987). Bootstrapping operations in child language. In K. E. Nelson & A. van Kleeck (Eds.), *Children's language* (Vol. 6, pp. 1–22). Hillsdale, NJ: Erlbaum.

Sigman, M., & Kasari, C. (1995). Joint attention across contexts in normal and autistic children. In C. Moore & P. Dunham (Eds.), *Joint attention: Its origins and role in development* (pp. 189–204). Hillsdale, NJ: Erlbaum.

Sigman, M., & Ruskin, E. (1999). Continuity and change in the social competence of children with autism, Down syndrome, and developmental delays. *Monographs of the Society for Research in Child Development, 64*(1).

Sigman, M., & Ungerer, J. A. (1984). Cognitive and language skills in autistic, mentally retarded, and normal children. *Developmental Psychology, 20*(2), 293–302.

Siller, M., & Sigman, M. (2002). The behaviors of parents of children with autism predict the subsequent development of their children's communication. *Journal of Autism and Developmental Disorders, 32*, 77–90.

Stone, W. L., Ousley, O. Y., Yoder, P. J., Hogan, K. L., & Hepburn, S. L. (1997). Nonverbal communication in two- and three-year-old children with autism. *Journal of Autism and Developmental Disorders, 27*(6), 677–696.

Taylor, B., & Harris, S. (1995). Teaching children with autism to seek information: Acquisition of novel information and generalization of responding. *Journal of Applied Behavior Analysis, 28*, 3–14.

Tomasello, M. (1995). Joint attention as social cognition. In C. Moore & P. J. Dunham (Eds.), *Joint attention: Its origins and role in development* (pp. 103–130). Hillsdale, NJ: Erlbaum.

Wetherby, A., & Prizant, B. (1993). *Communication and Symbolic Behavior Scales: Normed edition*. Chicago: Riverside.

Wetherby, A., & Prutting, C. (1984). Profiles of communicative and cognitive-social abilities in autistic children. *Journal of Speech and Hearing Research, 27*, 364–377.

Whalen, C., & Schreibman, L. (2003). Joint attention training for children with autism using behavior modification procedures. *Journal of Child Psychology and Psychiatry, 44*, 456–468.

Yoder, P. J., Kaiser, A. P., & Alpert, C. L. (1991). An exploratory study of the interaction between language teaching methods and child characteristics. *Journal of Speech and Hearing Research, 34*(1), 155–167.

Yoder, P. J., Kaiser, A. P., Goldstein, H., Alpert, C., Mousetis, L., Kaczmarek, L., et al. (1995). An exploratory comparison of milieu teaching and responsive interaction in classroom applications. *Journal of Early Intervention, 19*(3), 218–242.

Yoder, P. J., & Warren, S. F. (1993). Can developmentally delayed children's language development be enhanced through prelinguistic intervention? In A. P. Kaiser (Ed.), *Enhancing children's communication: Research foundations for intervention* (Vol. 2, pp. 35–61). Baltimore: Brookes.

Yoder, P. J., & Warren, S. F. (1998). Maternal responsivity predicts the prelinguistic communication intervention that facilitates generalized intentional communication. *Journal of Speech, Language, and Hearing Research, 41*(5), 1207–1219.

Yoder, P. J., & Warren, S. F. (1999a). Self-initiated proto-declaratives and proto-imperatives can be facilitated in prelinguistic children with developmental disabilities. *Journal of Early Intervention, 22*, 337–354.

Yoder, P. J., & Warren, S. F. (1999b). Maternal responsivity mediates the relationship between prelinguistic intentional communication and later language. *Journal of Early Intervention, 22*, 126–136.

Yoder, P. J., & Warren, S. F. (2001). Relative treatment effects of two prelinguistic communication interventions on language development in toddlers with developmental delays vary by maternal characteristics. *Journal of Speech, Language, and Hearing Research, 44*(1), 224–237.

Yoder, P. J., & Warren, S. F. (2002). Effects of prelinguistic milieu teaching and parent responsivity education in dyads with children with intellectual disabilities. *Journal of Speech, Language, and Hearing Research, 45*, 1158–1174.

Yoder, P. J., & Warren, S. F. (2004). Early predictors of language in children with and without Down syndrome. *American Journal on Mental Retardation, 109*, 285–300.

6

Evidence-Based Interventions for Language Development in Young Children with Autism

SALLY J. ROGERS

The abnormal development and use of spoken language is one of autism's most unusual and striking features. Kanner's (1943) first description of autism painted a very detailed picture of the two main subgroups of language symptoms in children with autism. One pattern involved children who did not develop spoken language, a group described in past years as including as many as 50% of persons with autism (Rutter, 1978). Unlike other diagnostic groups of children who for one reason or another do not develop speech, these children did not develop an alternative communication system using distal signals, either, but instead moved people around physically, manipulating hands, pushing and pulling on others' limbs and bodies when they needed adult help. These children appeared to understand little speech, and long-term follow-up revealed little change in their relatively noncommunicative status over many years (Kanner, 1971).

The second pattern involved children who produced speech that was markedly atypical. These children tended to mimic speech rather than generate their own sentences, with patterns of both immediate and delayed echolalia. Their ability to remember long strings of stories, songs, lists, and other memorized content was remarkable, and Kanner surmised that this was a sign of latent preserved intelligence. A second atypical feature was the lack of communicative content of their speech. These children did not use language to share their experiences with others or to gain information by asking questions. Other atypical features of the verbal children's language included unusual prosody and intonation, unusually mature syntax patterns given the children's ages, and the use of unusual words, or neologisms (Kanner, 1943).

Kanner described abnormal features in most areas of language use: semantics, or meanings; syntax, or grammatical form; and pragmatics, the social functions of language, as well as abnormalities of the supersegmental aspects of language—the additional information afforded by the rhythm, rate, intonation, and volume of speech. Only the phonology of language appeared spared, at least in the children who acquired speech. In the 40 years of published, empirically based intervention studies of autism, there is probably no aspect of autism that has received greater attention, and interventionists have attempted to treat every aspect of the atypical language development and usage patterns seen in autism.

The purpose of this chapter is to review the main types of empirically supported language interventions that have successfully taught preschool-age children with autism, age 5 or under, to use spoken language, and to consider the strengths and relative weaknesses of each approach. The distinction between the terms *language* and *speech* in this chapter defines *language* as an intentional communication system involving shared symbols, with *speech* as a specific type of symbol. The procedure for reviewing research studies involved a Web-based search in the PsycINFO data base, searching under the following key words: *autism, intervention, treatment,* and *language*. All studies that resulted from this search and that involved empirically based studies concerning teaching preschool-age children with autism to speak or to increase their speech that were published in peer-reviewed journals were examined. Studies involving older children were reviewed if a significant number of the participants were 5 years old or younger. References from those studies were also searched.

This chapter provides a comprehensive but not exhaustive review of the literature. It reviews the main findings from empirically based articles involving single-subject and group designs, both those that target improvement in spoken language as the primary outcome of the treatment and also those that involve many different goals of intervention, including spoken language gains. The chapter ends with some consideration of possible mechanisms that underlie the different language subgroups in autism and possible treatment implications.

THE DIDACTIC, OR MASSED-TRIAL, BEHAVIORAL APPROACH

History of This Approach

The first empirical reports of language interventions were published almost 40 years ago, by Wolf, Risley, and Mees (1964) and Risley and Wolf (1967), working at the University of Kansas, and Hewett (1965) and Lovaas, Berberich, Perloff, and Schaeffer (1966), working at the University of California, Los Angeles. At the time, there were two prevailing models of language development in the United States: the operant model of Skinner (1957) and the nativist model of Chomsky (1975). The first interventions, which specifically targeted development and remediation of spoken language, came from the operant tradition. Risley's initial two studies and Lovaas's first writing on language interventions provided the model of massed-trial, adult-directed teaching that continues today and that is often referred to as discrete trial teaching (DTT). This shorthand is inaccurate in that teaching episodes in many conditions contain planned antecedents, behaviors, and responses, and are, technically, discrete trials. For the purposes of this chapter, the term *didactic teaching* is borrowed from Warren and Kaiser (1988) to refer to this type of adult-directed teaching.

Characteristics of the Approach

The characteristics of didactic teaching are well known in the autism treatment world and represent applications of the laboratory studies of operant learning. All learning theory–based approaches rely on the teaching techniques involving shaping, prompting, and chaining to teach new behaviors and sequences of behaviors in response to specific antecedent events. Principles of reinforcement are used to increase the frequency and consistency of desired behaviors in response to antecedents, and principles of extinction and punishment (including time-out from reinforcement) are used to decrease unwanted behaviors (Cipani & Spooner, 1994). The didactic method applies these principles in teaching sessions that are marked by high levels of adult control and direction, massed-practice periods of preselected tasks, and precise antecedent, teaching, and reinforcement practices. The learner is in a responder role, and the teacher has a directive role.

Studies Supporting the Approach

Many published studies involving both single-subject and group designs have demonstrated the efficacy of the didactic model for teaching speech to nonverbal children with autism and increasing the use and complexity of speech and vocabulary size in verbal children with autism. Children who, at the start of treatment, were completely nonverbal, lacking even consonant sounds, have been taught to speak and to use increasingly complex syntax and vocabulary, including response to questions. (In most studies, the measurement system has involved behavioral frequency counts of specific words or word combinations.) In addition to focusing on building semantic knowledge and syntactic structures, the didactic approach has taught use of gestures and supersegmentals, such as intonation and volume. Various pragmatic functions have been addressed, such as requesting, commenting, negation, and asking questions. For examples, see Krantz, Zalenski, Hall, Fenske, and McClannahan (1981; teaching complex sentences), Ross and Greer (2003; vocal imitation), Williams, Perez-Gonzalez, and Vogt (2003; use of questions), Yoder & Layton (1988; development of first words), in addition to the early work of Hewett (1965) and Lovaas et al. (1966).

The early reports involved children in hospital settings, who received treatment all day long. When these children left the training setting, they lost many of their newly learned language skills. The fragility of their gains demonstrated the importance of ongoing environmental supports for speech (Lovaas, Koegel, Simmons, & Long, 1973). This finding led to a shift away from hospital-like treatment settings and toward explorations of treatment delivery in natural settings, where children's new learning could be constantly supported in their natural environments by the people in those settings.

Several studies examined parents' ability to master the didactic approach and deliver the treatment at home. Howlin and Rutter (1989) and Sandra Harris (Harris, Wolchik, & Weitz, 1981; Harris, Wolchik, & Milch, 1983) reported that a combination of weekly group parent-training classes combined with individual weekly or biweekly home visits resulted in child gains, with two important caveats. First, language gains were almost completely confined to children who already had some speech at the start of treatment. Nonverbal children made minimal gains, perhaps because the shaping of speech in nonspeaking children requires more intensity, clinical training, or treatment precision than parents can easily implement. Second, most gains occurred in the first 6 months, during which time parents received both group and individual instruction, with little progress beyond this. Undergraduate college students have also been trained to carry out this type of teaching at high levels of fidelity, resulting in child improvement (Lovaas, 1987; Smith, Groen, & Wynn, 2000), as long as ongoing training and support are provided to the students. Thus the didactic approach can be used successfully to teach children with autism spoken language by people without advanced educational degrees, as long as ongoing monitoring, training, and oversight of nonprofessionals are provided by sophisticated therapists who are directing the individualized treatment of the child.

Most of the studies cited previously have involved single-subject designs, which tend to demonstrate short-term changes in very specific behaviors. However, group studies examine child progress over somewhat longer periods of time, use more general measures of progress, and use comparison groups to determine the effect of the treatment. Several group studies have also demonstrated the ability of the didactic method to increase language development. Lovaas (1987) reported significantly greater gains in expressive and receptive language by children with autism who had received his treatment model at a high level of intensity during the preschool period than by a comparison group who received the same model at a low level of intensity. Similarly, Eikeseth, Smith, Jahr, and Eldevik (2002) reported greater language progress on standardized tests by a group of somewhat older children receiving Lovaas's treatment model than by children receiving an eclectic model involving the same intensity of treatment. Although Smith et al. (2000) originally reported greater gains made by children receiving Lovaas's method than those in a randomly assigned parent treatment comparison group, they later indicated that the difference was not significant (Smith, Groen, & Wynn, 2001).

Strengths and Weaknesses of the Approach

The didactic behavioral approach has several strengths. First and foremost, it has demonstrated efficacy in many studies from a variety of independent researchers, using a variety of treatment settings and treatment deliverers, with both single-subject and group designs, including one randomly controlled trial. It has demonstrated efficacy in teaching a number of skills involving spoken language, including the development of speech in children who were completely mute, and the improvement in all three main aspects of speech: semantics, the meanings of words; syntax, the structuring of multiword utterances; and pragmatic, or social effects of an utterance. The teaching approach involves a general method for building and altering behavioral repertoires, and treatment givers who master the general principles of this approach generalize them to other teaching goals as well (Koegel, Russo, & Rincover, 1977; Koegel, Glahn, & Nieminen, 1978).

Second, it is accessible to a wide range of consumers. Its teaching *method* is highly specified and rule bound, and the behaviors associated with the teaching practices are relatively easily mastered. The method is readily available to the public through published instruction manuals that target teachers, therapists, and parents. Finally, the *content* of the teaching, or the specific teaching programs and curricula, has been published for the lay audience and is widely available (Maurice, Green, & Luce, 1996;

Lovaas, Freitag, Gold, & Kassorla, 1965; Lovaas, 1981; Lovaas, 2002; Leaf & McEachin, 2001). This general manualization of both the process and the content of the teaching approach is a great strength.

Warren and Kaiser (1988) provided an excellent summary of this approach. There are many teaching situations in which bouts of drill and practice can be extremely useful in rapidly establishing a new behavior pattern or in developing speed or fluency, and massed-practice periods with tight instructional control accomplish this. Its strengths are in establishing initial skills—those with zero baseline—and for teaching imitation, initial sound–label repertoire, articulation and phonology, as well as initial teaching of linguistic rules such as plurals and verb tense.

"However, the advantages offered by didactic instruction for teaching basic discriminations may become liabilities to promoting functional generalized language" (Warren & Kaiser, 1988, p. 93). Limitations to this approach as a comprehensive language-training method were recognized from very early on. A core problem described by Lovaas and colleagues concerned the children's lack of generalization. They did not use their trained language behaviors in other contexts or with other people, and they lacked communicative initiative (Lovaas et al., 1973). Several researchers described alterations of the basic techniques to deal with problems involving learning rates, maintenance and generalization, and behavior outbursts (Dunlap, 1984; Matson, Sevin, Box, Francis, & Sevine, 1993; Charlop, Schreibman, & Thiebodeau, 1985). These problems point to a fundamental limitation of this particular approach, and that is the very atypical communicative framework that surrounds the teaching situation. The teaching approach focuses on language as one of many learned behaviors, following the same learning rules as other operant behaviors. By targeting semantics, syntax, and pragmatics in adult-directed, rote-teaching drills, the main purpose of communication is bypassed, and the opportunity to associate new skills with functional, real-life settings and communicative experiences is lost. All communication, including speech, is a form of social interaction, with the main function of meeting social needs. This pragmatic understanding of communication has been most fully developed in the past 20–30 years, after the initial operant teaching approaches were first developed. The teaching approach and the teaching curriculum initially described in writings from the 1960s and the 1970s remain the core of didactic treatment as it is delivered today, even though the children who now receive the treatment vary considerably from the original group (in their younger age; in their multiple intervention experiences; in the wider, especially milder, range of symptoms recognized to be part of autism; and in having the benefit of much more community know-how and expectations of response to intervention). The treatment settings differ greatly from the original settings, and the field of communication science has developed enormously in the past 30 years. The limitations of the didactic model are clearly recognized by experts in the operant approach. Both Smith (2001) and Sundberg and Partington (1999) caution users that didactic treatment approaches need to be combined with the naturalistic teaching in order to foster spontaneity and generalization.

THE PRAGMATIC REVOLUTION
IN UNDERSTANDING EARLY LANGUAGE

The current scientific understanding of communication and language development stems from the pragmatics revolution of the 1970s and 1980s, in which infant language was demonstrated to develop from the preverbal social exchanges of infants involving facial expressions, gestures, and vocalizations with important others (Bates, 1976). Two types of interactions were described as particularly important for ushering in the use of spoken language: ritualized infant games involving movements, sounds, and shared pleasurable emotion (Ratner & Bruner, 1978); and gestures that coordinated child and adult attention on objects, used by the infant to achieve goals concerning regulation of the adult's behavior, joint attention (Bates, 1976), or social interaction and dyadic exchange.

These early communicative exchanges are marked by reciprocity and emotion sharing between the partners and by the use of preverbal behaviors involving eye contact, gestures, vocalizations, and facial expressions to accomplish social coordination. As infant phonation and receptive word learning develop, infants add words to these already established communicative exchanges. Thus the typical preverbal infant who has mastered the use of gesture to share intention and attention is already an accomplished communicator who understands and uses the power of communication to share subjective experiences and to affect others' behavior (Stern, 1985).

Current research has demonstrated that young children with autism lack these early building blocks of communication. The seminal work of Wetherby (Wetherby & Prutting, 1984), and Sigman and Mundy (Mundy, Sigman, & Kasari, 1990; Mundy, Sigman, Ungerer, & Sherman, 1986, 1987) demonstrated that young children with autism tend not to use nonverbal communication behaviors, nor do they seem aware of them, interested in them, or able to comprehend their meaning, compared with both typical and atypical groups well matched for cognitive development. These studies demonstrated that very young children with autism lacked social initiative, joint attention, social and emotional reciprocity, and the use of early gestures to coordinate social exchanges—behaviors now known to be essential features of language development.

This pattern of low social initiative and lack of shared control of interactions is continued and further reinforced in the didactic approach to communication training, with its emphasis on an atypical level of adult directiveness and control of the interaction, paired with a quiet, attending student who responds when requested and slowly builds up a semantic store of object labels and memorized responses to questions. Whereas later aspects of the didactic curriculum do focus on teaching communicative initiative and use of speech to accomplish various communicative functions, in normal development communication and language are, from their very beginning, focused on social exchanges with others and coordination of interactions with people and objects. The pragmatic use of language is not one aspect of language, like verb forms or pronoun use. It is the foundation of language. Difficulties of the didactic approach in achieving generalization and spontaneity are likely due to: (1) its fundamental mismatch between the teaching approach and the nature of communication, (2) its reinforcement of atypical social patterns (didactic instruction and passive responding), especially in combination with the fundamentally deficient social repertoire seen in autism, and (3) the development of spoken language outside of a functional interactive social frame.

THE NATURALISTIC BEHAVIORAL
LANGUAGE INTERVENTIONS

History of the Approach

In 1968, a landmark study by Hart and Risley (1968) was published that described the application of operant teaching principles to teaching language using a different paradigm from the didactic model described previously. This study experimentally demonstrated the relative inefficiency of teaching a language form didactically and then "relying on unsystematic events to make that skill functional" (p. 119). In this study, the authors analyzed a particular type of language (descriptive speech) by its function and then deliberately structured the children's environments so that the function of that form was highlighted. They used children's self-initiated behavior toward an object as the vehicle for the intervention, inserting the "instruction," or prompt, *after the child initiated a communication* for the object but before giving them access to the object. Thus the children's requested item was the reinforcer for the new behavior. Even though previous attempts were made to teach the same skill didactically in the classroom with very little gain, this change to naturalistic teaching created rapid increases in spontaneous use of descriptive words in children's language to gain access to preschool materials. Furthermore, when the reversal condition began, in which all requirements for use of descriptive language to access materials were removed, the children maintained a greatly increased rate of

descriptive speech. Apparently, the natural environment contained sufficient reinforcers to maintain the new skill and even to support new learning.
This study made two great contributions to behavioral language intervention approaches. First, it focused on the pragmatic functions of language,
and it delivered the intervention within the natural social interactional
frame in which the communication occurred. Second, by respecting the
pragmatic goal of the communication, the intervention preserved the inherent reinforcement underlying a motivated interaction, in this case using
children's desired objects and events in the natural environment as the reinforcers for learning. The authors suggested that such "intrinsic" reinforcers
might provide stronger reinforcement than "external" reinforcers selected
by adults and might help to maintain the new behavior in the environment
because they are the same class of reinforcers that maintain behavior in everyday situations.

Hart and Risley (1968) labeled the approach *incidental teaching* to
draw the comparison with the didactic, or directive, style of teaching. Both
the efficacy of the intervention and the unexpected maintenance and generalization effects that resulted stimulated a wave of research on new methods of stimulating language development, using typical environments and
the people in those environments: parents, teachers, and others (as reviewed by Warren, McQuarter, & Rogers-Warren, 1984). Whereas the initial incidental teaching intervention began from child initiations, Warren
and colleagues (1984) demonstrated that similar effects could be gained in
classroom environments for children with very low rates of initiating by
training teachers to initiate certain types of communication prompts using
child-selected activity reinforcers (the "mand-model" approach). The first
references to this type of teaching in the autism literature occurred in the
mid-1980s in research by behaviorists who had already achieved recognition for their work using the didactic teaching approach and were now
moving to new kinds of intervention models (Koegel, O'Dell, & Koegel,
1987; Carr & Kologinsky, 1983; McGee, Krantz, Mason, & McClannahan,
1983).

Characteristics of the Approach

Although the teaching method used in each of these studies varied somewhat (Hepting & Goldstein, 1996), the approaches shared a number of
common elements, particularly the delivery of the intervention in natural
environments, the use of intrinsic reinforcers, a focus on child initiation of
communication, and pragmatically functional social interactions. Warren
and Kaiser (1988) classified these approaches as "naturalistic teaching"
and suggested that the common elements included (1) teaching the form
and content of language in naturally occurring exchanges, (2) using dis-

persed and intermittent trials; and (3) following the child's lead, rather than directing the child to communicate. Warren and Kaiser (1988) attributed the rapid development of this approach to the convergence of behaviorists, who were following an inductive approach to achieving improved generalization and initiation of speech, and developmentalists, who followed a deductive approach, applying current theories and research regarding typical language development to children with atypical communication development.

McGee et al. (1983) defined the key differences that are core elements of naturalistic behavioral teaching and that do not characterize didactic teaching:

1. Teaching episodes are initiated by child behavior via requests or gestures for preferred items.
2. Teaching takes place in the context of ongoing activities, with items of child interest as part of the naturally occurring stimuli of the space.
3. The teaching stimuli are child selected, and contingent access to them is the reinforcement.
4. Prompt strategies for elaborated language vary according to the child's initiating behavior.

Studies Supporting the Approach

Empirical support for this approach to language training in autism is substantial. A number of studies, virtually all using single-subject designs, have demonstrated the efficacy of this approach in teaching many linguistic responses to children with autism. Work by Koegel et al. (1987) demonstrated that completely nonverbal children could learn to speak using this approach. As described in excellent reviews by Delprato (2001), Lynn Koegel (2000), and Howard Goldstein (2000), children with autism have demonstrated increases in frequency, spontaneity, and syntactic sophistication of their language through naturalistic approaches (Laski, Charlop, & Schreibman, 1988). Examples of the use of naturalistic approaches to successfully teach various aspects of language include: teaching prepositions (McGee et al., 1983), using grammatical morphemes (Carter, 2001), improving articulation (Koegel, Camarata, Koegel, Ben-Tall, & Smith, 1998), teaching use of *yes* and *no* (Neef, Walters, & Egel, 1984), and using questions appropriately (Koegel, Camarata, Valdez-Menchaca, & Koegel, 1998). All aspects of language—pragmatics, semantics, syntax, and phonation— have been successfully treated using naturalistic approaches. Furthermore, direct comparisons between didactic and naturalistic approaches have demonstrated some advantages, including improved behavior (Koegel, Koegel,

Hurley, & Frea, 1992; Koegel, Koegel, & Surratt, 1992) and greater progress (especially maintenance and generalization of newly learned skills) using naturalistic strategies than using didactic strategies (see Delprato, 2001, for a review of the comparative studies).

All the aforementioned studies involve individual treatment, but several studies have also demonstrated delivery of this approach in group treatment. Both Peck (1985) and McBride and Schwartz (2003) trained classroom teaching staff to use naturalistic teaching to increase the opportunities for child initiation and responding embedded inside ongoing classroom activities, with resulting increases in children's communications, including speech. Similarly, McGee's current use of incidental teaching is being delivered in the integrated, inclusive Walden Preschool at Emory University, though the outcome data have been provided in descriptive rather than empirical studies (McGee, Morrier, & Daly, 1999; Strain, McGee, & Kohler, 2001).

The effectiveness of this approach most likely results from four aspects of the technique. First, child language functions to achieve child-chosen goals and child-chosen reinforcers, which apparently strengthens the power of the reinforcers. (See Carter [2001], for a nicely designed experiment demonstrating that child choice, by itself, is reinforcing. Children showed more positive learning rates and behavior when they actively chose between two rewards than when they were given a reward by an adult, even though they had previously chosen the reward.) Second, the teaching style heavily emphasizes child initiation, either verbal or nonverbal, and the exchanges involve reciprocity of child and adult. Active child initiation is fostered and rewarded, and the interactions and the reinforcers that occur in the intervention approach are typical child–adult verbal exchanges in natural environments. Thus teaching focuses on child communication skills that are functional in all settings. Third, the social functions of language that lead to reinforcers are highlighted, so the core pragmatic aspects of language permeate the intervention. Finally, the emphasis on child motivation and natural reinforcers adds a positive affective element to the interactions, which may enhance memory for learning.

Strengths and Weaknesses of the Approach

The strengths of the naturalistic approach have been clearly demonstrated in maintenance, generalization, child gains, and child behavior. It has been demonstrated to develop useful, spontaneous speech in completely nonspeaking children. It has been used successfully to teach semantics, syntax, and pragmatics of spoken language. However, there are also several weaknesses in the literature on naturalistic teaching. First of all, most of the published empirical studies involve one-to-one teaching using a highly trained therapist. Some of the promise of the naturalistic teaching approaches is in its application in typical environments, as described in the original Hart and Risley (1968) study. Although McGee and colleagues (1999) developed a method for applying naturalistic teaching for children with autism in an inclusive preschool classroom setting, empirical studies using comparative group designs are not yet available to demonstrate the amount of gain children make in group settings due to this technique. Second, because the teaching technique is (purposely) looser than the didactic method, it involves more degrees of freedom, and more adult choices, than does didactic instruction. Thus it may require more therapist training and sophistication than the didactic method. However, two studies demonstrate the ability of parents to learn naturalistic techniques (though in neither study were the children preschoolers; Laski et al., 1988; Charlop & Trasowech, 1991). McGee has described an effective procedure for teaching typical preschool peers to deliver incidental teaching (McGee, Almeida, Sulzer-Azaroff, & Feldman, 1992). Thus, although naturalistic teaching approaches may require more moment-to-moment decision making than didactic methods, it is clear that ordinary people, including children, can learn the techniques successfully.

Finally, unlike the available publications that describe the didactic behavioral approach, there are no treatment manuals in the public domain that lay out either the process of naturalistic teaching or the content (curriculum) of such teaching in such a way that others could independently learn from the materials. Without the ready availability of treatment manuals that allow others ready access to test this model, the approach currently remains in the hands of the few people who have developed the technique and are publishing work about it.

Whether naturalistic techniques are always preferred over didactic teaching is a matter of current debate. Whereas several literature reviews have maintained that naturalistic teaching is always advantageous (Koegel, 2000; Delprato, 2001), others have suggested that comparative data are insufficient to support this conclusion (Goldstein, 2000; Smith, 2001). Smith (2001) states that only didactic teaching approaches are able to develop a completely new behavior. However, this position does not seem tenable, given that naturalistic methods have demonstrated that children who lack all speech and imitative capacity have been shown to acquire speech in this method after failing to acquire speech through the didactic method (Koegel et al., 1987). Furthermore, the actual teaching techniques used in the two methods involve the same behavioral teaching repertoire: prompting, shaping, and chaining, as well as reliance on imitation, once it is learned, to shape new behaviors. As Goldstein (2000) points out, problems with generalization that occurred in the didactic teaching approach, described so carefully by Stokes and Baer (1977), stimulated behaviorists to incorporate the same teaching procedures used in didactic teaching in a novel way that maximized generalization, including embedding instruction in natural contexts and interspersing different types of trials, so as to apply discrete trial teaching in more natural contexts.

Schreibman's current work involving learner profiles is applicable to the question of choice of one approach over another (Ingersoll, Schreibman, & Stahmer, 2001). In this study, Schriebman and colleagues demonstrated that pretreatment profiles involving characteristics such as motivation for objects and tolerance for social interaction predicted progress in their naturalistic treatment approach. Furthermore, the children who did not fit the profile and did not make progress in naturalistic instruction nevertheless benefited greatly when moved to didactic instruction. The didactic and naturalistic teaching approaches should probably not be considered as either–or, but rather as both–and. Every treatment technique with demonstrated utility represents an additional tool in the toolbox of interventionists. Teaching children with autism is a complex process, and the more tools available to an individual therapist, the more choices the therapist has in constructing an intervention approach that is effective for an individual child.

In summary, there is considerable promise in the naturalistic teaching approaches, and their efficacy has been demonstrated in individual treatment and in group interventions, using single-subject designs. The work in this area may be held back somewhat by the many different variations of these techniques that exist, with resultant lack of standardization of both the process and the content of the teaching. Widespread public use will require widespread training availability and publication of treatment manuals that define both the content (curriculum) and the process (instructional techniques) of the approach. This area is in need of research that demonstrates broader applications of the method in order to test its full promise. Nevertheless, from the variety of publications already available, it is clear that naturalistic behavioral teaching, like didactic teaching, is a powerful and important treatment method with demonstrated efficacy for teaching many aspects of spoken language to children with autism.

DEVELOPMENTAL LANGUAGE APPROACHES

History of the Approach

As was stated at the beginning of this chapter, the behavioral approaches to teaching initially developed from the operant model of language development provided by Skinner (1957). However, that model of language development has been replaced by research findings in communication development over the past 30 years. As described earlier, children's development of spoken language is now understood to follow earlier use of nonverbal communicative behaviors involving eye contact, voice, and gesture that support several communicative functions, especially behavior regulation, social interaction, and joint attention. Joint-attention behaviors and use of intentional communicative gestures have been found to predict development of spoken language use and understanding in typical development. Imitation of speech appears to be a necessary skill, but not sufficient, for development of typical spoken language. Detailed studies of early language learning in typically developing infants and toddlers in several different languages described the timing and pattern of developments in all these areas, and relations to cognitive accomplishments as well, across the toddler and preschool period (Bates, Bretherton, Snyder, Shore, & Volterra, 1980).

This social pragmatics revolution in understanding development of spoken language has parallels in autism research and treatment theory. The finding that nonverbal communication was a better predictor than was early speech for predicting later verbal ability (Mundy et al., 1990) led to the third main paradigm for language intervention discussed here: a model built directly from literature on normal language development, referred to here as the *developmental pragmatics approach.* The current understanding of the communicative deficits of children with autism from the developmental pragmatics viewpoint has been most clearly articulated by Amy Wetherby and Barry Prizant in a substantial body of theoretical writings over the past 20 years.

The developmental pragmatics approach to understanding the communication difficulties in autism represents the merging of the scientific study of normal language development with the most current findings concerning the social-communicative impairments seen in autism. Excellent recent descriptions of this line of thinking have been provided by Wetherby, Prizant, and Schuler (2000) and Peter Mundy (Mundy & Crowson, 1997; Mundy & Markus, 1997). This line of theorizing focuses on early autism-specific deficits in sharing affect and in social orienting as the initial social-communicative deviations from the typical trajectory, deficits that interfere with the development of intersubjectivity as demonstrated by the presence of joint-attention behavior, intentional communication, and social referencing in the 9–12 month period. Delays in symbolic development in the second year of life further impede the process of acquiring a symbolic communication system. The patterns of communication that develop in preschoolers with autism—both the nonverbal child's limited repertoire of direct actions on other people's bodies and the young verbal child's extensive use of immediate and delayed echolalia as a starting point for deconstructing speech—are understood as direct reflections of the barriers caused by lack of intersubjective understanding of others that is a core feature of autism.

Characteristics of the Approach

The most elaborated description of this kind of treatment has been provided by Prizant, Wetherby, and Rydell (2000) as the SCERTS model of intervention, with its focus on social-communication, emotional regulation, and transactional support as both the major components of the intervention and the treatment priorities. Principles of this approach include the following:

1. The focus is on enhancing spontaneous social communication within a flexible structure and varied and motivating activities.
2. Emphasis is placed on building multimodal communicative repertoires (including alternative communication systems) to give children a range of strategies for expressing intention.
3. Interactions are characterized by shared control, turn taking, and reciprocity.
4. Context involves meaningful activities or events chosen for their interest and motivation.
5. Child behavior, including unconventional behavior, is interpreted within the communicative framework.
6. A variety of social groupings and interactions are used.
7. Treatment goals and progress assessment are derived from the overall developmental profile of the individual child.
8. Rather than simplifying interactions to make them more understandable to the child, scaffolds and supports are added to provide meaning.
9. Conventional means of controlling others are provided to preclude behavioral problems.
10. Sharing affect is central to the learning process.

Thus this approach emphasizes the development of the full range of interpersonal communicative behaviors, including eye contact, shared affect, intentional vocalization, and manual gestures, as well as speech, to achieve reciprocal communicative exchanges regarding interactions involving objects and social games. Functional communication, rather than speech, is the primary goal. The adult seeds the environment with desired objects and activities that lend themselves to dyadic interactions, including objects that require adult assistance to reach or operate and objects that allow for the construction of joint activity routines. These activities provide multiple communicative opportunities and presses for the child. The adult responds to child behaviors that initiate or continue interactions, with the desired activity reinforcing the child's communicative behavior. The affective quality of the exchanges, the amount of child control over the interaction, and the development of nonverbal gestures prior to speech are crucial aspects of the approach.

This approach bears many resemblances to the behavioral naturalistic teaching methods described earlier, as observed 20 years ago by Warren and Kaiser (1988) and recently reviewed by Prizant and Wetherby (1998), thus providing the potential for an unusual convergence between developmentalists and behaviorists. Kaiser and her colleagues continue to work in this kind of merged developmental–behavioral approach and have published two studies concerning the efficacy of their model, enhanced milieu teaching, for children with autism. Both studies used a single-subject design to test the effectiveness of this approach in increasing language use and social communication for 6 children in a parent-training model (Kaiser, Hancock, & Nietfeld, 2000) and for 4 children in a therapist-delivered model (Hancock & Kaiser, 2002). Developmental pragmatics work differs in several ways from the naturalistic teaching approaches described previously. First, the developmental approaches place more emphasis on developing nonverbal communicative behaviors prior to verbal communication than do the behavioral approaches, because the developmentalists observe continuity between nonverbal and verbal communications both in typical development and in autism. Second, the developmental approach easily includes alternative and augmentative symbol systems as alternatives to speech for both expressive and receptive language development, because symbolic communication is the goal. Third, the goals of therapy are broader and more general than in the naturalistic behavioral approaches, including affect sharing and play development. Fourth, the treatment approach, in terms of the therapist's behavior, is more loosely defined and would likely include a wider range of behaviors and interventions than the naturalistic behavioral approaches. In the developmental approach, symbolic communication in any form is the goal, with the assumption that children who are able to learn to speak will do so with appropriate treatment and that supporting nonverbal communication will always assist development of verbal communication. This approach to language development reflects the theory taught in the majority of university programs today. Communication scientists and practitioners, early educators, and special educators are trained in the pragmatics approach to communication development, and this is generally the disciplinary viewpoint of education and speech and language professionals who are new to autism. Although this knowledge is crucial for treating children with autism, professionals new to autism also need exposure to the language-teaching methods from the behavioral literatures, as reviewed in this chapter.

The line being drawn here between developmental and behavioral approaches regarding alternative/augmentative supports is not meant to be rigid, and there are points of crossover. Bondy and Frost's (1994) Picture

Exchange Communication System (PECS) is a well-known behavioral approach that focuses quite heavily on augmentative/alternative communication supports. The PECS approach uses careful shaping techniques to teach children to hand picture icons to adults to initiate requests. Adults verbalize the child's request using simple, repetitive language, and a significant subgroup of children later begins to speak, apparently through imitating the adult responses. The approach known as verbal behavior (Sundberg & Michael, 2001), solidly based on Skinnerian theory of language acquisition (Skinner, 1957), focuses on the functionality of communication. It shapes children's use of natural gestures, conventional gestures, and manual signs in functional, naturalistic, and reciprocal communicative exchanges for preverbal children, later shaping a verbal repertoire to accompany the nonverbal communicative behaviors. Both of these behavioral approaches also emphasize the function of communication for children in terms of requesting and supports for spontaneity of child communication. However, both approaches are solidly behavioral rather than developmental, and this difference permeates their approaches to teaching speech, the theoretical concepts underlying them, therapist behavior in the treatment, and the goals and objectives that are developed for the treatment.

Studies Supporting the Approach

Unlike the bodies of work already reviewed, empirical studies of the efficacy of interventions based on the developmental pragmatics approach are few in number and involve group studies rather than single-subject designs. This is likely because the single-subject model focuses on behavioral changes seen during brief periods of time, whereas the developmental pragmatics approach is more focused on multiple developmental changes that would involve longer periods of time. Kaiser and colleagues' work (Hancock & Kaiser, 2002; Kaiser et al., 2000) is an empirically based developmental model. Rogers and colleagues published several studies describing the Denver model and its use of one version of the developmental pragmatics approach to treatment, known as the INREAL approach (Weiss, 1981), developed at the University of Colorado in the 1970s and 1980s. These studies involved relatively large groups of 30 or more preschoolers with autism in a pre–post design over a 6-month period. Pre–post standardized measures revealed a doubling of developmental rates and significant gains for a large group of children in expressive and receptive language beyond that which would have been expected from the children's initial developmental rates, as well as increases in a variety of positive social interactions in dyadic exchanges with parents. Furthermore, of the completely nonverbal children, 50% acquired useful, multiword utterances, with the end result that 75% of children with autism had useful multiword speech by age 5. These results were independently replicated in four different settings (Rogers, Herbison, Lewis, Pantone, & Reis, 1986; Rogers & Lewis, 1989; Rogers & DiLalla, 1991; Rogers, Lewis, & Reis, 1987). However, lack of comparison or control groups and lack of blind raters limit conclusions that can be drawn. Furthermore, the Denver model has since added behavioral components to the language intervention in order to improve success rate further for developing speech in completely nonverbal children (Rogers et al., in press).

Mahoney and Perales (2003, 2005) described a developmental intervention in a study that demonstrates the relationships between maternal sensitive and responsive interventions and child language development in both typically and atypically developing toddlers. Training mothers to use a sensitive, responsive interaction style with their toddlers with autism in one clinical session per week resulted in significant gains in child language development across a year of treatment. Furthermore, the amount of gain was directly linked to the level of maternal sensitivity measured in the mother's communicative behavior, as reported in a pre–post study. A similar parent-training study using the developmental pragmatics approach was recently reported by Chandler, Christie, Newson, and Prevezer (2002). Parents of 10 toddlers with autism received weekly home visits, individualized home programs for their children, and a variety of teaching supports (booklets, a toy lending library, music therapy sessions). In 18 months, all the children were using communicative gestures and expressive speech according to parental report, though there was no control group and no independent assessment of the children. Greenspan and Weider (1997) described an intervention model that embraced the developmental pragmatics view and its strong affective base. A report of clinical outcomes of 200 children receiving this model described development of affectively rich, communicative behavior. A final model from the developmental pragmatics tradition is the Hanen Early Childhood Educators Program. The Hanen approach is well known as a developmental language intervention method taught to parents and therapists. However, the only empirical study that was found had significant design problems and reported no positive effects of the method as applied by preschool teachers in generic preschool classrooms (Coulter & Gallagher, 2001).

Strengths and Weaknesses of the Approach

Even with the sparseness of supportive data, the developmental approach is a very popular treatment model with a strong basis in the science of communication development, which is its clear strength. A second strength of the model is similar to the naturalistic approaches in that the interactional exchanges are built on more typical models of communication, and thus teach communication in terms of its natural functions and social interactions, and are readily delivered in natural environments and by a variety of adults. However, the lack of controlled studies of the approach is a major weakness at this time. Furthermore, the treatment model is built from models of language development in typically developing toddlers and young children (though it accommodates to the different communicative trajectory that autism often creates in early childhood). Whether moving children with autism through a typical developmental sequence is the best approach is an open question. We have very little information concerning developmental patterns of language in autism. The only detailed language study done (Tager-Flusberg et al., 1990) compared 6 children with autism with those with Down syndrome, a group that also has difficulties developing expressive speech. It may be that the typical sequence of skills is the best sequence for teaching spoken language to children with autism, but it is not necessarily so. Another problem, similar to the naturalistic approaches, is the lack of treatment manuals in the public domain that lay out the process of intervention and the content or sequence of skills to be taught. The developmental pragmatics approach contains even more therapeutic techniques and approaches than the naturalistic model because of the many communicative behaviors that are treatment targets, and thus it represents an even more complex therapy to deliver. Furthermore, it requires a considerable body of knowledge on the part of the therapist. Nevertheless, parents and classroom staff members, including paraprofessionals, have been taught to carry out the method with high levels of treatment fidelity (Mahoney & Perales, 2003, 2005; Rogers et al., 1987) and thus the approach can be taught to a wide range of adults.

Finally, the extensive use of augmentative or alternative supports for communication has not been documented to assist acquisition of spoken language. Bondy and Frost's (1994) data suggesting that children using PECS spontaneously acquired some speech have been confirmed by a recent replication by Charlop-Christy, Carpenter, Le, LeBlanc, and Kellet (2002). However, there is no way to evaluate whether speech development was actually enhanced by the PECS model in comparison with other models. The only experiment in the literature that examined that question is the elegant experimental design by Yoder and Layton (1988), who demonstrated no advantage to speech acquisition for children with autism when a visual system was included—in this case, sign language. Given the widespread use of PECS and other visual systems in programs for young children with autism, this is a very important empirical question and needs scientific attention. While use of visual systems may not inhibit the learning of speech, they may not enhance the learning of speech, either, and enhancement of use of spoken language has to be a main goal of early intervention for autism, given its role in better outcomes.

The importance of the pragmatics of communication is unmistakable, and all the approaches described here have focused on teaching children with autism to use spoken language to accomplish a variety of interpersonal functions. What is not clear is whether nonverbal communication needs to be a precursor to other kinds of language teaching for nonverbal children with autism. It may be that simultaneous interventions in pragmatics of nonverbal communication, understanding of spoken language, and development and shaping of spoken language can be carried out and may result in more rapid acquisition of useful communicative speech. A summary of the main characteristics of these three approaches is provided in Table 6.1.

CURRENT ISSUES

Several issues that are currently points of conflict in the field appear to have considerable influence on decisions concerning language treatment for young children with autism. Some of these are as follows:

1. *Capacity for spoken language.* One continuing description of autism appears to need drastic revision, and that is the statement that 50% of persons with autism will not acquire useful speech. The lessons from the published studies across many designs and many approaches suggest that a more accurate statement is that 75–90% of young children with autism will acquire functional spoken language if they receive appropriate treatment during the preschool years (Smith et al., 2000; McGee et al., 1999). In contrast, no study of any alternative language system reveals improved general outcomes or even mastery of an alternative system at a more than rudimentary level. Because functional spoken language predicts better outcomes for preschoolers with autism, and because the large majority of young children with autism apparently can master speech, should teaching children to understand and use speech be a main priority of every early-intervention program for children with autism?

2. *Is there a preferred choice of treatments?* As reviewed by Goldstein (2000), the data do not support the conclusion that there is one best approach for *all* children, to teach *all* skills. There is a body of work demonstrating efficacy of both didactic and naturalistic behavioral models, with a few comparative studies. There is no comparable set of studies from the developmental pragmatics model. The published data from several of the group studies, and also from some single-subject designs, suggest that child characteristics interact with treatment outcomes. Those children with some speech appear to progress more rapidly than those without, and those with certain profile characteristics may respond better to one type of treatment

TABLE 6.1. Characteristics of Three Main Approaches for Language Interventions for Young Children with Autism

Characteristics	Didactic behavioral approach	Naturalistic behavioral approaches	Developmental language approaches
Some well-known approaches that use the technique	Lovaas's approach; discrete trial teaching (DTT)	Incidental teaching; pivotal response training (PRT); milieu teaching	Prizant and Wetherby's SCERTS model; Denver model; Greenspan and Wieder's DIR model
Underlying theory	Skinner's operant learning model	Skinner's operant learning model	Current pragmatics-based language development theory
Setting	Specific teaching location. Limited stimuli available. Child and adult generally sitting and facing each other.	Natural or naturalistic settings with attractive materials to draw children's interest and motivate communication.	Natural or naturalistic settings involving meaningful activities or events chosen to elicit children's interest and motivate communication.
Style of teaching	Adult directed. Massed trials of preselected tasks with set rules for determining "mastery."	Adult–child interactions are pragmatically functional. Trials are dispersed. Mastery trials interspersed with new skills. Child interest and engagement is a main target for adult.	Interactions involve shared control, turn taking, and reciprocity. Interactions are affectively rich and positive in nature. Shared affect is central to the teaching process. Nonverbal conventional communication is developed prior to or alongside of speech.
What initiates the teaching interaction	Adult directs and the child responds as directed. Child follows adult lead.	Adult creates a situation in which the child indicates desire for an object or activity. Adult then follows the child's lead with a prompt for a more mature communication.	Adult creates a situation in which the child indicates desire for an object or activity. Adult assures that the child's communication is successful by delivering desired object. Adult may prompt or model an additional communication before allowing access to desired activity.

(continued)

TABLE 6.1. (*continued*)

Characteristics	Didactic behavioral approach	Naturalistic behavioral approaches	Developmental language approaches
Teaching techniques	Precise teaching with set ABC. Begins with vocal imitation and prompts, shapes, and chains desired speech behaviors in response to specific stimulus and language model.	Prompt, shape, and chaining procedures to shape or elaborate speech. Many different behaviors may be reinforced. Focus on form and content of language in typical communicative contexts.	A wide range of communicative behaviors, both verbal and nonverbal, and a wide range of pragmatic functions are targeted. Child behavior is interpreted within the communicative framework.
Therapeutic goal	Production of appropriate speech in response to multiple types of stimuli	Initiation of speech for communicative purposes	Effective communication for varied pragmatic functions
Choice and use of reinforcers	Extrinsic to the teaching task; chosen based on reinforcer strength; targeted behavior is reinforced by adult delivery of reinforcer.	Intrinsic to the teaching task; chosen based on child motivation for the activity/objects; child efforts and attempts, as well as mastered target behaviors, are reinforced with access to desired objects.	Intrinsic to the teaching task; chosen based on child motivation for the activity/objects; child efforts and attempts, as well as mastered target behaviors, are reinforced with access to desired objects.
Research base	Substantial base in single subjects and some group designs.	Substantial single-subject research base; some group designs.	Limited number of studies thus far; both single-subject and group designs.
Specificity of the targeted behavior	Extremely specific. There is one targeted behavior per trial.	Several different behaviors may be reinforced.	Wide range of nonverbal and verbal productions may be rewarded.
Knowledge needed to deliver the treatment	Precise nature of the teaching allows for a wide range of people to be trained but requires ongoing direction from master behavior therapist.	Requires greater therapist judgment than didactic teaching but can be learned by many different deliverers.	Because of the multiple targets for communication, requires considerable therapist decision making and judgment; typically delivered by developmentally trained therapists who train parents.

TABLE 6.1. (*continued*)

Characteristics	Didactic behavioral approach	Naturalistic behavioral approaches	Developmental language approaches
Strengths of the approach	Efficacious approach. Teaching approach generalizes to other teaching targets easily. The precision of the instruction makes it deliverable by a wide range of people. Teaching manuals and curricula are published. Drill and practice methods lead to rapid mastery of new skills and development of speed and fluency in responding.	Efficacious approach. Use of naturalistic teaching settings and interactional styles lead to maintenance and generalization of learned behaviors across natural settings. Use of highly motivating materials and activities promotes child positive behaviors; reduces unwanted behaviors. Children initiate communication at high frequencies. Highlights the pragmatic functions of language and thus is in line with current communication science.	Uses pragmatically typical interaction exchanges. Fits easily into natural routines and settings. Use of highly motivating materials and activities should promote child positive behaviors; reduces unwanted behaviors. Highlights the pragmatic functions of language and thus is in line with current communication science.
Weaknesses of the approach	Artificial learning environment and interactional style limit generalization without additional teaching to transfer skills. Does not foster communicative initiative. Not based in current science of communicative development. Is not, by itself, a comprehensive language intervention approach.	More degrees of freedom in the approach make for a more difficult therapy to learn. No systematic treatment manuals available to the public. No published curriculum. Technique is not appropriate for teaching skills for which there is no intrinsic reinforcement.	Lacks a large body of effectiveness data. Model is based on normal development; may or may not be most effective route for autism. Lacks published treatment manuals and curricula. Most complex therapy to deliver because of the multiple communicative behaviors and functions that are targeted.

than another at a particular point in time. Additionally, specific skills may show different outcomes depending on treatment. For instance, increase in spontaneous communications will probably occur more rapidly when the teaching trial follows the child's initial act rather than when it precedes it. In that case, the naturalistic approach may be the more powerful intervention. On the other hand, if one is trying to increase consistency of the use of the plural form of nouns, massed trials using a variety of material sets will likely result in faster increases initially than spaced, naturalistic teaching. As stated earlier, several authorities in the field are calling for blended approaches that offer the benefits of both didactic and naturalistic approaches, and McDonnell (1996) has demonstrated advantages of the combined approach over both of the single approaches.

For children who do not speak, naturalistic behavioral approaches may be the most powerful for teaching functional communication and shaping speech with spontaneity, generalization, and motivation to communicate. The few comparative studies that exist support this conclusion (see Delprato, 2001, for a review). In addition, many national leaders in communication and learning sciences, including those initially trained in the didactic models, have moved to naturalistic models. However, as Ingersoll et al. (2001) have discussed, the didactic teaching method may be a more powerful initial teaching approach for some very avoidant children who initially lack much motivation for objects. Furthermore, didactic approaches may be usefully combined with naturalistic behavioral approaches for some specific reasons, such as teaching a particularly difficult syntactic form such as pronouns or other deictic constructions.

It is a truism that no single approach can best meet the needs of all children with autism and that individualization of approach to maximize progress will be necessary to attain the best outcome for an individual child. This means that interventionists need to monitor progress frequently and carefully and change intervention strategies when progress on specific objectives is poor. This also means that interventionists need to master several different intervention approaches, so that they are able to individualize for specific children, drawing from the approaches that have some empirical support. Speech and language pathologists are the communication experts on most children's teams, but they may lack a breadth of expertise in the multiple, empirically supported approaches described here. Clinicians without special autism training need to seek out the approaches that have empirical support and learn them, rather than relying on general disciplinary therapeutic practices. This would be easier to do if treatment manuals and curricula were more readily available.

3. *Should all nonverbal children with autism immediately have alternative communication systems taught to them?* Although studies have demonstrated that some children will develop speech while using alternative

systems (Charlop-Christy et al., 2002), there is currently no empirical evidence that the use of alternative systems will *accelerate* the development of spoken language compared with the published approaches that focus completely on developing spoken language. The few studies that demonstrate development of speech after visual systems show much longer timelines for speech development than those intervention studies that teach speech directly to nonverbal children. Additionally, time spent on augmentative training is time not spent on learning to use and understand speech, and the alternative systems take considerable time to teach. Our knowledge is limited by the lack of studies targeting this question; only one true comparative study (Yoder & Layton, 1988) exists. We need empirical research that specifically examines the usefulness of alternative/augmentative systems in accelerating speech acquisition for children with autism. The existing research suggests that augmentative systems have a crucial role as a primary communication system for some children with autism, but they have not yet been demonstrated to be a necessary or even an important step in developing useful, communicative speech.

4. *Parent training.* Parent training is considered a necessary practice for intervention with young children with autism (National Research Council, 2001). Several studies have demonstrated that parents can learn all the major interventions described herein: didactic and naturalistic behavioral language therapy techniques and developmental pragmatic approaches. Parents can learn these techniques at high levels of fidelity, can deliver them at home, and can improve their children's language abilities, even when parental interventions are the main interventions occurring. Furthermore, there is a plethora of evidence that certain parental styles encourage language and communication development in children with and without diagnoses, including those with autism (Siller & Sigman, 2002). These styles, considered to represent a "sensitive and responsive" interaction style, resemble the naturalistic and developmental pragmatics approaches in that they follow children's leads, are sensitive to children's goals, use intrinsic reinforcers that are inherent to the situation, and use modeling and expansion. Parents trained in didactic teaching have also facilitated language gains in their children (Howlin & Rutter, 1989) However, the studies also make clear that parents have to receive ongoing individual training and frequent, regular support if child progress is to occur and to continue. Parent-training groups are efficient and economical, but ongoing individual coaching sessions must be part of the package. Thus language treatment for children with autism should include enough parent training and support so that parents are delivering the method in the child's home environment. Interventions that embed instruction in natural family routines and child-care practices may be especially effective.

5. *Language subgroups in autism.* The variety of language patterns

seen in toddlers and preschoolers with autism who first come to treatment seems to fall into several clinical clusters. The first involves children who have some speech, however echolalic and unusual it seems. These children appear to have no difficulty with phonology or auditory memory. They can imitate speech (though they may not be able to imitate body movements or actions on objects), and there may be some pragmatic functions to their echolalic speech (Rydell & Mirenda, 1994), but they seem unable to deconstruct the language they hear and to infer the underlying meanings. A hypothesis is that, for this subgroup, the primary language problem is at the level of pragmatics. One of the core difficulties for those with autism is understanding others' mental states: the intersubjectivity problem. "The child's major task in learning language is to infer the relationships between language content, form, and use" (Warren & Kaiser, 1988, p. 91). Young children with autism lack the pragmatic and intersubjective tools needed to deconstruct others' language and infer the relationships among language form, content and use that is the basic language learning challenge for toddlers.

Treatment for this group requires that the meanings underlying word use have to become very simple and clear for them. Clinical experience has taught us that, as tempting as it is to use children's auditory memory ability to prompt them to use correct phrase speech, going this route seems to reinforce echolalia. A better language treatment approach is to simplify the language environment for these children and make the relationships between forms, functions, and meanings very transparent by using and stimulating single-word utterances or very short phrases in functional communicative situations, so that these children can map out semantics and functions of single words. As they spontaneously begin to use single words appropriately for various functions, then the model increases to two-word and their longer utterances. For these children, many of the studies reviewed here describe approaches that expand their vocabularies, develop syntax, teach pragmatic use of language, and target spontaneity and initiative. The focus on pragmatics is crucial for this group, which probably has the potential for the very best outcomes (see Koegel, Camarata, et al., 1998; Williams, Donley, & Keller, 2000, for examples of teaching procedures that teach the pragmatic intent behind complex language structures). The naturalistic approaches seem a particularly good choice for these children because of better generalization and initiative that accompanies this approach to teaching.

The remaining children, those without speech or imitative vocalizations, are often seen as a homogeneous group—the nonverbal group—and the term *oral dyspraxia* is currently being used to characterize them. These children do not imitate adult behavior, whether movements or sounds. Research in our lab has demonstrated strong relationships between imitation of motor movements, facial movements, and simple sounds in preverbal toddlers with autism (Rogers, Hepburn, & Stackhouse, 2003). Many studies have demonstrated success at teaching this group to imitate actions and movements using a variety of methods (Kamps, Walker, Locke, Delquadri, & Hall, 1990; Bernard-Opitz, Sriram, & Sapuan, 1999; Smith et al., 2000; Garfinkle & Schwartz, 2002; Lovaas et al., 1966; Lovaas, Freitas, Nelson, & Whalen, 1967; Metz, 1965), after which a subgroup of them proceed rapidly to imitation of facial movements and speech sounds. Once they are imitating speech sounds, they are on the road to learning spoken language. There are also alternative approaches to developing speech that do not rely on motor imitation but instead shape vocalizations into imitative responses (Ross & Greer, 2003; McGee et al., 1999; Koegel et al., 1987), and children have developed speech using these routes as well.

For the subgroup of initially nonverbal children who learn through treatment to imitate speech, the underlying mechanisms preventing language development may involve both (1) the intersubjective deficit described either, and (2) a second general deficit involving intentional imitation of motor movements, including oral movements and vocal imitation. Although the underlying neurocognitive mechanisms for general imitation are not yet known, brain-imaging studies are converging to identify activation in the parietal and inferior frontal lobes, suggested to indicate the presence of "mirror neurons" that fire both when an individual movement is seen and when it is made, thus providing a neural representation of that movement to be acted on (for a review, see Rizzolatti, Fadiga, Fogassi, & Gallese, 2003). This "resonance mechanism" may be at the source of imitation of motor movements. Current mirror neuron research suggests that certain of these neurons are specific for facial movements (see Bekkering, 2002). We conjecture that further work in humans may reveal mirror neurons that resonate specifically to the sound and sight of movements associated with speech. Although the concept of a generalized "dyspraxia" resulting in generalized motor planning and execution problems of all sorts is often applied to these children, initial findings from our lab suggest that this group's difficulty appears to be specifically in making intentional, imitative body movements (Rogers et al., 2003). This group can learn to imitate body movements well through intensive and rigorous training. To develop meaningful speech, these children need to be taught to imitate speech, whether through didactic teaching approaches or through prompting and shaping techniques inside naturalistic approaches. Extrapolating from existing intervention studies, one could hypothesize that the imitation deficit is more remediable than the intersubjective deficit. (In fact, the two may be related [Rogers et al., 2003; Rogers & Pennington, 1991], and mirror neurons may underlie this relationship [Williams, Whiten, Suddendorf, & Perrett, 2001]). With appropriate treatment, these children can learn to imitate motor and vocal behavior and can learn functional spoken language. The two main foci of their language intervention, then, are (1) imitation and (2) the pragmatics of social interactions and shared meanings of language.

However, there is a third subgroup, and these are the initially nonverbal children who do not progress into vocal imitation even after they have learned to understand some words and phrases, who have learned to imitate body movements, including novel acts (and thus have learned the underlying "do as I do" rule that defines imitation), and who may have developed impressive sight-word vocabularies and other nonverbal cognitive skills through intensive treatment. They have often learned to produce an intentional vocalization, but they cannot learn to imitate speech phonemes. For this group, a true underlying speech dyspraxia may prevent them from gaining intentional control of the speech–motor mechanisms for phoneme production.

These children desperately need alternative communication systems to develop awareness of symbolic communication. Some of them will develop speech as they use signs, PECS, and other visual systems, according to existing research. Mastery of spoken language for this group may depend on adding to their general treatment a specific intervention that can develop intentional control of the speech–motor mechanisms. One approach that may hold promise for this group involves the PROMPT approach (Square-Storer & Hayden, 1989), a technique that provides manual facilitation of the speech–motor mechanisms during episodes of naturalistic communication therapy. An initial pilot study of the PROMPT approach has demonstrated considerable promise for rapid development of verbal imitation and spontaneous speech in nonverbal preschoolers with autism (Rogers et al., in press). Thus some or many children in this subgroup may also have the potential for spoken language given appropriate treatment for dyspraxia of speech. Interestingly, in Lovaas's first study on teaching language, he refers to using motor prompts to shape oral–facial movements (Lovaas et al., 1966).

There is probably a fourth subgroup: those preschoolers who do not have the necessary cognitive maturity to support language development (those with nonverbal performance skills well below the 12 month level). This is likely a small number of children, and this group will need to be taught gestural and simple alternative communication systems initially.

6. *The gap is immense between the language treatments most young children with autism receive and what connotes the state of the science in language intervention for children with autism.* Speech–language pathologists represent the professional group with the greatest knowledge of language development. However, most young children with autism have, at best, only a few hours of speech–language therapy per week and thus may not be

receiving a rigorous enough intervention to make the most rapid gains possible. Furthermore, training in speech–language pathology alone may not equip a therapist with the special knowledge needed to optimally serve children with autism.

Many young children in the United States currently receive didactic behavioral teaching, both because of the empirical reports of outcomes from Lovaas's method and because of the readiness of treatment manuals and relative ease of delivery. However, the well-documented difficulties of this approach in developing initiative, spontaneity, generativity, a wide range of communicative functions, and generalization to natural settings and interactions too often result in children whose speech consists primarily of echoic or rotely trained phrases. Smith (2001) reminds users of the didactic intervention approaches to incorporate the use of naturalistic approaches and generalization techniques early rather than late in the speech acquisition process in order to achieve spontaneous, functional communicative speech.

The naturalistic behavioral approaches provide both a solid empirical base and bridges to current communication science, but the area is hampered by multiple similar approaches, and the most rigorous approaches have not been made easily available to the public. The plethora of models and terminology in various articles (Warren & Kaiser, 1988), combined with the lack of treatment manuals that clearly lay out either the process or the content of the treatment, make it hard to access by those outside of the circles in which it is taught. It would be of great benefit to the field for the leaders of the naturalistic approaches to foster a convergence, similar to the way that those working in the area of positive behavior supports have converged on terminology, process, and content, yielding treatment manuals, journals, and accessibility (Carr et al., 2002). It would be of even greater benefit if this convergence could create a true wedding of learning science and communication science, with professionals trained in current communication science, the science of human learning, and the use of single-subject designs to examine treatment efficacy.

It is clear that, whatever approach is used, effective language teaching involves ongoing individual interactions with a child using carefully planned and sequenced strategies and clear reinforcement practices in natural environments. Such interventions are being delivered effectively in many settings: home, inclusive and specialized preschool group programs, therapy sessions. Is there a best setting? We know that teaching in natural settings fosters maintenance and generalization in those settings. Carrying out this kind of successful teaching in group classroom situations is nicely described by Peck, Killen, and Baumgart (1989) and McBride and Schwartz (2003). Whether or not initial teaching occurs in those settings, skills have to be practiced and reinforced in those settings if they are ever to become part of the child's permanent repertoire. The behavioral model of collecting ongoing data and using it for decision making is crucial here. The bottom line is skill development and skill generalization. Whatever decisions are made regarding the style of language training, if children are not progressing and learned skills are not being used spontaneously in natural environments, the treatment is not succeeding, and changes need to be made. The intervention research is clear about this: Given appropriate treatment, children with autism progress. Lack of progress requires revision of the treatment.

7. *Research needs*. Given all that has been written about language intervention in autism, there are a relatively small number of empirical studies that describe well-controlled research involving young children with autism, and most of these are single-subject designs examining one specific language skill. We continue to need these studies to describe successful methods for teaching individual skills that have not yet been examined. Single-subject designs that document initial treatment failures and the alterations that were made to finally yield success provide strong models for clinicians.

The few comparative studies that exist have been quite helpful, but there are too few. There are big decisions to be made at the start of treatment. Will it help the child to use augmentative visual systems? Should we begin with a didactic or a naturalistic approach? Do we begin with one-to-one treatment sessions exclusively, or can excellent progress be accomplished by adding group treatment? If so, how? Parents and practitioners need answers to these questions from comparative group studies in which the children's initial communication and imitation abilities are spelled out in detail and in which language progress is measured quite frequently. Measures that examine pragmatics, semantics, and syntax independently will provide more information than standardized summary scores of receptive and expressive language.

Measurement systems for assessing language progress in the published research have been criticized as being too restricted. Prizant and colleagues have made important recommendations in this regard:

"In measuring efficacy of intervention, researchers need to go beyond traditional measures of communicative and language skills such as improvement on standardized tests and include broader characteristics, such as degree of success in communicative exchange, related dimensions of emotional expression and regulation, sociocommunicative motivation, social competence, peer relationships, and the child's competence in natural environments" (Prizant et al., 2000, p. 218).

Finally, we need to understand more about the nature of language development in autism. Replication and extension of the work begun by Tager-Flusberg and colleagues in 1990 are needed to examine autism-specific differences in timing, sequencing, and learning strategies underlying specific aspects of language development so that we can construct intervention models that maximize the breadth, depth, and rate of language learning in children with autism.

ACKNOWLEDGMENTS

Work on this chapter was partially supported by Grant Nos. NICHD U19 HD35468, NIDCD R21 DC05574, NIMH R21 067363, and MHR01 068398. Debra Galik provided invaluable assistance.

REFERENCES

Bates, E. (1976). *Language and context: The acquisition of pragmatics*. New York: Academic Press.

Bates, E., Bretherton, I., Snyder, L., Shore, C., & Volterra, V. (1980). Vocal and gestural symbols at 13 months. *Merrill–Palmer Quarterly, 26*, 407–423.

Bekkering, H. (2002). Common mechanisms in the observation and execution of finger and mouth movements. In A. N. Meltzoff & W. Prinz (Eds.), *The imitative mind: Development, evolution, and brain bases* (pp. 163–182). Cambridge, UK: Cambridge University Press.

Bernard-Opitz, V., Sriram, N., & Sapuan, S. (1999). Enhancing vocal imitations in children with autism using the IBM Speech Viewer. *Autism, 3*, 131–147.

Bondy, A. S., & Frost, L. A. (1994). The Picture Exchange Communication System. *Focus on Autistic Behavior, 9*, 1–19.

Carr, E. G., Dunlap, G., Horner, R. H., Koegel, R. L., Turnbull, A. P., Sailor, W., et al. (2002). Positive behavior support: Evolution of an applied science. *Journal of Positive Behavior Interventions, 4*, 4–16.

Carr, E. G., & Kologinsky, E. (1983). Acquisition of sign language by autistic children: II. Spontaneity and generalization effects. *Journal of Applied Behavior Analysis, 16*, 297–314.

Carter, C. M. (2001). Using choice with game play to increase language skills and interactive behaviors in children with autism. *Journal of Positive Behavior Interventions, 3*, 131–151.

Chandler, S., Christie, P., Newson, E., & Prevezer, W. (2002). Developing a diagnostic and intervention package for 2- to 3-year-olds with autism: Outcomes of the frameworks for communication approach. *Autism, 6*, 47–69.

Charlop, M. H., Schreibman, L., & Thiebodeau, M. G. (1985). Increasing spontaneous verbal responding in autistic children using a time delay procedure. *Journal of Applied Behavior Analysis, 18*, 155–166.

Charlop, M. H., & Trasowech, J. E. (1991). Increasing autistic children's daily spontaneous speech. *Journal of Applied Behavior Analysis, 24*, 747–761.

Charlop-Christy, M. H., Carpenter, M., Le, L., LeBlanc, L. A., & Kellet, K. (2002). Using the picture exchange communication system (PECS) with children with autism: Assessment of PECS acquisition, speech, social-communicative behavior, and problem behavior. *Journal of Applied Behavior Analysis, 35,* 213–231.

Chomsky, N. (1975). *Reflections on language.* New York: Pantheon.

Cipani, E., & Spooner, F. (1994). *Curricular and instructional approaches for persons with severe disabilities.* Boston: Allyn & Bacon.

Coulter, L., & Gallagher, C. (2001). Evaluation of the Hanen Early Childhood Educators Programme. *International Journal of Language and Communication Disorders, 36,* 264–269.

Delprato, D. J. (2001). Comparisons of discrete-trial and normalized behavioral language intervention for young children with autism. *Journal of Autism and Developmental Disorders, 31,* 315–325.

Dunlap, G. (1984). The influence of task variation and maintenance tasks on the learning and affect of autistic children. *Journal of Experimental Child Psychology, 37,* 41–64.

Eikeseth, S., Smith, T., Jahr, E., & Eldevik, S. (2002). Intensive behavioral treatment at school for 4- to 7-year-old children with autism: A 1-year comparison controlled study. *Behavior Modification, 26,* 49–68.

Garfinkle, A. N., & Schwartz, I. S. (2002). Peer imitation: Increasing social interactions in children with autism and other developmental disabilities in inclusive preschool classrooms. *Topics in Early Childhood Special Education, 22,* 26–38.

Goldstein, H. (2000). Communication intervention for children with autism: A review of treatment efficacy. *Journal of Autism and Developmental Disorders, 32,* 373–396.

Greenspan, S. I., & Wieder, S. (1997). Developmental patterns and outcomes in infants and children with disorders in relating and communicating: A chart review of 200 cases of children with autism spectrum diagnoses. *Journal of Developmental and Learning Disorders, 1,* 87–141.

Hancock, T. B., & Kaiser, A. P. (2002). The effects of trainer-implemented enhanced milieu teaching on the social communication of children with autism. *Topics in Early Childhood Special Education, 22,* 29–54.

Harris, S. L., Wolchik, S. A., & Milch, R. E. (1983). Changes in the speech of autistic children and their parents. *Child and Family Behavior Therapy, 4,* 151–173.

Harris, S. L., Wolchik, S. A., & Weitz, S. (1981). The acquisition of language skills by autistic children: Can parents do the job? *Journal of Autism and Developmental Disorders, 11,* 373–384.

Hart, B. M., & Risley, T. R. (1968). Establishing use of descriptive adjectives in the spontaneous speech of disadvantaged preschool children. *Journal of Applied Behavior Analysis, 1,* 109–120.

Hepting, N. H., & Goldstein, H. (1996). What's natural about naturalistic language intervention? *Journal of Early Intervention, 20,* 249–265.

Hewett, F. M. (1965). Teaching speech to an autistic child through operant conditioning. *American Journal of Orthopsychiatry, 35,* 927–936.

Howlin, P., & Rutter, M. (1989). Mothers' speech to autistic children: A preliminary causal analysis. *Journal of Child Psychology and Psychiatry, 30,* 819–843.

Ingersoll, B., Schreibman, L., & Stahmer, A. (2001). Brief report: Differential treatment outcomes for children with autistic spectrum disorder based on level of peer social avoidance. *Journal of Autism and Developmental Disorders, 31,* 343–350.

Kaiser, A. P., Hancock, T. B., & Nietfeld, J. P. (2000). The effect of parent-implemented enhanced milieu teaching on the social communication of children who have autism. *Early Education and Development, 11,* 423–446.

Kamps, D. M., Walker, D., Locke, P., Delquadri, J. C., & Hall, R. V. (1990). A comparison of instructional arrangements for children with autism served in a public school setting. *Education and Treatment of Children, 13,* 197–215.

Kanner, L. (1943). Autistic disturbances of affective contact. *Nervous Child, 2,* 217–250.

Kanner, L. (1971). Follow-up study of eleven autistic children originally reported in 1943. *Journal of Autism and Childhood Schizophrenia, 1,* 119–145.

Koegel, L. K. (2000). Interventions to facilitate communication in autism. *Journal of Autism and Developmental Disorders, 30,* 383–391.

Koegel, L. K., Camarata, S. M., Valdez-Menchaca, M., & Koegel, R. L. (1998). Setting generalization of question-asking by children with autism. *American Journal on Mental Retardation, 102,* 346–357.

Koegel, L. K., Koegel, R. L., Hurley, C., & Frea, W. D. (1992). Improving social skills and disruptive behavior in children with autism through self-management. *Journal of Applied Behavior Analysis, 25,* 341–353.

Koegel, R. L., Camarata, S., Koegel, L. K., Ben-Tall, A., & Smith, A. E. (1998). Increasing speech intelligibility in children with autism. *Journal of Autism and Developmental Disorders, 28,* 241–251.

Koegel, R. L., Glahn, T. J., & Nieminen, G. S. (1978). Generalization of parent-training results. *Journal of Applied Behavior Analysis, 11,* 95–109.

Koegel, R. L., Koegel, L. K., & Surratt, A. (1992). Language intervention and disruptive behavior in preschool children with autism. *Journal of Autism and Developmental Disorders, 22,* 141–153.

Koegel, R. L., O'Dell, M. C., & Koegel, L. K. (1987). A natural language teaching paradigm for nonverbal autistic children. *Journal of Autism and Developmental Disorders, 17,* 187–199.

Koegel, R. L., Russo, D. C., & Rincover, A. (1977). Assessing and training teachers in the generalized use of behavior modification with autistic children. *Journal of Applied Behavior Analysis, 10,* 197–205.

Krantz, P. J., Zalenski, S., Hall, L. J., Fenske, E. C., & McClannahan, L. E. (1981). Teaching complex language to autistic children. *Analysis and Intervention in Developmental Disabilities, 1,* 259–297.

Laski, K. E., Charlop, M. H., & Schreibman, L. (1988). Training parents to use the natural language paradigm to increase their autistic children's speech. *Journal of Applied Behavior Analysis, 21,* 391–400.

Leaf, R., & McEachin, J. (2001). *A work in progress.* New York: DRL Books.

Lovaas, O. I. (1981). *Teaching developmentally disabled children: The me book.* Baltimore: University Park Press.

Lovaas, O. I. (1987). Behavioral treatment and normal educational and intellectual functioning in young autistic children. *Journal of Consulting and Clinical Psychology, 55,* 3–9.

Lovaas, O. I. (2002). *Teaching individuals with developmental delays: Basic intervention techniques.* Austin, TX: PRO-ED.

Lovaas, O. I., Berberich, J. P., Perloff, B. F., & Schaeffer, B. (1966). Acquisition of imitative speech by schizophrenic children. *Science, 151,* 705–707.

Lovaas, O. I., Freitag, G., Gold, V. J., & Kassorla, I. C. (1965). Experimental studies in child schizophrenia: Analysis of self-destructive behavior. *Journal of Experimental Child Psychology, 2,* 67–84.

Lovaas, O. I., Freitas, L., Nelson, K., & Whalen, C. (1967). The establishment of imitation and its use for the development of complex behavior in schizophrenic children. *Behaviour Research and Therapy, 5,* 171–181.

Lovaas, O. I., Koegel, R. L., Simmons, J. Q., & Long, J. S. (1973). Some generalization and follow-up measures on autistic children in behavior therapy. *Journal of Applied Behavior Analysis, 6,* 131–166.

Mahoney, G., & Perales, F. (2003). Using relationship-focused intervention to enhance the social-emotional functioning of young children with autism spectrum disorders. *Topics in Early Childhood Special Education, 23,* 77–89.

Mahoney, G., & Perales, F. (2005). The impact of relationship-focused intervention on young children with autism spectrum disorders: A comparative study. *Journal of Developmental and Behavioral Pediatrics, 26,* 77–85.

Matson, J. L., Sevin, J. A., Box, M. L., Francis, K. L., & Sevine, B. M. (1993). An evaluation of two methods for increasing self-initiated verbalizations in autistic children. *Journal of Applied Behavior Analysis, 26,* 389–398.

Maurice, C., Green, G., & Luce, S. C. (1996). *Behavioral intervention for young children with autism.* Austin, TX: PRO-ED.

McBride, B. J., & Schwartz, I. S. (2003). Effects of teaching early interventionist to use discrete trials during ongoing classroom activities. *Topics in Early Childhood Special Education, 23,* 5–17.

McDonnell, A. P. (1996). The acquisition, transfer, and generalization of requests by young children with severe disabilities. *Education and Training in Mental Retardation and Developmental Disabilities, 31,* 213–234.

McGee, G. G., Almeida, M. C., Sulzer-Azaroff, B., & Feldman, R. S. (1992). Promoting reciprocal interactions via peer incidental teaching. *Journal of Applied Behavior Analysis, 25,* 117–126.

McGee, G. G., Krantz, P. J., Mason, D., & McClannahan, L. E. (1983). A modified incidental-teaching procedure for autistic youth: Acquisition and generalization of receptive object labels. *Journal of Applied Behavior Analysis, 16,* 329–338.

McGee, G. G., Morrier, M. J., & Daly, T. (1999). An incidental teaching approach to early intervention for toddlers with autism. *Journal of the Association for Persons with Severe Handicaps, 24,* 133–146.

Metz, J. R. (1965). Conditioning generalized imitation in autistic children. *Journal of Experimental Child Psychology, 2,* 389–399.

Mundy, P., & Crowson, M. (1997). Joint attention and early social communication: Implications for research on intervention with autism. *Journal of Autism and Developmental Disorders, 27,* 653–676.

Mundy, P., & Markus, J. (1997). On the nature of communication and language impairment in autism. *Mental Retardation and Developmental Disabilities Research Reviews, 3,* 343–349.

Mundy, P., Sigman, M., & Kasari, C. (1990). A longitudinal study of joint attention and language development in autistic children. *Journal of Autism and Developmental Disorders, 20,* 115–128.

Mundy, P., Sigman, M., Ungerer, J., & Sherman, T. (1986). Defining the social deficits of autism: The contribution of non-verbal communication measures. *Journal of Child Psychology and Psychiatry, 27,* 657–669.

Mundy, P., Sigman, M., Ungerer, J., & Sherman, T. (1987). Nonverbal communication and play correlates of language development in autistic children. *Journal of Autism and Developmental Disorders, 17,* 349–364.

National Research Council. (2001). *Educating children with autism.* Washington, DC: National Academies Press.

Neef, N. A., Walters, J., & Egel, A. L. (1984). Establishing generative yes/no responses in developmentally disabled children. *Journal of Applied Behavior Analysis, 17,* 453–460.

Peck, C. A. (1985). Increasing opportunities for social control by children with autism and severe handicaps: Effects on student behavior and perceived classroom climate. *Journal of the Association for Persons with Severe Handicaps, 10,* 183–193.

Peck, C. A., Killen, C. C., & Baumgart, D. (1989). Increasing implementation of special education instruction in mainstream preschools: Direct and generalized effects of nondirective consultation. *Journal of Applied Behavior Analysis, 22,* 197–210.

Prizant, B. M., & Wetherby, A. M. (1998). Understanding the continuum of discrete-trial traditional behavioral to social-pragmatic developmental approaches in communication enhancement for young children with autism/PDD. *Seminars in Speech and Language, 19,* 329–353.

Prizant, B. M., Wetherby, A. M., & Rydell, P. (2000). Communication intervention issues for children with autism spectrum disorders. In A. M. Wetherby & B. M. Prizant (Eds.), *Autism spectrum disorders: A transactional developmental perspective* (pp. 193–224). Baltimore: Brookes.

Ratner, N. B., & Bruner, J. (1978). Games, social exchange, and the acquisition of language. *Journal of Child Language, 5,* 391–401.

Risley, R., & Wolf, M. (1967). Establishing functional speech in echolalic children. *Behaviour Research and Therapy, 5,* 73–88.

Rizzolatti, G., Fadiga, L., Fogassi, L., & Gallese, V. (2003). From mirror neurons to imitation: Facts and speculations. In A. Meltzoff & W. Prinz (Eds.), *The imitative mind: Development, evolution, and brain bases* (pp. 247–266). Cambridge, UK: Cambridge University Press.

Rogers, S. J., & DiLalla, D. (1991). A comparative study of the effects of a developmentally based instructional model on young children with autism and young children with other disorders of behavior and development. *Topics in Early Childhood Special Education, 11,* 29–48.

Rogers, S. J., Hepburn, S., Hayden, D., Charlifue-Smith, R., Hall, T., & Perkins, A. (in press). Teaching young nonverbal children with autism useful speech: A pilot study of the Denver model and PROMPT interventions. *Journal of Autism and Developmental Disorders.*

Rogers, S. J., Hepburn, S. L., & Stackhouse, T. (2003). Imitation performance in toddlers with autism and those with other developmental disorders. *Journal of Child Psychology and Psychiatry and Allied Disciplines, 44,* 763–781.

Rogers, S. J., Herbison, J., Lewis, H., Pantone, J., & Reis, K. (1986). An approach for enhancing the symbolic, communicative, and interpersonal functioning of young children with autism and severe emotional handicaps. *Journal of the Division of Early Childhood, 10,* 135–148.

Rogers, S. J., & Lewis, H. (1989). An effective day treatment model for young children with pervasive developmental disorders. *Journal of the American Academy of Child and Adolescent Psychiatry, 28,* 207–214.

Rogers, S. J., Lewis, H. C., & Reis, K. (1987). An effective procedure for training early special education teams to implement a model program. *Journal of the Division of Early Childhood, 11,* 180–188.

Rogers, S. J., & Pennington, B. (1991). A theoretical approach to the deficits in infantile autism. *Development and Psychopathology, 3,* 137–162.

Ross, D. E., & Greer, R. D. (2003). Generalized imitation and the mand: Inducing first instances of speech in young children with autism. *Research in Developmental Disabilities, 24,* 58–74.

Rutter, M. (1978). Diagnosis and definition. In M. Rutter & E. Schopler (Eds.), *Autism: A reappraisal of concepts and treatment* (pp. 1–25). New York: Plenum Press.

Rydell, P., & Mirenda, P. (1994). Effects of high and low constraint utterances on the production of immediate and delayed echolalia in young children with autism. *Journal of Autism and Developmental Disorders, 24,* 719–735.

Siller, M., & Sigman, M. (2002). The behaviors of parents of children with autism predict the subsequent development of their children's communication. *Journal of Autism and Developmental Disorders, 32,* 77–89.

Skinner, B. F. (1957). *Verbal behavior.* Englewood Cliffs, NJ: Prentice Hall.

Smith, T. (2001). Discrete trial training in the treatment of autism. *Focus on Autism and Other Developmental Disabilities, 16,* 86–92.

Smith, T., Groen, A. D., & Wynn, J. W. (2000). Randomized trial of intensive early intervention for children with pervasive developmental disorder. *American Journal on Mental Retardation, 105,* 269–285.

Smith, T., Groen, A. D., & Wynn, J. W. (2001). Erratum. *American Journal on Mental Retardation, 106,* 208.

Square-Storer, P., & Hayden, D. (1989). PROMPT treatment. In P. Square-Storer (Ed.), *Acquired apraxia of speech in aphasic adults: Theoretical and clinical issues* (pp. 190–219). Hillsdale, NJ: Erlbaum.

Stern, D. N. (1985). *The interpersonal world of the human infant.* New York: Basic Books.

Stokes, T. F., & Baer, D. M. (1977). An implicit technology of generalization. *Journal of Applied Behavior Analysis, 10,* 349–367.

Strain, P. S., McGee, G. G., & Kohler, F. W. (2001). Inclusion of children with autism in early intervention environments. In M. J. Guralnick (Ed.), *Early childhood inclusion: Focus on change* (pp. 337–363). Baltimore: Brookes.

Sundberg, M. L., & Michael, J. (2001). The benefits of Skinner's analysis of verbal behavior for children with autism. *Behavior Modification, 25,* 698–724.

Sundberg, M. L., & Partington, J. W. (1999). The need for both discrete trial and natural environment language training for children with autism. In P. M.Ghezzi, W. L. Williams, & J. E. Carr (Eds.), *Autism: Behavior-analytic perspectives* (pp. 139–156). Reno, NV: Context Press.

Tager-Flusberg, H., Calkins, S., Nolin, T., Baumberger, T., Anderson, M., & Chadwick-Dias, A. (1990). A longitudinal study of language acquisition in autistic and Down syndrome children. *Journal of Autism and Developmental Disorders, 20,* 1–21.

Warren, S. F., & Kaiser, A. P. (1988). Research on early language intervention. In S. L. Odom & M. A. Karnes (Eds.), *Early intervention for infants and children with handicaps: An empirical base* (pp. 84–108). Baltimore: Brookes.

Warren, S. F., McQuarter, R. J., & Rogers-Warren, A. K. (1984). The effects of mands and models on the speech of unresponsive language-delayed preschool children. *Journal of Speech and Hearing Disorders, 49,* 43–52.

Weiss, R. (1981). INREAL intervention for language handicapped and bilingual children. *Journal of the Division of Early Childhood, 4,* 40–51.

Wetherby, A. M., Prizant, B. M., & Schuler, A. L. (2000). Understanding the nature of communication and language impairments. In A. M. Wetherby & B. M. Prizant (Eds.), *Autism spectrum disorders: A transactional developmental perspective* (pp. 109–142). Baltimore: Brookes.

Wetherby, A. M., & Prutting, C. A. (1984). Profiles of communicative and cognitive-social abilities in autistic children. *Journal of Speech and Hearing Research, 27,* 364–377.

Williams, G., Donley, C. R., & Keller, J. W. (2000). Teaching children with autism to ask questions about hidden objects. *Journal of Applied Behavior Analysis, 33,* 627–630.

Williams, G., Perez-Gonzalez, L. A., & Vogt, K. (2003). The role of specific consequences in the maintenance of three types of questions. *Journal of Applied Behavior Analysis, 26,* 285–296.

Williams, J. H. G., Whiten, A., Suddendorf, T., & Perrett, D. I. (2001). Imitation, mirror neurons and autism. *Neuroscience and Biobehavioral Reviews, 25,* 287–295.

Wolf, M., Risley, T., & Mees, H. (1964). Application of operant conditioning procedures to the behaviour problems of an autistic child. *Behaviour Research and Therapy, 1,* 305–312.

Yoder, P. J., & Layton, T. L. (1988). Speech following sign language training in autistic children with minimal verbal language. *Journal of Autism and Developmental Disorders, 18,* 217–229.

7

Promoting Social Reciprocity and Symbolic Representation in Children with Autism Spectrum Disorders

Designing Quality Peer Play Interventions

Pamela J. Wolfberg
Adriana L. Schuler

The distinct problems that children on the autism spectrum encounter in play and peer relations pose significant challenges for practitioners and family members who want to help them. Difficulties in peer play directly speak to the core impairments in reciprocal social interaction, communication, and imagination that have come to define the syndrome of childhood autism (American Psychiatric Association, 2000). In a recent examination of early diagnosis in autism spectrum disorders (ASD), Charman and Baird (2002, p. 289) include "a lack of varied and imaginative or imitative play" and "a failure to develop peer relationships" as key features. In sharp contrast to the rich social and imaginary play lives of typically developing children, the play of children with ASD is strikingly detached and stark. Spontaneous, diverse, flexible, and interactive qualities are all noticeably lacking. The fact that children with ASD are commonly excluded from their peer culture exacerbates their disabilities. Without intervention, their play lives are likely to remain impoverished.

Looking at children from both a psychological and sociocultural perspective, Vygotsky (1933/1966, 1932/1978) attributes a most active role to play as a primary social activity for acquiring symbolic capacities, interpersonal skills, and social knowledge. According to his view, play's significance extends beyond that of merely reflecting development to that of leading development. To quote Vygotsky (1932/1978):

> In play a child always behaves beyond his average age, above his daily behavior; in play it is as though he were a head taller than himself. As in the focus of a magnifying glass, play contains all developmental tendencies in a condensed form and is itself a major source of development. (p. 102)

Play is thus seen as a driving force rather than just a mirror of development. It is through active participation in play that children construct shared meanings and transform their understanding of the skills, values, and knowledge inherent to society and culture at large. Vygotsky even considers independent play as social activity, because children's themes, roles, and scripts are a reflection of these larger sociocultural worlds. Not only does such a view have powerful implications for our understanding of autistic symptomatology, but it also provides a powerful testimony to the importance of play interventions.

Despite its therapeutic potential, play, and particularly peer play, has not received the attention it deserves in the education and treatment of children with ASD. The relative neglect of play has had unfortunate repercussions for these children. Without the interpersonal skills and flexible modes of representation that manifest themselves in the context of play, it is difficult to develop friendships or nurture social relations. Without the benefits of participation in play culture, many children with ASD remain isolated. From a transactional perspective, the neglect of peer play comes at a high price. Research and clinical experience lead us to believe that the pervasive dynamics of social exclusion impose a secondary level of disability over a more basic deficit in the processing of social information (for discussions, see Jordan, 2003; Schuler & Wolfberg, 2000). The ever-decreasing opportunities to socialize serve to amplify the skill deficits already encountered. If unmitigated, this dynamic leads to ever-increasing social deficits. There is growing evidence to further suggest that many children with ASD are much more capable of play (both symbolic and social forms) than is typically assumed (for further discussion, see Boucher & Wolfberg, 2003). We believe that it is the lack of access to and support for peer play that is primarily responsible for the skill deficits encountered. Even if only secondary in nature, the dynamic of exclusion may be more pervasive and disabling than

the more primary, biologically based impairments in the processing of social information.

There are numerous reasons why play has not received its due attention in the education and treatment of children with ASD. Besides the
implicit challenge of addressing the defining features of the syndrome of
early childhood autism, intervention efforts are further complicated by conflicting views regarding the function and value of play. Particularly when
dealing with children whose behaviors defy developmental expectations,
play is more likely to be viewed as a luxury to be targeted only when more
basic deficiencies have been remedied. Moreover, the current emphasis on
accountability, quantification, and empirically validated programs may
have inadvertently discouraged the pursuit of play in a broader developmental and cultural context. Because play at large is characterized by initiation, innovation, and novelty, advances in play are not readily assessed by
commonly used measures, such as percentages of correct responding.

Additional pitfalls undermine the validity of program development
and research when play is pursued as a discrete set of skills. First of all,
when precisely operationalized scripts and training sequences are adopted,
their very use threatens the essence of play. Second, the type of adult-
directed training sequences that have documented their effectiveness in
teaching compliance through the use of reinforcement of prompted behaviors and explicit modeling may not lend themselves well to the realm of
play. Finally, the pursuit of correct literal repetition of targeted skills
sequences is hardly compatible with the thematic variation that is the very
cornerstone of play and symbolic thinking.

Given all of the preceding, it is not surprising that Williams (2003) recently reported that only 7% of 161 studies making reference to play in autism actually focused on play. The majority of studies only touched on play
as a context for other, more specific aims or in relation to other developmental phenomena and/or treatment goals. However, recent advances in
our understanding of early social communication in typical development as
they relate to the skills deficits in autism have underscored the value of play
and peer interactions in early intervention (see, for example, Prizant,
Wetherby & Rydell, 2000). Following an extensive review of educational
interventions, the National Research Council (2001) ranked the teaching of
play skills with peers among the six types of interventions that should have
priority in the design and delivery of effective educational programs for
young children with ASD.

As the importance of play interventions is increasingly acknowledged,
the closer examination of current theoretical knowledge of play and
early social-communicative development is timely. Similarly, a review of
evidence-based intervention practices seems warranted to optimize treatment outcomes. The purpose of this chapter is to enhance the quality of

play interventions designed to promote social reciprocity and symbolic representation in children on the autism spectrum. In order to accomplish this, we:

1. Highlight the nature of play development in typical children as related to the challenges encountered by children with autism within their sociocultural context.
2. Review a variety of promising play-related interventions in search of common themes, practices, and measurement strategies that allow for documentation of meaningful changes.
3. Describe a peer play intervention model (Integrated Play Groups) that draws from a range of practices that have demonstrated their value in advancing both the reciprocal and representational aspects of play in autism.

DEVELOPMENTAL PLAY PATTERNS
AND VARIATIONS IN CHILDREN WITH ASD

Tracking the course of symbolic and social play in typical childhood development provides a context for understanding play patterns and variations in children with ASD. Typical play development reflects the child's growing understanding of objects, social awareness of self and others, and emotional attachments to and relationships with adults and peers. As play develops in children, its forms, functions, and levels of complexity are radically transformed. Various kinds of play emerge, peak and interweave at different cross points of development, building on, extending, and transforming each other throughout the lifespan.

Although it is commonly accepted that play follows a universal developmental sequence (Garvey, 1977; Piaget, 1962; Rubin, Fein, & Vandenberg, 1983), variations are observed, as they pertain to cultural background, attachment history, language acquisition style, and personality types. What also needs to be kept in mind is that play does not develop as a discrete set of skills independent of other developmental attainments, nor does play develop in a step-by-step manner along a linear path. Rather, different layers of play become ever more intertwined, incorporating increasingly differentiated and decontextualized units of behavior that evolve from more basic reflexive interactions with surrounding objects and people. To quote Bloom and Tinker (2001; pp. 5–6), play, like other aspects of behavior and development, "depends on and emerges out of a nexus of closely connected developments in [language], cognition, emotion, and social interaction."

An underlying feature of play development in children with ASD is that people- and object-focused lines of development fail to merge at around 9 months. This merger, which normally provides for the emergence of communicative intent as first described by Sugarman (1982), lays the foundation for increasingly abstract levels of representation and, ultimately, for *decontextualized*, symbolic thought and action. Williams, Costall, and Reddy (1999) articulate this point as they highlight the reciprocal nature of the interactions between the child, other people, and objects:

> Given the evidence that other people play an important role in introducing objects to children . . . an impairment in interpersonal relations should itself lead us to expect corresponding disruption in the autistic child's use of objects. Conversely, an unusual use of objects is likely to manifest itself in disturbances in relating to other people, given the importance of a shared understanding and use of objects in facilitating interaction. (p. 367)

Recognizing that this merger is missing or incomplete, we have found it useful to describe and assess levels of play development in children with ASD according to the contributing social dimensions (i.e., levels of reciprocity and social coordination) juxtaposed to cognitive dimensions (levels of object use and representation).

Levels of Representational Play: Cognitive Dimensions

Compared with typical children, children on the autism spectrum present unique profiles of play in terms of the levels of representation involved (for reviews, see Jarrold, Boucher, & Smith, 1996; Jarrold, 2003; Williams, 2003). When given opportunities to play freely, for example, they tend to spend excessive amounts of time pursuing repetitive activities in isolation (Frith, 1989; Wing, Gould, Yeates, & Brierly, 1977). Many children get stuck on one or a few activities, which they may literally repeat over and over. Some children are attracted to conventional toys, activities, and themes that reflect the play preferences of younger children as well as agemates. Others develop unique fascinations or preoccupations that revolve around objects and unusual interests. What is missing across these activities is the systematic variations along a theme, thus making activities appear void of purpose other than to provide sensory feedback. Because of the apparent lack of intent, the behaviors involved may be described as self-stimulatory. A description of typical levels of play development compared with those of children with ASD follows and is summarized in Table 7.1.

   Play involving the *manipulation* or sensory exploration of objects and/or space occurs in children on the autism spectrum at higher rates than functional or symbolic play and is less diversified than that of children of a similar maturational age (Libby, Powell, Messer, & Jordan, 1998; Sigman & Ungerer, 1984; Tilton & Ottinger, 1964). Children with autism are often fascinated by play activities and materials that involve sensory experiences. Many young children spontaneously seek out physical or rough-and-tumble forms of play, such as running, jumping, or skipping. Manipulating toys and other objects in a stereotyped fashion is a frequently cited characteristic of autism (Tiegerman & Primavera, 1981). Objects are often the focal point of sensory exploration. Stereotyped play routines range from undifferentiated acts—such as indiscriminate mouthing, banging, or spinning (e.g., the wheels of a toy car) to more elaborate routines and rituals, such as lining up objects according to size and/or color. The extraordinary feats of balance and coordination performed by some children when they manipulate objects in unconventional ways speak to their refined grasp of the inanimate properties of the physical world that surround them.

Functional play, defined as the conventional use of an object or association of two or more objects according to common functions and sociocultural conventions, is less likely to spontaneously emerge in children on the autism spectrum as compared with developmentally matched age-mates (Jarrold et al., 1996; Lewis & Boucher, 1988; Williams, Reddy, & Costall, 2001). Nevertheless, some children do display this capacity; for instance, by demonstrating the function of common objects—placing a cup to their mouths or using a spoon to stir in a cup. Functional play schemes may range from simple to complex acts that may be directed to objects, self, and others. Overall, children with autism spend less time in functional play and produce fewer functional play acts. In addition, they display qualitative differences in their functional play in terms of diversity, elaboration, and integration of play schemes. Showing their limited appreciation of sociocultural conventions, they exhibit fewer doll-directed functional play acts (Sigman & Ungerer, 1984; Williams et al., 2001).

Symbolic pretend play, defined as the capacity to purposefully engage in imaginative activity or advanced pretense, is least likely to surface spontaneously in children with ASD (Baron-Cohen, 1987; Lewis & Boucher, 1988). Pretend play in typical development reflects the child's capacity to substitute and transform, as well as invent imaginary objects, roles, and/or events as if they were present (Leslie, 1987). At a more sophisticated level, children demonstrate capacities to act out roles and scripts with people, as well as with dolls and other inanimate objects (McCune-Nicolich, 1981; Westby, 2000). When children with ASD show evidence of pretend play, it is often at a rudimentary level, with qualities of diversity, flexibility, and creativity noticeably lacking. Compared with children of similar developmental levels, they tend to incorporate fewer novel acts in their pretend play (Charman & Baron-Cohen, 1997; Jarrold, Boucher, & Smith, 1996). In addition, they have difficulty planning, organizing, and integrating play scripts. Play scenarios are often carried out as rituals with little variation; they appear to be well-rehearsed scenes prompted by a predictable situation or context rather than spontaneously generated (Harris, 1993). Similarities between these forms of play and the types of verbal rituals observed in children with high rates of echolalic speech have led us to coin the term "echoplaylia" (Wolfberg & Schuler, 1993).

Levels of Reciprocity and Coordination: Social Dimensions

Children on the autism spectrum present distinct variations with respect to the social dimensions of play, that is, not what objects represent but how objects are shared and incorporated into social interactions (for further review, see Jordan, 2003; Williams et al., 1999). When it comes to these social dimensions, such as coordinating play themes, toys, and space with their peers, children with ASD are notably challenged.

Whereas joint attention, spontaneous imitation, and emotional responsiveness characterize the early social play interactions between typically developing infants and their caregivers (Eckerman & Stein, 1982; Ross & Kay, 1980), it is the lack of, or compromised emergence of, these very features that constitute the early signs of atypical development in autism. In sharp contrast to the apparent ease with which infants typically learn to share action, attention, and affect, the vast majority of children with ASD show developmental delays or differences in these areas (Baron-Cohen, 1989; Mundy, Sigman, Ungerer, & Sherman, 1987; Sigman & Ruskin, 1999). Deficits or delays in such social signaling further inhibit their capacity to engage in reciprocal interactions with siblings and peers.

Peer play can be characterized along a continuum of social complexity and cohesiveness that traverses the age span. With growing exposure to peers, typically developing children progressively learn how to coordinate their play activity and social behavior (Parten, 1932). Rather than following a strict sequence of developmental stages, children tend to cycle back and forth among a range of social play behaviors as they gain experience and skill.

In the absence of explicit structure and support, children with ASD are likely to remain isolated or on the fringes of peer groups. Overall, children with autism make fewer overt initiations to peers. When they do attempt to interact, their initiations tend to be subtle, obscure, or poorly timed, and therefore not acknowledged. By the same token, limitations in joint attention make children with ASD less likely to consistently respond to the social advances of peers (Lord & Magill, 1989).

Wing and Gould (1979) describe three qualities of social behavior—aloof, passive, and active–odd—that are consistent with our clinical observations of children with autism at play with peers. Some children present patterns of social play that reflect a distinct social style that is consistent over time. Others present social styles that change over time. Still others present overlapping characteristics that may shift according to the social play context. Children who seem to be withdrawn or avoidant of peers are considered aloof. Passive children appear indifferent to peers but are more easily led into social situations and will go along with their peers when the latter take the initiative to play. Children considered active–odd show an interest in being with peers but do so in socially awkward or peculiar ways. Some active–odd children have an idea of what to say and do to initiate or join peers in play but have a poor sense of timing.

Taking into consideration these individual differences, the following descriptions build on the work of Parten (1932), who documented the progression along the key parameters of social play in typical development. These are summarized and compared with children with ASD in Table 7.1.

It is quite natural for children to spend some of their time in solitary or independent play while in the company of peers. Solitary play is often a natural extension of social play with peers, as it enables children to imitate, practice, consolidate, and appropriate newly acquired skills. This selective engagement in solitary play differs sharply from the nonelective play activities often exhibited by children with ASD, which may be more accurately described as *isolate* play behavior.

The fact that children with ASD are predisposed toward ritualistic activity involving preoccupations with objects, themes, or pedantic interests may partially explain this tendency toward isolate play. On the one hand, it may be the attraction to the ritual itself that is especially compelling. On the other hand, because typically developing peers are not likely to relate to such unconventional interests and behavior, there is even less of an incentive for social play to occur.

When typically developing children first encounter peers in a childcare or preschool setting, many spend a significant amount of time as *onlookers*, observing peers at play before actually entering into the play. This often helps in orienting them to choosing a particular activity or playmate to join. Older children, in contrast, spend time watching peers in group situations in order to become familiar with the rules, roles, and social patterns of the play culture (Dodge, Schlundt, Schocken, & Delugach, 1983). Although it is not uncommon for children with ASD to spend time watching peers at play, for many this is the extent to which they exhibit a social interest. Moreover, some children exhibit onlooker behavior in rather subtle as opposed to more obvious ways. For instance, some children indicate that they are observing peers and their play activities by wandering among them rather than directly watching them. Similarly, some children indicate that they are watching peers by using a peripheral gaze as opposed to direct eye gaze while facing them.

TABLE 7.1. Typical Play Patterns and Play Variations in Children with Autism

Play domain	Typical play patterns	Play variations in autism
Symbolic dimension	Spontaneous progression along developmental continuum *Sensory exploration/manipulation* play progressing from undifferentiated, repeated acts to varied acts and combinations *Functional play* progressing from simple to complex and diverse play schemes reflecting deferred imitation *Symbolic/pretend play* progressing from simple to complex and cohesive play scripts by transforming objects, self, and others and creating imaginary roles and situations	Delayed and/or atypical progression within developmental continuum High rates of stereotyped sensory exploration/manipulation play involving fewer novel acts and combinations Spontaneous functional play less common—play schemes less integrated, incorporate fewer different novel acts and doll-directed acts Spontaneous symbolic/pretend play least common—play scripts inflexible, literal, disjointed, reflecting difficulties in generating novelty, planning, and organizing
Social dimension	Joint attention, spontaneous imitation, emotional responsiveness evident in early social exchanges with adults and peers Play with peers spontaneously develops along a continuum of social complexity and cohesiveness across the age span, surfacing as *solitary, onlooker/ orientation, parallel/proximity, common focus,* and *common goal* Individual variations in social play styles as signs of increased social differentiation and social competence Children perceived as socially competent more readily accepted and included within peer play culture	Problems in joint attention, spontaneous imitation, emotional responsiveness emerging in early development and persisting in social play Delayed and/or atypical development along social continuum of play with peers, surfacing as high rates of *solitary (isolate), onlooker/orientation,* and *parallel/proximity* and low rates of socially coordinated play characterized by *common focus* and *common goal* Individual variations in social play styles described as aloof, passive, active–odd Children perceived as lacking social competence, increases likelihood of peer neglect or rejection from play culture

Playing in *parallel* or proximity to peers is also a consistent feature of typical childhood development. In this type of play, the child plays independently alongside or nearby other children. While playing with similar play materials and in the same play space, the children do not join one another in play. They may occasionally look over, imitate, show an object, and alternate actions with peers, but they do not interact in any apparent way. This type of play persists throughout childhood, offering ongoing opportunities for learning through modeled behavior. There are children with ASD who display this behavior by spending time playing in parallel or proximity to peers; however, this is where their social development in play typically plateaus without the benefit of explicit guidance or support. Parallel play ordinarily is a stepping-stone to more socially coordinated forms of play, which require reciprocal communication and present much greater obstacles for this population.

The capacity to establish a *common focus* in play emerges as children engage in interactions that are loosely organized around mutually enjoyed play activities. In the preschool years, play interchanges gradually increase in length, frequency, and complexity as children establish a common focus by actively sharing materials, taking turns, giving and receiving assistance, asking questions, giving directions, and generally conversing about the play. Common focus is also reflected in sociodramatic play as children jointly construct imaginative play sequences. At a more sophisticated level are cooperative forms of play involving complex social organization with shared *common goals*. The play is directed for the purpose of making a product, dramatizing an event, or playing a formal game. The children determine the agenda by generating rules or roles through explicit planning, negotiation, and division of labor. The efforts of one child supplement those of another, thereby establishing a sense of cooperation and belonging to a group.

PEER INFLUENCES ON PLAY IN CHILDREN WITH ASD

Developmental play patterns (along both cognitive and social dimensions) are further shaped by the child's experiences with others and the social, cultural, and societal contexts in which they participate (Hanson et al., 1998; Meyer, Park, Grenot-Scheyer, Schwartz, & Harry, 1998). Peers, in particular, perform a distinct role in offering opportunities for learning and development that adults essentially cannot duplicate (Hartup, 1979). Through shared experiences in play with peers, children acquire many interrelated skills that are necessary for attaining social competence and forming mutual friendships (Hartup & Sancilio, 1986; Parker & Gottman, 1989). Particularly within a social pretend framework, children practice and assimilate these skills while developing their imaginations. Moreover, the peer group or *peer culture* has an especially profound influence on whether children gain access to and reap the benefits of such play experiences.

Peer culture is defined as the unique social worlds that children construct out of their everyday experiences with one another apart from adults (Corsaro, 1992; Wolfberg et al., 1999). It is based on children's active participation in those social activities that are most valued by the peer group. A vital feature of their peer culture is that children develop a sense of collective identity in which they recognize themselves as members of a group created exclusively by and for children. Although the adult world may be represented within the content of the peer culture, children pursue social activities on their own terms regardless of adult expectations.

Because play is, for all intents and purposes, the leading social activity in children's lives, it is the very essence of their peer culture. As such, *play culture* more precisely describes that realm in which children create and live out their social and imaginary worlds (Mouritsen, 1996; Selmer-Olsen, 1993). Like living folklore, play culture manifests itself in the rituals, narratives, and creations children produce and pass on to one another.

The reality for many children with ASD is that they are frequently excluded from their peer groups simply because their behavior does not conform to the conventions of the play culture. Unconventional attempts to socialize and play are commonly perceived as signs of deviance, limited social interest, or even rejection. As a consequence, many children with ASD become targets of bullying, teasing, and taunting by intolerant peers (Heinrichs, 2003), whereas others are simply ignored or overlooked by peers who might otherwise be open-minded to the differences of others (Wolfberg et al., 1999). The transactional nature of these influences poses a dilemma—with limited capacities to socialize and play with peers, children with ASD are likely to be excluded from participating in their play culture; yet without such participation, they are unlikely to develop the capacities to socialize and play that would be needed to escape their isolation. Thus the developmental play patterns of children with ASD are characterized not only by delays or deficits in cognitive complexity but also by the effects of social isolation. In order to break this vicious cycle, intervention efforts would need to carefully consider the role of the peer culture as it interacts with the child's overall development and experience within the context of play as socially meaningful activity.

PLAY-RELATED INTERVENTION RESEARCH

A review of play and play-related interventions reveals a wide assortment of theoretical orientations, methods, and contexts used to promote play in children with ASD. A first complication in reviewing this literature is that studies differ in terms of their objectives and measurement tools. Whereas some studies specifically evaluate the effectiveness of a particular intervention, others focus on the manipulation of single experimental variables. The fact that some studies emphasize the cognitive dimensions of play and others the social dimensions of play constitutes another complication. There is also variability in degree of structure—whether the intervention is adult-directed as opposed to child-centered and involves play with adults as opposed to play with peers. In terms of context, play interventions also differ in their settings—clinical as opposed to natural—and in the kinds of activities and materials that are provided. For our purposes, we highlight adult-directed, child-centered, peer-mediated, and ecological approaches, as follows.

Adult-Directed Practices

Adult-directed play interventions are primarily behavioral in orientation, following principles of applied behavior analysis (for a review, see Stahmer, Ingersoll, & Carter, 2003). Such practices involve systematic reinforcement to increase desired low-frequency behaviors while reducing the frequency of undesirable behaviors. Adult-structured interventions involving the use of extraneous contingencies and direct prompting typify early efforts (Koegel, Firestone, Kramme, & Dunlap, 1974; Romancyzk, Diament, Goren, Trunell, & Harris, 1975). When applied to play, the inherent emphasis placed on response topographies reduces play to a series of operationally defined behaviors, which are taught in a step-by-step fashion. Associated with the work of Lovaas (1987), discrete trial training is one such approach that continues to be in practice today (Leaf & McEachin, 1999; Maurice, Green, & Luce, 1996; Smith, 2001). In discrete trial training, the play is broken down and taught as subskills through a series of repeated teaching trials. The environment is highly structured and controlled by the adult, who relies on prompting, shaping, and reinforcement to elicit the target response. Although a number of studies document varying degrees of success in teaching "play skills" to children with ASD through discrete trial training (Nuzzolo-Gomez, Leonard, Ortiz, Rivera, & Green, 2002; Santarcarangelo, Dyer, & Luce, 1987), as previously discussed, the high degree of structure and adult control calls into question issues of validity when one considers play in a broader developmental and cultural context.

Current innovations that have evolved within a behavioral framework reveal a greater appreciation of developmental contributions with respect to adult-directed play (Lifter, Sulzer-Azaroff, Anderson, & Cowdery, 1993; Stahmer et al., 2003). This appreciation may surface in the selection of instructional targets based on developmental criteria and broader definitions of play, as well as active use of stereotypic behavior to establish reciprocity and expand the child's play repertoire. For instance, Koegel, Dyer, and Bell (1987) enhanced the social interaction of children with autism by allowing them to select preferred play activities. Similarly, children with ASD showed improved toy play skills while directed by an adult using pivotal response training (Stahmer, 1995; Thorp, Stahmer, & Schreibman, 1995). This approach is specifically designed to capitalize on the child's motivation by presenting the child with choices for play; modeling the desired action; reinforcing reasonable, purposeful attempts at correct responding; and directly prompting the correct response (Koegel, Koegel, Harrower, & Carter, 1999).

In vivo modeling techniques, involving the presence of live models who perform a predictable sequence of desired behaviors, have also been shown to be effective in increasing independent toy play (Tryon & Keane, 1986) and engagement in scripted cooperative play sequences (Jahr, Eldevik, & Eikeseth, 2000) in preschool children with ASD. Video modeling has similarly been shown to increase the frequency and duration of toy play, as well as play-related statements, which generalized to novel settings and toys (Schwandt et al., 2002; Taylor, Levin, & Jasper, 1999). Self-management training teaches the child to self-monitor and deliver self-reinforcement for appropriate behavior in the absence of an adult. This type of training has been used to support children with ASD in higher levels of independent play (Stahmer & Schreibman, 1992), as well as more diverse forms of play (Newman, Reinecke, & Meinberg, 2000).

Child-Centered Practices

Child-centered practices are primarily developmental in orientation, whereby the adult follows the child's lead, as opposed to directing the child, to stimulate, expand, and scaffold play along the lines of a progression that mirrors typical development. The child's spontaneous initiations in play with objects, self, and others are guided by a careful appraisal of the child's developmental status.

Van Berckelaer-Onnes (2003) developed a program in which an adult offers and models toy play that is matched to the child's interest and developmental level. Research indicates that the children with autism showed increased interest in toys, a broader range of object manipulations, and evidence of relational and functional object use (Van Berckelaer-Onnes & Kwakkel-Scheffer, 1996). Hauge (1988) further demonstrated higher rates of social interaction between children with autism and typically developing peers when the toys were selected according to developmental levels and prevailing object initiations, such as banging, twisting, stacking, and turning.

A number of child-centered practices involve adults in deliberately imitating the child's spontaneous behavior to build imitation and reciprocity. For instance, Tiegerman and Primavera (1981) documented increased eye contact and play in children with autism by imitating their object manipulations. Dawson and Adams (1984) demonstrated increased social attentiveness and imitative behavior in children with autism by imitating their actions in play. Ingersoll and Schreibman (2002) similarly found that very young children with autism learned imitative pretend play with an adult imitating the child's actions and vocalizations to elicit an imitative response. It is interesting to note that a variety of radically different treatment approaches have reported success in stimulating social responsiveness in children with ASD using similar imitative procedures (e.g., Kalmanson & Pekarsky, 1987; Kaufmann, 1976; Mahler, 1952).

A number of early childhood intervention models incorporate child-centered practices to elicit a joint focus in play routines through the use of rich affect, mutual imitation, and drama. Greenspan and Wieder (1997a) developed the "floor time" approach for enhancing reciprocal play between an adult and child as a part of a more comprehensive developmental and relationship-based model (Wieder & Greenspan, 2003). In "floor time" sessions, the adult follows the child's lead, utilizing gestures, words, and affect to establish joint attention and increasingly complex social-communicative exchanges (Greenspan & Wieder, 1997b). The Denver model, a comprehensive educational approach developed by Rogers and colleagues (Rogers, Hall, Osaki, Reaven, & Herbison, 2000) uses a similar method to teach social play and toy play skills by engaging the child in "sensory social exchanges" that revolve around the child's toy preferences and social initiations with an adult. Sherrat (2002) utilized a systematic classroom-based approach involving elements of structure, affect, and repetition to stimulate symbolic play in children with ASD. In a study using this approach, children generated spontaneous and novel forms of play. The SCERTS model (Social Communication, Emotional Regulation and Transactional Support) provides another example of evidence-based child-centered practices for overcoming core deficits in autism, leading to growing capacities for social and symbolic forms of play (Prizant, Wetherby, Rubin, Rydell, & Laurent, 2003).

Peer-Mediated Practices

Although studies have demonstrated that interactions established between children with ASD and adults do not easily generalize to peer partners, peers are increasingly being included in play-related interventions (National Research Council, 2001). Odom and Strain (1984) were among the first to document peer-mediated approaches. Following a behavioral orientation, peers are trained, prompted, and reinforced by adults to increase the social initiations and responses of the children with autism. Although early studies resulted in increased frequency and duration of social interaction, critics point out that improvements did not generalize beyond the peer tutor (Lord & Hopkins, 1986) and that interventions did not correspond to contexts in which social behavior would naturally occur (Lord & Magill, 1989).

Subsequent intervention efforts have made attempts to remediate problems of generalization and the artificial role of peers. Extensions of earlier approaches include a dual focus on training the typical peers and the children with autism to increase interactive play (Haring & Lovinger, 1989; Oke & Schreibman, 1990). Self-monitoring has been used to increase play interactions between children with ASD and their typically developing peers (e.g., Sainato, Goldstein, & Strain, 1992; Shearer, Kohler, Buchan, & McCullough, 1996). In vivo and video modeling have also been used to increase play with peers and siblings (Taylor et al.,1999). Interventions are also more commonly being carried out in inclusive settings where play with typically developing peers naturally occurs (e.g., preschool settings; Pierce & Schreibman, 1997; Roeyers, 1996; Strain & Kohler, 1998). Further, there is more of an emphasis on supporting the children in play activities that are common among typically developing children. For instance, Goldstein and Cisar (1992) used modeling, prompting, and reinforcement procedures to train triads, consisting of one child with autism and two typically developing peers, to act out specific roles in sociodramatic play scripts.

Although these types of adult-directed practices involving peer-mediated play are documented to be effective, it is well established that there is a heavy reliance on explicit and precise adult control to effectively deliver the intervention (National Research Council, 2001). This type of adult-imposed structure defies the inherent qualities of children's play as intrinsically motivated, governed by a self-imposed structure.

Systematic comparisons of low versus high levels of adult intrusion on children's spontaneous play (Meyer et al., 1987) speak to a growing trend toward less adult-imposed structure consistent with child-centered practices. A number of investigators report the use of naturalistic approaches whereby children with ASD had repeated exposure to familiar peers and their play activities with minimal adult support (e.g., Casner & Marks, 1984; Lord & Hopkins, 1986; McHale, 1983). These interventions yielded both quantitative and qualitative improvements in the social interaction, language, and play of the children with ASD. In a recent study, Kok, Kong, and Bernard-Opitz (2002) compared structured versus facilitated peer play in children with ASD and found that communication and play increased with both techniques; however, the facilitated approach was more effective in eliciting spontaneous communication and play in children with more advanced skills.

Ecological Considerations

Child-centered approaches closely interface with ecological considerations in the selection of suitable play partners and contexts. Several investigations examined the developmental status of peers as a variable in promoting play and playful interactions. Studies that have included younger, typically developing peers closely matched in developmental age to children with autism revealed improvements in specific social play behaviors that did not occur with adults or same-age peers (Lord & Hopkins, 1986). Bednersh and Peck (1986) also report that children with autism displayed more conventional object play while interacting with older, typically developing peers and more sensory–motor object play while interacting with younger peers. Consistent with Vygotsky's (1932/1978) claims, these findings suggest that same-age or older peers may be more capable of structuring and scaffolding the play event to facilitate higher levels of cognitive performance.

High degrees of predictability and consistency in the social and physical environment have long been recognized as beneficial for children with ASD (Rutter, 1978). Lord and Magill (1989) suggest that providing children with autism with opportunities to interact, develop experience, and become familiar with peers contributes to advances in social play. The positive influences of setting variables, such as arranging and limiting the size of the physical play space (Phyfe-Perkins, 1980; Smith & Connolly, 1980) and providing specific play materials on the basis of social potential (Beckman & Kohl, 1984), structure (Dewey, Lord, & Magill, 1988), and complexity (Ferrara & Hill, 1980), are also noteworthy considerations.

Prizant et al. (2000) further suggest a transactional approach that incorporates both developmental and ecological features into the design of peer and sibling play interventions. They highlight a number of key principles that reflect a blending of practices, including: (1) engineering environments so that naturally occurring interactions and play routines are consistent, predictable, and familiar; (2) controlling for novelty within interactions and the environment; (3) fostering shared control and reciprocity among social partners; (4) acknowledging unconventional verbal and social play behaviors as purposeful and intentional; (5) enhancing intrinsic motivation through highly predictable joint action routines; (6) creating multiple opportunities for expressing communicative intent to establish joint attention and social interaction; and (7) systematically transferring active participation and support from the adult to peers.

The intervention efforts reviewed have been helpful in that they have yielded a wide range of promising practices that promote various aspects of play in children with ASD. Nevertheless, what may be discouraging is that the methods reported seem contradictory; adult-imposed modes of behavioral training are not easily reconciled with more loosely structured child-centered approaches of a developmental variety. Whereas highly directive adult-structured approaches might be overly controlling, approaches that attempt to acknowledge the child's state of mind and follow his or her lead might be too subtle to draw the child into play. One of the challenges in the design of effective interventions thus lies in the creation of child-centered structures that are neither too lax nor too rigid. Such conceptual, as well as procedural, differences make it difficult to articulate a coherent approach to intervention to guide practitioners and parents in their efforts to help children with ASD.

What may be more encouraging to note is that among the interventions reported there appear to be some common themes and trends emerging. For instance, recognition is growing of the inherent value of more naturalistic approaches to support children with ASD in play. Play interventions are increasingly taking place in natural settings, with more involvement of typically developing peers. Many interventions share a focus on identifying and responding to what is intrinsically motivating for the child. Similarly, there is a greater acknowledgement of individual differences among children, as early intervention programs incorporate strategies that are tailored to each child's developmental level and style of learning. Further, evidence exists of a growing trend in which such programs are more amenable to a blending of approaches and practices, as opposed to strictly adhering to a particular paradigm or method.

To arrive at a broader conceptual foundation that can incorporate complementary perspectives and help guide practitioners in deciding which techniques and training contexts to use when and where, a closer understanding is needed of the different layers and configurations of support that invite play. In doing so, it is important to realize that a sole focus on single contributions may not be productive; all these components may be better combined into a more powerful multidimensional approach. Thus, to provide children with ASD sufficient and contextually relevant support, all of the factors known to affect play (both from a developmental and sociocultural perspective) must be carefully weighed and considered when designing a comprehensive peer play intervention.

INTEGRATED PLAY GROUPS MODEL

The concept of Integrated Play Groups (IPG) grew in an effort to address the distinct problems that children on the autism spectrum experience in play (for detailed descriptions, see Wolfberg, 1999, 2003). The IPG model draws on current theory, research, and evidence-based practices, incorporating parameters pertinent to the development of social interaction, communication, play, and imagination in children with ASD. The most striking feature of the IPG model is that it is multidimensional in its conception. As discussed earlier, most reported interventions address single aspects of play. The current model is more broadly based, as it encompasses developmental, as well as ecological, features that are embedded within a sociocultural framework (Vygotsky, 1933/1966; 1932/1978).

The IPG model embraces Vygotsky's theory, focusing on "guided participation" in play, a concept described by Rogoff (1990) as the process by which children develop through their active participation in culturally valued activity with the guidance, support, and challenge of companions who vary in skill and status. This process is also similar to Heath's (1989) conception of "the learner as cultural member," to Brown and Campione's (1990) "community of learners," and to Lave and Wenger's (1991) "legitimate peripheral participation." Novices thus gain expertise while playing with other, more competent players under the guidance of a skilled practitioner.

From a practical standpoint, the IPG model is explicitly designed to support children of diverse ages and abilities on the autism spectrum (novice players) in mutually enjoyed play experiences with typical peers or siblings as playmates (expert players) within school, home, and community settings. Through a carefully tailored system of support, the intervention seeks to maximize each child's developmental potential, as well as intrinsic desire to play, socialize, and form meaningful relationships with peers. An equally important focus is on teaching the peer group to be more accepting of and responsive to the children with ASD in spite of their atypical behavior.

Program and Environmental Design

IPG are customized for children (ages 3 to 11 years) as a part of an individualized educational or therapeutic program. Play groups are facilitated by a trained adult, referred to as a *play guide*. Each group is made up of a consistent group of three to five children, with a higher proportion of expert (typical peers and/or siblings) to novice players (children on the autism spectrum). Expert players are recruited from places where children ordinarily have contact with peers (e.g., school, other families, neighborhood, community). Playmates ideally have some familiarity and attraction to one another and the potential for developing long-lasting friendships. Groups may vary with respect to children's gender, ages, developmental status, and play interaction styles, offering different types of beneficial experiences. Prior to the first session, the players participate in an orientation that includes awareness and friendship activities. A major focus is on preparing the expert players to be accepting of and responsive to novice players' unique ways of relating, communicating, and playing.

IPG take place in natural play environments within school, home, therapy, or community settings (e.g., inclusive classrooms, after-school programs, recreation centers, or neighborhood parks). Play groups generally meet twice a week for 30- to 60-minute sessions over a 6- to 12-month period. Times may vary depending on the ages and developmental stages of the participating children.

Play spaces are specially designed based on a consideration of multiple factors, including size, density, organization, and thematic arrangements. Play materials include a wide range of highly motivating sensory–motor, exploratory, constructive, and sociodramatic props with high potential for interactive and imaginative play. Play materials vary in degree of structure and complexity to accommodate children's diverse interests, learning styles, and developmental levels. Intrinsic motivation for peer participation derives from identifying play activities that will be mutually enjoyed by novice and expert players.

Play sessions are structured by establishing consistent schedules, routines, and rituals and incorporating visual supports that foster familiarity, predictability, and a cohesive group identity. Personalized visual calendars and schedules help children anticipate the days and times of meetings. Basic rules for fair and courteous behavior and appropriate care of materials are presented at the outset of play groups. Play sessions begin and end with an opening and closing ritual (e.g., greeting, song and brief discussion of plans and strategies). Group membership is established by creating play group names and associated rituals, which also serve to provide the intrinsic motivation for true peer participation.

Assessment Approach

Play guides are well versed in the range of assessment tools and techniques specifically developed for use with this model. Systematic observations provide a basis for setting realistic and meaningful goals, guiding decisions on how best to intervene on behalf of the novice players, and systematically documenting and analyzing the children's progress. Thus our assessments include a focus on cognitive–symbolic and social dimensions of play, communication functions and means, play preferences, and diversity of play.

Cognitive–symbolic dimensions of play refer to play acts that the child directs toward objects, self, or others and that signify events (adapted from McCune-Nicholich, 1981; Piaget, 1962; and Smilansky, 1968). These include exploratory play (manipulation), conventional object use and simple pretense (functional), and advanced pretense (symbolic–pretend). *Social dimensions of play* focus on the child's distance to and involvement with one or more children (adapted from Parten, 1932). These include playing alone (isolate), watching peers (onlooker/orientation), playing beside peers (parallel/proximity), playing with peers in joint activity (common focus), and collaborating with peers in an organized fashion (common goal). Although each set of play characteristics appears to follow a relatively consistent developmental sequence, they are not considered mutually exclusive stages of development.

Communicative functions describe what the child communicates within the context of peer play activities (e.g., requests for objects or peer interaction, protests, declarations, and comments). The functions of communication may be accomplished through a variety of verbal and nonverbal *communicative means* (e.g., facial expressions; eye gaze; proximity; manipulating another's hand, face, or body; showing or giving objects; gaze shift; gestures; intonation; vocalization; nonfocused or focused echolalia; and one-word or complex speech or sign) (adapted from Peck, Schuler, Tomlinson, Theimer, & Haring, 1984).

Documenting the *play preferences* of both novice and expert players in play groups offers a means by which to identify and match children's play interests. Play preferences include a child's attraction to toys or props (e.g., preferring round objects, toys that move, realistic replicas), interactions with toys or props (e.g., preferring to spin toys, line up toys, conventional object use), choice of play activities (e.g., preferring roughhousing, quiet play, constructive play), choice of play themes (e.g., preferring familiar routines, invented stories, fantasy play), and choice of playmates (preferring no one in particular, one or more peers). Documenting the play preferences of the children with ASD further provides a means to assess *diversity of play*.

Intervention Approach

Guided by the assessment process, the intervention, *guided participation*, translates into a carefully tailored system of support that is responsive to each child's underlying difference and unique developmental profile while also being sufficiently intensive to maximize the child's developmental potential. The idea is to enhance opportunities that allow novice and expert players to initiate and incorporate desired activity into socially coordinated play while challenging novice players to practice new and increasingly complex forms of play. The adult methodically guides novice and expert players to engage in mutually enjoyed play activities that encourage social interaction, communication, play, and imagination—such as pretending, constructing things, art, music, movement, and interactive games. Gradually the adult weans herself out as the children learn to mediate their own play activities. Play guides apply the following set of practices, which may be understood as multiple layers of support.

1. *Monitoring play initiations* focuses on uncovering novice players' meaningful attempts to socialize and play by recognizing, interpreting, and responding to the subtle and idiosyncratic ways in which they express intentions to play in the company of peers. Spontaneous, self-generated play

initiations represent present interests and capacities, whereas imitative and socially guided play acts represent emerging capacities in play. Play initiations may take many conventional and unconventional forms, including unusual fascinations with materials, events, or people and idiosyncratic forms of communication. Child initiations, even if they take unusual forms, serve as indices of present and emerging capacities in play. The adult's capacity to recognize, interpret, and respond to play initiations is critical if support is to be offered commensurate with the level of comprehension and ability of the individual novices within their "zone of proximal development," as described by Vygotsky (1932/1978).

2. *Scaffolding play* involves building on the child's play initiations by systematically adjusting assistance to match or slightly exceed the level at which the child is independently able to engage in play with peers within the child's zone of proximal development. Scaffolding refers to the provision of adjustable and temporary support structures. In facilitating play, the amount of external support provided needs to be adjusted based on child signals. Initially, the play guide acts as an interpreter to help expert and novice players understand each other and/or as a coach who structures the amount and type of support provided by the peers. At a more intensive level, the adult directs the play event and models behavior, much like the director of a stage performance, by identifying and/or narrating common themes, arranging props, and assigning roles and play partners that ensure everyone a satisfying part. At a less intensive level, the adult guides the children to set the stage for their own play by posing leading questions, commenting on activities, offering suggestions, and giving subtle reminders using verbal and visual cues. As the children grow increasingly comfortable and competent in their play, the support is withdrawn. Eventually, the adult remains on the periphery of the group, offering the children a "secure base" from which to explore and try out new activities.

3. *Social-communication guidance* focuses on promoting the children's use of conventional verbal and nonverbal communicative cues to elicit each other's attention and sustain joint engagement in mutually enjoyed play activities. Directed to both experts and novices alike, social-communication guidance strategies encourage *extending invitations* to each other to play, *persisting* in enlisting reluctant players to play, *responding* to each other's cues and initiations in play, *maintaining and expanding* interactions with each other, and *entering* or joining each other in an established play event. Experts learn to interpret even subtle, nonverbal cues of novice players as meaningful and purposeful acts. By the same token, novices learn to better understand and fully participate in the play context by breaking down the complex social cues of expert players.

To guide these social exchanges, the adult presents the children with nonverbal and/or verbal behavior scripts or strategies that serve to elicit and sustain another child's attention in play when natural occasions arise. For this purpose, we developed (and encourage others to develop their own) posters and corresponding cue cards depicting picture–word combinations of *what children can do* (e.g., look, stand close, tap shoulder, take hand, point, give [toy], take turns, do what your playmate is doing) and *what children can say* (e.g., Say name of playmate, "Come on, let's play," "Do you want to play?" "What do you want to play?" "What are you doing?" "Can I play with you?" "Whose turn is it?" "Can I have a turn?" "My turn/Your turn" "Follow me"). For instance, if an expert player calls the name of a novice player who has not yet learned how to respond, the adult can prompt the peer to stand close to the other child, say the child's name, take the child's hand, and say, "Come on, let's play." These types of cues are especially useful for starting an interaction. Once the interaction is in progress, children may look to these cues as a way to fill in the blanks when they feel uncertain as to what to say or do next. The intent is for children to naturally incorporate these strategies into their repertoires, and to no longer rely on adult guidance or the presence of visual cues.

4. *Play guidance* encompasses a set of strategies that support novice players in peer play experiences that are slightly beyond the child's capacity while fully immersed in the whole play experience at his or her present level, even if participation is minimal. Thus novices may carry out play activities and roles that they may not as yet fully comprehend. For example, a child inclined to bang objects may incorporate this scheme into a larger play theme of constructing a building with blocks. With the assistance of more capable peers, the child may take the role of a construction worker and hammer the blocks with a play tool. By building on play initiations and encouraging participation in activities that are just slightly beyond the child's present abilities, peers may encourage novices to begin to explore and diversify existing play routines.

Play guidance strategies range from *orienting* (watching peers and activities), *mirroring* (mimicking the actions of a peer), *parallel play* (playing side by side in the same play space with similar materials), and *joint focus* (active sharing and informal turn taking in the same activity) to socially coordinated activity involving *joint action* (formal turn taking), *role enactment* (portraying real-life activities through conventional actions), and *role playing* (taking on pretend roles and creatively using objects while enacting complex scripts).

Case Illustration of an Integrated Play Group

Table 7.2 illustrates the play guide's application of multiple layers of support in an IPG (Wolfberg, 2003, pp. 204–206). The novice player, Luna, is a 4-year-old girl who was diagnosed with autism at the age of 3. She con-

TABLE 7.2. Illustration of the Play Guide's Application of Multiple Layers of Support in an Integrated Play Group

Play scenario	Monitoring play initiations	Scaffolding play	Social-communication guidance	Play guidance
The session opens with a ritual greeting and song. Luna's mother says, "It is sunny today, so let's play outside." She leads the children to the patio, where a water table is prominently displayed. Floating in the water are several baby dolls, sponges, plastic bottles, and containers of various sizes.	Recognize play initiation	Maximum support: directing and modeling		Orienting
Pointing to the water table, Mother asks, "What do you want to play?" Melanie and Katie (expert players) immediately head to the water table and begin exploring the materials. Luna starts to head back inside to the kitchen sink.	Recognize play initiation	Intermediate support: verbal and visual cueing		Orienting
Mother says, "It looks like everyone wants to play with water. "Melanie and Katie, I think Luna might like to join you. Remember what we can do to get our friends to join us. Say 'Luna, look at the water in the tub.' " Melanie and Katie repeat this in unison, but Luna does not respond.	Interpret and respond to play initiation	Intermediate support: verbal and visual cueing	Reinforce cue: what to say— "Look"	Orienting
Mother holds up a picture cue, "take hand," and models this by taking Luna by the hand and leading her to the water table and saying, "Look at the water." Katie follows by taking Luna's hand and leading her the rest of the way to the water table. Melanie calls out, "Look," while pouring water from a container.	Interpret and respond to play initiation	Maximum support: directing and modeling	Reinforce cue: what to do— "Take hand"— and what to say—"Look"	Orienting
Luna immediately gravitates to the water table and grabs the container from Melanie's hand and begins pouring water over her fingers.	Recognize play initiation	Minimum support: standing by		

(continued)

TABLE 7.2. (*continued*)

Play scenario	Monitoring play initiations	Scaffolding play	Social-communication guidance	Play guidance
Mother says, "That's Luna's way of telling you that she likes playing in the water with you. Maybe you can get a different container and pour it over a baby doll—to wash the doll's hair."	Interpret and respond to play initiation	Intermediate support: verbal and visual cueing		Parallel play/joint focus
Melanie and Katie both pick up baby dolls and pretend to wash them. Luna looks over and reaches out and touches Katie's doll.	Recognize play initiation	Minimum support: standing by		
Mother hands a doll to Luna and says, "Here's a doll for you. Do you want to wash the doll, too?"	Interpret and respond to play initiation	Maximum support: directing and modeling		Parallel play/joint focus
Luna picks up the doll and dunks it head first in the water and repeats this action several times.	Recognize play initiation	Minimum support: standing by		
Mother says, "Look, the baby is diving in the water. Let's all make our baby dolls dive in the water like that."	Interpret and respond to play initiation	Intermediate support: verbal and visual cueing		Imitation: mirroring
Katie and Melanie imitate Luna's actions. Luna takes notice and begins to giggle, which catches on—the three girls all giggle in unison as they dunk their baby dolls in and out of the water.		Minimum support: standing by		
Katie extends the script by saying that her baby is hungry. She pretends to feed the doll with a baby bottle. Melanie imitates Katie and feeds her doll with a second bottle. A moment later, Luna picks up a third baby bottle and holds it to her doll's lips.				

Note. From Wolfberg (2003). Copyright 2003 by Autism Asperger Publishing Co. Reprinted by permission.

currently receives special education support services in an integrated pre-school and home-based program. She is described as having an aloof social style. She tends to ignore or avoid peers in social situations. She generally wanders on the periphery of peer groups when they congregate around play activities.

Luna has a particular fascination with water. She enjoys spending time in the bathtub pouring water in and out of containers. She also plays for long periods at the sink, running water through her fingers and over objects. Luna is nonverbal, but she is beginning to use pictures to express her needs and make simple requests.

Luna participates in an IPG at home with two expert players from her preschool class. The play groups meet twice a week for an hour in a play area set up in the living room. On sunny days they often move the group outdoors. Luna's mother and home-based therapist alternate days taking the lead as play guide.

The focus of the intervention is on maximizing Luna's development in the following areas: (1) representational play with an emphasis on functional object play, (2) social play with an emphasis on establishing parallel play with peers, (3) social-communicative competence with an emphasis on establishing joint attention by initiating and responding more effectively, and (4) expanding and diversifying her repertoire of play interests.

RESEARCH SUMMARY AND FUTURE DIRECTIONS

A series of experimental and exploratory studies have been carried out to evaluate the efficacy of the IPG model (see Table 7.3 for a summary of selected studies that support IPG practices). Much of this research has focused on documenting the effect of the intervention on the novice players' (i.e., children with ASD) development of play along social and cognitive dimensions, as well as the possible influences that shaped their experiences (Lantz, Nelson, & Loftin, 2004; Mikaelian, 2003; O'Connor, 1999; Wolfberg, 1988, 1994, 1999; Wolfberg & Schuler, 1992, 1993; Yang, Wolfberg, Wu, & Hwu, 2003; Zercher, Hunt, Schuler, & Webster, 2001). In addition to evaluating outcomes for novice players, we have examined expert players' attitudes, perceptions, and experiences participating in IPG (Gonsier-Gerdin, 1993; Wolfberg, 1994, 1999; Yang et al., 2003), practitioner (teachers and therapists) perceptions and experience of facilitating IPGs for the children, as well as themselves (Lantz et al., 2004; O'Connor, 1999; Wolfberg & Schuler, 1992), and parent perceptions of the impact of the intervention on their children with ASD (Lantz et al., 2004; Mikaelian, 2003; Wolfberg & Schuler, 1993; Yang et al., 2003; Zercher et al., 2001).

General findings and hypotheses educed from the accumulated data support the efficacy of the IPG model in promoting social and representational forms of play in children of various ages and abilities on the autism spectrum. Although progress varied relative to participants' initial developmental levels, the evidence suggests that the children generated more spontaneous, diverse, and complex forms of play along social and cognitive dimensions than they had exhibited prior to the implementation of the intervention. Specifically, decreases in isolate and stereotypic play were noted, along with collateral gains in increasingly socially coordinated play (parallel and common focus/goal) and representational play (functional and symbolic/pretend). Qualitative analyses of amassed language samples also indicate that substantive gains were made by those children who entered our play groups with largely stereotypic speech. Although it is not feasible to determine which components of the intervention model were most pertinent to the observed changes (because the IPG model specifically incorporates a selection of evidence-based practices), the collected data further suggest that the intervention as a whole yielded generalized and socially valued gains.

Consistent with the play-related intervention studies reviewed in this chapter, these cumulative findings suggest that children with ASD are capable of improving their social interaction, communication, and play with explicit adult guidance and peer-mediated support. The system of support provided through guided participation in play with typical peers apparently helped to arouse and nurture the children's social and symbolic growth. Immersion in joint play with more competent peers allowed for the fine-tuning of imitation skills, the practice of more advanced forms of play and language, and the contextualization of stereotypic behavior (including echolalic speech) that might otherwise have been perceived as deviant.

Commensurate with claims made by Vygotsky (1932/1978) and Bruner (1982), one might speculate that social reciprocity propels symbolic growth within the context of culturally relevant activity. The IPG model created a cultural milieu with the potential to counteract the deficits in imagination and symbolic thinking that may be secondary to limited social experience in children with ASD. As addressed earlier in this chapter and discussed in detail by Jordan (2003), one might infer that cognitive deficiencies are an outgrowth of the social isolation rather than intrinsic to the autistic syndrome. To quote Jordan (2003): "The possibility that social play can be both a result of, and a means towards, imaginative play, suggests the ontology of autism involves a transactional relationship between social and cognitive difficulties rather than a single primary root" (p. 356).

The collected studies reported here are limited in terms of both sample size and methodologies. First, six of the seven reported studies focus on a relatively small number of children with ASD who participated in IPGs. The one study that reports on larger numbers of participants does not fea-

TABLE 7.3. Summary of Selected Studies Focused on Integrated Play Groups

Investigation	Focal participants	Play group composition	Setting	Methods	Findings
Wolfberg (1988) (pilot study)	4 novice players—2 boys/2 girls (ages 9 to 10 years) with mild to severe autism	2 play groups of 5 children (2 novices/3 experts per group), mixed ages ranging from 8 to 10 years	30-minute IPG sessions/2 x per week for school term (9 months) in elementary school; led by special educator	Preliminary videotape observational analysis of social interaction and play with peers	Initial observations: • Gains in social interaction and play detected for each novice within first 3 months • Generalization to other social settings involving peers noted at end of school year *Note:* Tentative findings inspired large-scale investigation to field-test and refine the IPG model.
Wolfberg & Schuler (1992) (large-scale investigation)	38 novice players—(ages 5 to 11 years) with mild to severe autism	20+ play groups of 3 to 5 children (varied combinations novice and expert players), ages 5–11 years	IPG sessions with varied time frames carried out in 10 elementary school sites; led by teachers and speech and language therapists	Evaluation of 3-year model demonstration project using quantitative (see Wolfberg & Schuler, 1993) and qualitative (survey/interview) methods to validate IPG model and its impact on children with autism	Teachers/speech–language–pathologists reported: • Children interacted more naturally in IPGs than in other integrated situations • Novice and expert players become like a family • Greater reciprocity among novice and expert players • Certain novice players required extra support to "fit in" • Rituals are an important part of the play group experience for children • Play groups are therapeutic • Play groups offer children a "safe haven" to play with little outside pressure • Play groups provide more opportunities for social relationships than simply mainstreaming students in general education classes

Wolfberg & Schuler (1993)	3 novice players—boys (age 7 years) with moderate to severe autism	3 play groups of 5 children (2 novices/3 experts per group), all similar in age	30 minute IPG sessions/2 x per week for school term (9 months) in elementary school; led by special educator	Combined quantitative (multiple-baseline) and qualitative (observation/interview) measures to evaluate impact on social and cognitive dimensions of play, language, and social validity	Within first 3 months, each novice exhibited: • Decreases in isolate and stereotyped play • Increases in social play levels • Increases in functional and symbolic play • More diversified play End of term: • Language gains noted in two of the three children • Skills maintained when adult support withdrawn • Skills generalized to other peers, settings, and social activity contexts • Parents noted carryover of skills to home setting
Wolfberg (1994, 1999)	3 novice players—1 girl/ 2 boys (ages spanned 9 to 11 years while participating in IPG) with mild to moderate autism	2 play groups of 5 children (2 novices/3 experts per group), mixed ages ranging from 8 to 11 years	30-minute IPG sessions/2 x per week for 2 school terms (18 months) in elementary school; led by special educator	Longitudinal ethnographic case analyses of social relations with peers and symbolic representation in play, language, writing, and drawing	Novices showed similar developmental progression over time: • From isolate to more interactive/reciprocal peer play • From stereotyped/presymbolic to representational (functional/pretend) play • Parallel symbolic transformations in language, writing, and drawing • More diverse/complex forms of play in social vs. independent activity • Higher level social capacities emerged before higher level symbolic capacities • Combination of child characteristics (novice and expert) and social factors influenced changes

(continued)

TABLE 7.3. (*continued*)

Investigation	Focal participants	Play group composition	Setting	Methods	Findings
O'Connor (1999)	10 practitioners (7 preschool–kindergarten and 3 elementary special educators and speech and language therapists)	10+ play groups of 3 to 5 children (varied combinations novice and expert players), ages 3–11 years	IPG sessions with varied time frames carried out in preschool and elementary schools	As a part of a larger study, questionnaire/ interviews included focus on play guide perceptions of benefits for novice players	Play guide perceptions of novice players: • Showed outward signs of sheer enjoyment while participating in IPG • Increases in eye contact, watching, and imitating peers • Increases in social initiation and responsiveness • Increases in symbolic play levels • Increases in communication • Greater diversity of spontaneous play interests
Zercher et al. (2001) (replication of 1993 study)	2 novice players—twin boys (6 years) with mild to moderate autism	1 group of 5 children (2 novices/3 experts), mixed ages ranging from 5 to 11 years	30-minute weekly sessions for 20 weeks in community-based setting (Sunday School class) led by doctoral student	Quantitative (multiple-baseline) and qualitative (observation/ interview) measures to evaluate impact on social interaction, communication/ language and play	Novices exhibited: • Increases in shared social attention to objects • Increases in symbolic play acts • Increases in verbal utterances • Skills maintained when adult support withdrawn • Skills generalized to home setting • Results socially validated by parents

Study	Participants	Setting/Dosage	Measures	Outcomes
Mikaelian (2003)	3 novice—2 boys/1 girl (ages 3–5 years) players with moderate autism	3 groups of 3 children (1 novice/ 2 experts, including 1 sibling) mixed ages ranging from 3 to 7 years	30–60 minute sessions/1x per week for 19 weeks in home	Quantitative (multiple-baseline) measures to evaluate impact on social communication and language and qualitative (interview) social validation measure	Novice players exhibited: • Increases in frequency of communicative utterances • Increases in verbal interactions • Increases in diversity of functions of communication • Increases in nonverbal and verbal interactions between novices and experts • Skills maintained when adult support withdrawn • Results socially validated by parents
Yang et al. (2003)	2 novices—1 girl/1 boy (ages 6–7 years) with mild to moderate autism	2 groups of 5 children (2 novices/3 experts, including 1 sibling) mixed ages ranging from 6 to 8 years	40–60 minute sessions/2x per week for 6 months/1 group in home/1 group in school in Tapei, Taiwan	Combined quantitative (multiple-baseline) and qualitative (observation/ interview) measures to evaluate impact on social and cognitive dimensions of play and social validity	Novices exhibited: • Decreases in isolate play • Increases in social play levels (parallel and common focus) • Increases in cognitive play levels (functional and symbolic/pretend) • Skills maintained when adult support withdrawn • Parents noted generalized improvements in their children's social and symbolic play • Cross-cultural implications with IPG implemented in Taiwan where dominant language culture is Mandarin/Chinese

ture the tight levels of control needed for empirical validation. Finally, those studies that do apply formalized controls employ single-subject methodologies. The limitations of these methodologies lie in the fact that they reduce the complexities of play into a single measure, as described in our introduction dealing with the challenges of measuring play. The rich complexities of play are better captured by qualitative methods, which, however, do not provide direct evidence of the kinds of causal links required in traditional empirical studies. Nevertheless, such methods serve to complement and extend findings through triangulation of multiple data sources. The strength of combined methods opens up new research questions and avenues of study.

In future research, it would be pertinent to carry out larger scale replications. In doing so, a number of questions warrant further investigation through multiple modes of quantitative and qualitative inquiry. A first set of questions deals with determining the feasibility of establishing similar patterns of social and representational play development within the context of the play intervention. It would be relevant to examine the timing and order in which the social and symbolic behavior changes occur. For instance, do social gains precede, parallel, or follow the gains that can equally be found in functional and symbolic play? The answer may help to elucidate whether the child needs to learn to play in order to socialize or to socialize in order to play.

Future research might also address questions pertaining to the extent to which speech, language, and overall communication skills can be advanced through guided participation in peer play. Closely related to this is a need to focus on matters of affect. Although we informally noted improvements in communicative initiations, spontaneous language use, and overall affect in many participants, these changes would need to be validated through systematic investigations in a larger sample of children. A phenomenon that deserves special attention pertains to transformations from nonfocused and delayed forms of echolalia to more communicative and mitigated forms and, eventually, into true language (for a more in-depth discussion, see Schuler, 2003). It seemed as if the peer interactions served to remove the literal and rigid edges from the echoing behaviors, which allowed for more functional communication within a meaningful context.

Future research might also examine whether observed gains in both the social and cognitive dimensions of play are paralleled by changes in mentalizing skills. Our own clinical impressions suggest that the participating children with ASD became more aware of and displayed a greater sensitivity to the perspectives of others. Is it possible that the coconstruction of pretend-play scenarios allows for the formation of a theory of mind? Formalized tests specifically designed to assess such mentalizing skills could be supplemented by other, more naturalistic measures.

Another set of questions deals with identifying configurations of support, guidance, and/or instruction needed to bring about optimal levels of play in children with ASD. A closer examination of how adults and peers effectively scaffold with individual children who present differing developmental profiles may help to elucidate the type and amount of structure that is needed at different points in a child's development. Future investigations are also needed to further our understanding of which configurations of support best facilitate opportunities for children with ASD to more fully participate in their peer culture. The extent to which guided peer play experiences contribute to long-term peer relationships, particularly friendships, would be especially important to establish. More extensive research would also be needed to answer questions concerning the interdependence of social mediated support, children's play culture, and various domains of social and symbolic growth. Further clarification of these interrelationships would enhance our theoretical understanding of autism and the design of meaningful interventions in education, psychology, and related therapies.

REFERENCES

American Psychiatric Association. (2000). *Diagnostic and statistical manual of mental disorders* (4th ed., text rev.). Washington, DC: Author.

Baron-Cohen, S. (1987). Autism and symbolic play. *British Journal of Developmental Psychology, 5*(2), 139–148.

Baron-Cohen, S. (1989). Joint-attention deficits in autism: Towards a cognitive analysis. *Development and Psychopathology, 1*, 185–189.

Beckman, P. J., & Kohl, F. L. (1984). The effects of social and isolate toys on the interactions and play of integrated and nonintegrated groups of preschoolers. *Education and Training of the Mentally Retarded, 19*, 169–175.

Bednersh, F., & Peck, C. A. (1986). Assessing social environments: Effects of peer characteristics on the social behavior of children with severe handicaps. *Child Study Journal, 16*(4), 315–329.

Bloom, L., & Tinker, E. (2001). The intentionality model and language acquisition: Engagement, effort, and the essential tension in development. *Monographs of the Society for Research in Child Development, 66*(4, Serial No. 267).

Boucher, J., & Wolfberg, P. J. (2003). Play [Special issue]. *Autism: The International Journal of Research and Practice, 7*(4).

Brown, A. L., & Campione, J. C. (1990). Communities of learning and thinking: A context by any other name. *Human Development, 21*, 108–125.

Bruner, J. S. (1982). The organization of action, and the nature of adult–infant transaction. In E. F. Tronick (Ed.), *Social interchange in infancy: Affect, cognition, and communication* (pp. 25–35). Baltimore: University Park Press.

Casner, M. W., & Marks, S. F. (1984, April). *Playing with autistic children.* Paper presented at the annual convention of the Council for Exceptional Children, Washington, DC.

Charman, T., & Baird, G. (2002). Practitioner review: Diagnosis of autistic spectrum disorder in 2- and 3-year-old children. *Journal of Child Psychology & Psychiatry 43*, 289–305.

Charman, T., & Baron-Cohen, S. (1997). Brief report: Prompted pretend play in autism. *Journal of Autism and Developmental Disorders 27*, 325–332.

Corsaro, W. A. (1992). Interpretive reproduction in children's peer cultures. *Social Psychology Quarterly, 55*, 160–177.

Dawson, G., & Adams, A. (1984). Imitation and social responsiveness in autistic children. *Journal of Abnormal Child Psychology, 12*, 209–225.

Dewey, D., Lord, C., & Magill, J. (1988). Qualitative assessment of the effect of play materials in dyadic peer interactions of children with autism. *Canadian Journal of Psychology, 42*(2), 242–260.

Dodge, K. A., Schlundt, D. C., Schocken, I., & Delugach, J. D. (1983). Social competence and children's sociometric status: The role of peer group entry strategies. *Merrill–Palmer Quarterly, 29*, 309–336.

Eckerman, C. O., & Stein, M. R. (1982). The toddler's emerging interactive skills. In K. H. Rubin & H. S. Ross (Eds.), *Peer relationships and social skills in childhood* (pp. 41–71). New York: Springer-Verlag.

Ferrara, C., & Hill, S. (1980). The responsiveness of autistic children to the predictability of social and nonsocial toys. *Journal of Autism and Developmental Disorders, 10*, 51–57.

Frith, U. (1989). *Autism: Explaining the enigma.* Oxford, UK: Blackwell.

Garvey, C. (1977). *Play.* Cambridge, MA: Harvard University Press.

Goldstein, H., & Cisar, C. L. (1992). Promoting interaction during sociodramatic play: Teaching scripts to typical preschoolers and classmates with disabilities. *Journal of Applied Behavior Analysis, 25*, 265–280.

Gonsier-Gerdin, J. (1993). *Elementary school children's perspectives on peers with disabilities in the context of integrated play groups: "They're not really disabled. They're like plain kids."* Unpublished manuscript, University of California, Berkeley.

Greenspan, S. I., & Wieder, S. (1997a). An integrated developmental approach to interventions for young children with severe difficulties in relating and communicating. *Zero to Three, 17*, 5–18.

Greenspan, S. I., & Wieder, S. (1997b). Developmental patterns and outcomes in infants and children with disorders in relating and communication: A chart review of 200 cases of children with autistic spectrum diagnoses. *Journal of Developmental and Learning Disorders, 1*(1), 87–141.

Hanson, M. J., Wolfberg, P. J., Zercher, C., Morgan, M., Gutierrez, S., Barnwell, D., et al. (1998). The culture of inclusion: Recognizing diversity at multiple levels. *Early Childhood Research Quarterly, 13*(1), 185–209.

Haring, T. G., & Lovinger, L. (1989). Promoting social interaction through teaching generalized play initiation responses to preschool children with autism. *Journal of the Association for Persons with Severe Handicaps, 14*(1), 58–67.

Harris, P. (1993). Pretending and planning. In S. Baron-Cohen, H. Tager-Flusberg, & D. J. Cohen (Eds.), *Understanding other minds: Perspectives from autism* (pp. 228–246). Oxford, UK: Oxford University Press.

Hartup, W. W. (1979). The social worlds of childhood. *American Psychologist, 34,* 944–950.

Hartup, W. W., & Sancilio, M. F. (1986). Children's friendships. In E. Schopler & G. B. Mesibov (Eds.), *Social behavior in autism* (pp. 61–80). New York: Plenum Press.

Hauge, D. (1988). *Using child initiated object manipulations to develop social, communicative responsiveness in children with autism and severe disabilities.* Unpublished master's thesis, San Francisco State University.

Heath, S. B. (1989). The learner as cultural member. In M. L. Rice & R. L. Schiefelbusch (Eds.), *The teachability of language* (pp. 330–350). Baltimore: Brookes.

Heinrichs, R. (2003). *Perfect targets: Asperger syndrome and bullying: Practical solutions for surviving the social world.* Shawnee Mission, KS: Autism Asperger Publishing.

Ingersoll, B., & Schreibman, L. (2002, November). *The effect of reciprocal imitation training on imitative and spontaneous pretend play in children with autism.* Paper presented at the International Meeting for Research on Autism, Orlando, FL.

Jahr, E., Eldevik, S., & Eikeseth, S. (2000). Teaching children with autism to initiate and sustain cooperative play. *Research in Developmental Disabilities, 21,* 151–169.

Jarrold, C. (2003). A review of research into pretend play in autism. *Autism: The International Journal of Research and Practice, 7*(4), 379–390.

Jarrold, C., Boucher, J., & Smith, P. (1996). Generativity deficits in pretend play in autism. *British Journal of Developmental Psychology, 14,* 275–300.

Jordan, R. (2003). Social play and autistic spectrum disorders. *Autism: The International Journal of Research and Practice, 7*(4), 347–360.

Kalmanson, B., & Pekarsky, J. H. (1987, Winter). Infant–parent psychotherapy with an autistic toddler. *Infant Mental Health Journal, 8*(4), 330–355.

Kaufmann, B. N. (1976). *Son rise.* New York: Warner.

Koegel, L. K., Koegel, R. L., Harrower, J. K., & Carter, C. M. (1999). Pivotal response intervention: Overview of approach. *Journal of the Association for Persons with Severe Handicaps, 24,* 174–185.

Koegel, R. L., Dyer, K., & Bell, L. K. (1987). The influence of child-preferred activities on autistic children's social behavior. *Journal of Applied Behavior Analysis, 20,* 243–252.

Koegel, R. L., Firestone, P. B., Kramme, K. W., & Dunlap, G. (1974). Increasing spontaneous play by suppressing self-stimulation in autistic children. *Journal of Applied Behavior Analysis, 7,* 521–528.

Kok, A. J., Kong, T. Y., & Bernard-Opitz, V. (2002). A comparison of the effects of structured play and facilitated play approaches on preschoolers with autism: A case study. *Autism: The International Journal of Research and Practice, 6,* 181–196.

Lantz, J. F., Nelson, J. M., & Loftin, R. L. (2004). Guiding children with autism in play: Applying the integrated play group model in school settings. *Exceptional Children, 37*(2), 8–14.

Lave, J., & Wenger, E. (1991). *Situated learning: Legitimate peripheral participation.* Cambridge, UK: Cambridge University Press.

Leaf, R., & McEachin, J. (1999). *A work in progress: Behavior management strategies and a curriculum for intensive behavioral treatment of autism.* New York: DRL.

Leslie, A. M. (1987). Pretense and representation: The origins of "theory of mind." *Psychological Review, 94,* 412–426.

Lewis, V., & Boucher, J. (1988). Spontaneous, instructed and elicited play in relatively able autistic children. *British Journal of Developmental Psychology, 6*(4), 325–339.

Libby, S., Powell, S., Messer, D., & Jordan, R. (1998). Spontaneous play in children with autism: A reappraisal. *Journal of Autism and Developmental Disorders, 28,* 487–497.

Lifter, K., Sulzer-Azaroff, B., Anderson, S., & Cowdery, G. (1993). Teaching play activities to preschool children with disabilities: The importance of developmental considerations. *Journal of Early Intervention, 17,* 139–159.

Lord, C., & Hopkins, M. J. (1986). The social behavior of autistic children with younger and same-age nonhandicapped peers. *Journal of Autism and Developmental Disorders, 16*(3), 249–262.

Lord, C., & Magill, J. (1989). Methodological and theoretical issues in studying peer-directed behavior and autism. In G. Dawson (Eds.), *Autism: Nature, diagnosis, and treatment* (pp. 326–345). New York: Guilford Press.

Lovaas, O. I. (1987). Behavioral treatment and normal educational and intellectual functioning in young autistic children. *Journal of Consulting and Clinical Psychology, 55,* 3–9.

Mahler, M. (1952). On child psychosis in schizophrenia: Autistic and symbiotic infantile psychosis. In R. S. Eissler, A. Freud, H. Hartmann, & K. Kris (Eds.), *Psychoanalytic study of the child* (pp. 265–305). New York: International Universities Press.

Maurice, C., Green, G., & Luce, S. C. (1996). *Behavioral intervention for young children with autism: A manual for parents and professionals.* Austin, TX: PRO-ED.

McCune-Nicolich, L. A. (1981). Toward symbolic functioning: Structure of early pretend games and potential parallels with language. *Child Development, 52,* 785–797.

McHale, S. (1983). Social interactions of autistic and nonhandicapped children during free play. *American Journal of Orthopsychiatry, 53*(1), 81–91.

Meyer, L. H., Fox, A., Schermer, A., Ketelsen, D., Montan, N., Maley, K., et al. (1987). The effects of teacher intrusion on social play interactions between children with autism and their nonhandicapped peers. *Journal of Autism and Developmental Disorders, 17*(3), 315–332.

Meyer, L. H., Park, H., Grenot-Scheyer, M., Schwartz, I. S., & Harry, B. (Eds.). (1998). *Making friends: The influences of culture and development.* Baltimore: Brookes.

Mikaelian, B. (2003). *Increasing language through sibling and peer support play.* Unpublished master's thesis, San Francisco State University.

Mouritsen, F. (1996). *Play culture: Essays on child culture, play and narratives.* Unpublished manuscript, Odense University, Denmark.

Mundy, P., Sigman, M., Ungerer, J., & Sherman, T. (1987). Non-verbal communication and play correlates of language development in autistic children. *Journal of Autism and Developmental Disorders, 17,* 349–364.

National Research Council, Division of Behavioral and Social Sciences and Education. (2001). *Educating children with autism: Committee on educational interventions for children with autism.* Washington, DC: National Academies Press.

Newman, B., Reinecke, D. R., & Meinberg, D. L. (2000). Self-management of varied responding in three students with autism. *Behavioral Interventions, 15,* 145–151.

Nuzzolo-Gomez, R., Leonard, M. A., Ortiz, E., Rivera, C. M., & Greer, R. D. (2002). Teaching children with autism to prefer books or toys over stereotypy or passivity. *Journal of Positive Behavior Interventions, 4,* 60–67.

O'Connor, T. (1999). *Teacher perspectives of facilitated play in integrated play groups.* Unpublished master's thesis, San Francisco State University.

Odom, S., & Strain, P. (1984). Peer-mediated approaches to promoting children's social interaction: A review. *American Journal of Orthopsychiatry, 54*(4), 544–557.

Oke, N. J., & Schreibman, L. (1990). Training social initiations to a high-functioning autistic child: Assessment of collateral behavior change and generalization in a case study. *Journal of Autism and Developmental Disorders, 20,* 479–497.

Parker, J. G., & Gottman, J. M. (1989). Social and emotional development in a relational context: Friendship interaction from early childhood to adolescence. In T. J. Berndt & G. W. Ladd (Eds.), *Peer relationships in child development* (pp. 95–131). New York: Wiley.

Parten, M. B. (1932). Social participation among preschool children. *Journal of Abnormal and Social Psychology, 27,* 243–269.

Peck, C. A., Schuler, A. L., Tomlinson, C., Theimer, R. K., & Haring, T. (1984). *The social competence curriculum project: A guide to instructional communicative interactions.* Santa Barbara: University of California, Special Education Research Institute.

Phyfe-Perkins, E. (1980). Children's behavior in preschool settings: A review of research concerning the influence of the physical environment. In L. G. Katz (Eds.), *Current topics in early childhood education* (pp. 91–125). Norwood, NJ: Ablex.

Piaget, J. (1962). *Play, dreams, and imitation in childhood.* New York: Norton.

Pierce, K., & Schreibman, L. (1997). Using peer trainers to promote social behavior in autism: Are they effective at enhancing multiple social modalities? *Focus on Autism and Other Developmental Disabilities, 12,* 207–218.

Prizant, B., Wetherby, A., Rubin, E., Rydell, P., & Laurent, A. (2003). The SCERTS Model: A family-centered, transactional approach to enhancing communication and socioemotional abilities of young children with ASD. *Infants and Young Children, 16*(4), 296–316.

Prizant, B., Wetherby, A., & Rydell, P. J. (2000). Communication issues for young children with autism spectrum disorders. In A. Wetherby & B. Prizant (Eds.), *Autism spectrum disorders: A transactional developmental perspective* (pp. 193–224). Baltimore: Brookes.

Roeyers, H. (1996). The influence of nonhandicapped peers on the social interactions of children with a pervasive developmental disorder. *Journal of Autism and Developmental Disorders, 11,* 61–70.

Rogers, S. J., Hall, T., Osaki, D., Reaven, J., & Herbison, J. (2000). The Denver model: A comprehensive, integrated educational approach to young children with autism and their families. In J. S. Handleman & S. L. Harris (Eds.), *Preschool education programs for children with autism* (2nd ed., pp. 95–133). Austin, TX: PRO-ED.

Rogoff, B. (1990). *Apprenticeship in thinking.* New York: Oxford University Press.

Romanczyk, R. G., Diament, C., Goren, E. R., Trunell, G., & Harris, S. L. (1975). Increasing isolate and social play in severely disturbed children: Intervention and postintervention effectiveness. *Journal of Autism and Childhood Schizophrenia, 5*(1), 57–70.

Ross, H. S., & Kay, D. A. (1980). The origins of social games. In K. H. Rubin (Eds.), *Children's play* (pp. 17–31). San Francisco: Jossey-Bass.

Rubin, K. H., Fein, G. G., & Vandenberg, B. (1983). Play. In E. M. Hetherington (Eds.), *Handbook of child psychology: Socialization, personality, and social development* (pp. 694–759). New York: Wiley.

Rutter, M. (1978). Diagnosis and definition. In M. Rutter & E. Schopler (Eds.), *Autism: A reappraisal of concepts and treatment* (pp. 1–25). New York: Plenum Press.

Sainato, D. M., Goldstein, H., & Strain, P. S. (1992). Effects of self-evaluation on preschool children's use of social interaction strategies with their classmates with autism. *Journal of Applied Behavior Analysis, 25,* 127–141.

Santarcangelo, S., Dyer, K., & Luce, S. C. (1987). Generalized reduction of disruptive behavior in unsupervised settings through specific toy training. *Journal of the Association for Persons with Severe Handicaps, 12,* 38–44.

Schuler, A. L. (2003). Beyond echoplaylia: Promoting language in children with autism. *Autism: The International Journal of Research and Practice, 7*(4), 455–469.

Schuler, A. L., & Wolfberg, P. J. (2000). Promoting peer socialization and play: The art of scaffolding. In A. Wetherby & B. Prizant (Eds.), *Autism spectrum disorders: A transactional developmental perspective* (pp. 251–279). Baltimore: Brookes.

Schwandt, W. L., Pieropan, K., Glesne, H., Lundahl, A., Foley, D., & Larsson, E. V. (2002, May). *Using video modeling to teach generalized toy play.* Paper presented at the annual meeting of the Association for Behavior Analysis, Toronto, Ontario, Canada.

Selmer-Olsen, I. (1993). Children's culture and adult presentation of this culture. *International Play Journal, 1,* 191–202.

Shearer, D. D., Kohler, F. W., Buchan, K. A., & McCullough, K. M. (1996). Promoting independent interactions between preschoolers with autism and their nondisabled peers: An analysis of self-monitoring, *Early Education and Development, 7,* 205–220.

Sherrat, D. (2002). Developing pretend play in children with autism: A case study. *Autism: The International Journal of Research and Practice, 6*(2), 169–179.

Sigman, M., & Ruskin, E. (1999). Continuity and change in the social competence of children with autism, Down syndrome, and developmental delays. *Monographs of the Society for Research in Child Development, 64,* 1–114.

Sigman, M., & Ungerer, J. A. (1984). Cognitive and language skills in autistic, mentally retarded and normal children. *Developmental Psychology, 20,* 293–302.

Smilansky, S. (1968). *The effects of sociodramatic play on disadvantaged preschool children.* New York: Wiley.

Smith, M. J. (2001). *Teaching play skills to autistic children.* New York: DRL.

Smith, P. K., & Connolly, K. J. (1980). *The ecology of preschool behavior.* Cambridge, MA: Cambridge University Press.

Stahmer, A. C. (1995). Teaching symbolic play to children with autism using pivotal response training. *Journal of Autism and Developmental Disorders, 25,* 123–141.

Stahmer, A. C., Ingersoll, B., & Carter, C. (2003). Behavioral approaches to promoting play. *Autism: The International Journal of Research and Practice, 7*(4), 401–413.

Stahmer, A. C., & Schreibman, L. (1992). Teaching children with autism appropriate play in unsupervised environments: Using a self-management treatment package. *Journal of Applied Behavior Analysis, 25,* 447–459.

Strain, P., & Kohler, F. (1998). Peer-mediated social interventions for young children with autism. *Seminars in Speech and Language, 19,* 391–405.

Sugarman, S. (1982). Developmental change in early representational intelligence: Evidence from spatial classification strategies and related verbal expressions. *Cognitive Psychology, 14,* 410–449.

Taylor, B. A., Levin, L., & Jasper, S. (1999). Increasing play-related statements in children with autism toward siblings: Effects of video modeling. *Journal of Developmental and Physical Disabilities, 11,* 253–264.

Thorp, D. M., Stahmer, A. C., & Schreibman, L. (1995). Teaching sociodramatic play to children with autism using pivotal response training. *Journal of Autism and Developmental Disorders, 25,* 265–282.

Tiegerman, E., & Primavera, L. (1981). Object manipulation: An interactional strategy with autistic children. *Journal of Autism and Developmental Disorders, 11*(4), 427–438.

Tilton, J. R., & Ottinger, D. R. (1964). Comparison of toy play behavior of autistic, retarded and normal children. *Psychological Reports, 15,* 967–975.

Tryon, A. S., & Keane, S. P. (1986). Promoting imitative play through generalized observational learning in autistic-like children. *Journal of Abnormal Child Psychology, 14,* 537–549.

Van Berckelaer-Onnes, I. A. (2003). Promoting early play. *Autism: The International Journal of Research and Practice, 7*(4), 415–423.

Van Berckelaer-Onnes, I. A., & Kwakkel-Scheffer, J. C. (1996). Spelinterventies voor kinderen met een autistische stoornis. *Kinder en Jeugd Psychotherapie, 23*(2/3), 77–93.

Vygotsky, L. S. (1966). Play and its role in the mental development of the child. *Soviet Psychology, 12,* 6–18. (Original work published 1933)

Vygotsky, L. S. (1978). *Mind in society: The development of higher psychological processes.* Cambridge, MA: Harvard University Press. (Original work published 1932)

Westby, C. E. (2000). A scale for assessing development of children's play. In K. Gitlin-Weiner, A. Sandgrund, & C. E. Schaefer (Eds.), *Play diagnosis and assessment* (2nd ed., pp. 131–161). New York: Wiley.

Wieder, S., & Greenspan, S. I. (2003). Climbing the symbolic ladder in the DIR model through floor time/interactive play. *Autism: The International Journal of Research and Practice, 7*(4), 425–435.

Williams, E. (2003). A comparative review of early forms of object-directed play and parent–infant play in typical infants and young children with autism. *Autism: The International Journal of Research and Practice, 7*(4), 361–377.

Williams, E., Costall, A., & Reddy, V. (1999). Children with autism experience problems with both objects and people. *Journal of Autism and Developmental Disorders, 29*(5), 367–378.

Williams, E., Reddy, V., & Costall, A. (2001). Taking a closer look at functional play in children with autism. *Journal of Autism and Developmental Disorders, 31*(1), 67–77.

Wing, L., & Gould, J. (1979). Severe impairments of social interaction and associated abnormalities in children: Epidemiology and classification. *Journal of Autism and Developmental Disorders, 9*, 11–29.

Wing, L., Gould, J., Yeates, S. R., & Brierly, L. M. (1977). Symbolic play in severely mentally retarded and autistic children. *Journal of Child Psychology and Psychiatry, 18*, 167–178.

Wolfberg, P. J. (1988). *Integrated play groups for children with autism and related disorders.* Unpublished master's thesis, San Francisco State University.

Wolfberg, P. J. (1994). Case illustrations of emerging social relations and symbolic activity in children with autism through supported peer play (Doctoral dissertation, University of California at Berkeley with San Francisco State University). *Dissertation Abstracts International,* No. 9505068, *55*(11-A), 3476.

Wolfberg, P. J. (1999). *Play and imagination in children with autism.* New York: Teachers College Press.

Wolfberg, P. J. (2003) *Peer play and the autism spectrum: The art of guiding children's socialization and imagination.* Shawnee, KS: Autism Asperger Publishing.

Wolfberg, P. J., & Schuler, A. L. (1992). *Integrated play groups project: Final evaluation report* (Report No. HO86D90016). Washington, DC: Department of Education, Office of Special Education and Rehabilitation Services.

Wolfberg, P. J., & Schuler, A. L. (1993). Integrated play groups: A model for promoting the social and cognitive dimensions of play in children with autism. *Journal of Autism and Developmental Disorders, 23*(3), 467–489.

Wolfberg, P. J., Zercher, C., Lieber, J., Capell, K., Matias, S. G., Hanson, M., et al. (1999). "Can I play with you?": Peer culture in inclusive preschool programs. *Journal for the Association of Persons with Severe Handicaps, 24*(2), 69–84.

Yang, T., Wolfberg, P. J., Wu, S., & Hwu, P. (2003). Supporting children on the autism spectrum in peer play at home and school: Piloting the integrated play groups model in Taiwan. *Autism: The International Journal of Research and Practice, 7*(4), 437–453.

Zercher, C., Hunt, P., Schuler, A. L., & Webster, J. (2001). Increasing joint attention, play and language through peer supported play. *Autism: The International Journal of Research and Practice, 5*, 374–398.

8

Imitation

Some Cues for Intervention Approaches in Autism Spectrum Disorders

JACQUELINE NADEL
NADRA AOUKA

Although we agree easily with the general statement that imitation is not a unitary phenomenon, it is more difficult to take advantage of this perspective with respect to imitation interventions. Is there a developmental sequence that should be followed in designing interventions? Are there basic competencies that are required regardless of the type of imitation being considered? Should stimulation of imitation encourage the functional uses of everyday imitation, or rather focus on the training of complex imitation prompted by the open-sesame words: "Do like me"? Let us note that different aspects of executive functioning are involved in the two conditions: spontaneous imitation is done at will, which supposes the child is able to select specific actions for reproduction and inhibit the reproduction of others; whereas induced imitation does not involve taking such initiative but rather implies the capacity to plan an action without a personal motive (Nadel, 2006). This chapter explores aspects of this multidimensionality approach to understanding imitation with a view to providing pointers for future intervention studies in the imitation field.

Almost all studies of imitation use a "do like me" strategy, with an experimenter demonstrating gestures or actions to imitate. Only a few studies focus on spontaneous imitation and its functional uses. Because imitation is a social behavior with two different functions, those functional studies either deal with imitation in its acquisitive function or with imitation in its communicative function. This radical split does not take account of the fact that, depending on the context in which behaviors are embedded, depending on the partner, depending on the behavior itself, imitation may involve the reproduction of a new action resulting in an acquisitive benefit for the imitator or the reproduction of a familiar action resulting in a communicative benefit for both the imitator and the imitatee. A hierarchical relationship between a child and an adult will likely lead to a use of imitation for an acquisitive purpose, whereas a playful context between two peer partners is more likely to generate conversational turns by alternating imitating and being imitated (Nadel, 2002).

Such a distinction between spontaneous and induced imitation is relevant for typical development and is suggested to be so for the study of children with autism. Evaluations of imitation in children with autism have also more often been carried out with a "do like me" prompt (Dewey, 1993; Hill, 1998; O'Hare, 1999; Kools & Tweedie, 1975). These conditions, however, can be considered to hinder to some extent the evaluation of imitation. Whether or not children with autism show imitative impairments remains a controversial question (Charman & Baron-Cohen, 1994). Children with autism demonstrate capacities to imitate in rich and ecologically valid settings where they can select models to imitate (Nadel & Pézé, 1993), whereas they are often characterized by difficulties in imitation on request (Rogers, Bennetto, McEvoy, & Pennington, 1996; Smith & Bryson, 1998). Due to the executive impairments of these children, imitation without personal motives within such elicited contexts should be especially difficult to perform. A number of imitation scales propose an interesting procedure based on previous observation of children's interests in an attempt to model attractive actions (Schopler & Reichler, 1979; Stone, Ousley, & Littleford, 1997; Uzgiris & Hunt, 1975): Such procedures may lessen the differences between imitative skills displayed at will or demonstrated on request.

The capacity to imitate may also differ according to the kind of action observed. Actions involving objects facilitate imitation, especially when familiar actions are concerned: In this case, objects afford an automatic representation of their functional use (Grèzes & Decety, 2002). Depending on the meaning of the gestures that are imitated, different cerebral activations are found in healthy adults (Decety et al., 1997). Convergent with this finding, imitation by patients with apraxia is affected by the meaning of the task (Dewey, 1993; Goldenberg & Hagmann, 1997). These results support the view that the mechanisms underlying imitative performances are strongly influenced by the affordance of the object used and the meaning of the action observed.

Imitation that does not involve an object may be either meaningful or meaningless. When meaningful, an action without object consists more often in a symbolic or conventional gesture. The mime of an object use, or pantomime, requires the representation of objects and of their possible uses. It is the prototype of imitation tasks aimed at evaluating a child's praxis (Dewey, 1993; Hill, 1998; Kools & Tweedie, 1975; O'Hare, 1999; Rogers et al., 1996). Although it is informative about dyspraxic problems, pantomime taps a range of representational capacities that are not all required in everyday uses of imitation. The "overemphasis on symbolic processes in imitation" has been pointed out by Smith and Bryson (1998, p. 748). Young children, as well as children with developmental disorders or language impairment, perform significantly lower on pantomimes compared with imitation of meaningful actions with objects (Hill, 1998).

To sum up, induced imitation of action with objects involves different mechanisms according to the meaning of the actions performed, and imitation of the mime of an object's use requires additional involvement of symbolic representations. Finally, when induced imitation is concerned, a way to disambiguate imitative performance is to use meaningless gestures. Modeling meaningless gestures offers a unique opportunity to analyze the two important components of imitation that are body knowledge and visual–spatial capacity.

We take as examples of the many aspects of imitation two contrasted sets of studies conducted in our group. In the first set of studies, induced imitation of meaningless gestures was explored, whereas the second set depicts the use of spontaneous imitation in ecologically valid settings. We report on the development of these two aspects of imitation in typical children and in children with autism. We investigate whether children with autism have purposes that may be served by imitation, especially communicative purposes. We explore whether they perform differently when they are requested to imitate. Finally, we exploit these findings in an attempt to find key targets for intervention programs.

INDUCED IMITATION OF MEANINGLESS GESTURES: COMPARATIVE STUDIES

A set of studies was conducted in our group using meaningless hand movements that are without a reference to symbolic processes and that do not involve any object, be it real or evoked. Our first aim was to document the typical development of the capacities involved in the imitation of meaningless gestures. A second aim was to explore, with a population of children with autism, the hypothesis suggested by previous studies (Rogers, 1999; Rogers et al., 1996), according to which a degree of apraxia may account for imitation problems in autism.

Typically developing children and children with autism were presented a neuropsychological task of imitation developed by Goldenberg (1996, 1999). The task consists in imitating three categories of 10 hand movements: imitation of hand positions related to face, imitation of finger configurations, and imitation of finger configurations combined with hand positions (see Figure 8.1). The three categories of movements correspond to different capacities. Hand positions related to face do not allow a visual feedback and reveal body knowledge, the impairment of which is typical of patients with apraxia.

If an impaired representation of the human body is the mechanism that explains the difficulties showed by patients with apraxia when they have to imitate positions of hands relative to their faces (Goldenberg, 1996, 1999), then imitations performed by children of different ages should document the development of their body knowledge.

If a visual–spatial deficit is the mechanism underlying the defective imitation of finger configurations observed with right-brain damage, then this type of gesture may be considered a relevant tool to investigate the development of visual–spatial analysis in young children. Combined ges-

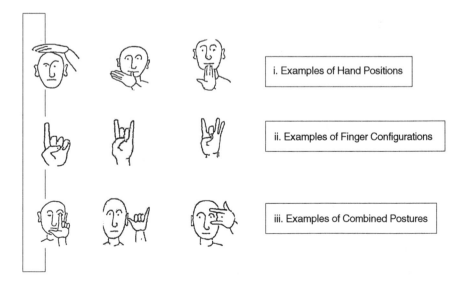

i. Examples of Hand Positions

ii. Examples of Finger Configurations

iii. Examples of Combined Postures

FIGURE 8.1. Examples of (i) hand positions, (ii) finger configurations, and (iii) combined postures in Goldenberg's task. From Goldenberg (1996). Copyright 1996 by BMJ Publishing Group. Reprinted by permission.

tures consisting of finger configurations allied to hand positions related to face require the coordination of the two capacities and thus the achievement of a complex planning of two different and co-occurring operations.

The development of planning has been explored by Bergès and Lézine (1972). The imitation of gestures that requires simple planning, such as opening both hands while facing the experimenter or raising an arm in vertical axis, was found to improve significantly between 3 and 5 years, but gestures that require complex planning, such as joining thumbs and index of both hands in order to frame a given shape, were not performed correctly before age 6. For children with autism, Smith and Bryson (1994, 1998) concluded that the complexity of motor planning may explain the divergence of their results from those of Rogers and colleagues (1996), who used motor sequences of three elements, whereas Smith and Bryson (1994, 1998) limited their modeling to two elements.

The dynamic versus static presentation of gestures is another important parameter in imitation evaluation. With Goldenberg's task, only the trajectories of the hand toward the face are demonstrated, finger configurations being already completed before their presentation. Smith and Bryson (1998) investigated dynamic versus static gestures with autistic children, who showed greater difficulty in imitating static postures compared with dynamic motor sequences. By contrast, Rogers and colleagues (1996) found that autistic children performed equally poorly on both positions and sequence gestures. The dynamic versus static parameter was also explored in the case of apraxia, with similarly divergent results. Sunderland and Sluman (2000) reported a higher frequency of errors in hand positions when their patients imitated static models, whereas the pattern of results of De Renzi, Fabrizia, and Nichelli (1980) showed great difficulties in both static and dynamic gestures for persons with apraxia.

Imitation of Meaningless Gestures by Typically Developing Children

Eighty-four typically developing children ages 2–8 years were presented with the task. They were sitting at a table, facing an experimenter, who modeled the movements twice, and a camera that filmed their imitation. Each of the 30 items was modeled twice, and the participants received a score of 0 when imitation was incorrect in the two trials, 1 when imitation was correct in the second trial, and 2 when imitation was correct in the first trial. This scoring led to a maximum global score of 60 and three maximum scores of 20 for each type of gesture.

Performance differed according to both age and type of gesture. For all types of gestures, performances improved significantly with age. Hand positions were the easiest task to imitate, followed by finger configurations, whereas combined postures received the lowest scores (see Figure 8.2).

As Figure 8.2 shows, the youngest children (mean age 2 years, 6 months) performed more accurately on the imitation of hand positions than they did in imitating finger configurations with visual feedback. This suggests that body knowledge is established very early on in development, as shown by other studies using different tasks. For instance, Heron and Slaughter (2002), exploring expectations about body shape, reported that infants are sensitive to body shape violations by 18–24 months. At 3 years of age, children are able to designate many parts of human body (Bergès & Lézine, 1972).

After 4 years, children performed equally in hand postures and finger configurations, although they did not reach the maximum score until age 7 for hand postures and age 8 for finger configurations. Children ages 6–7 years showed significant improvement in the imitation of combined postures, a task that requires complex planning. The ceiling score was not reached at 8 years, which is not surprising if we take account of the fact that not all healthy adults performed at ceiling in Goldenberg's studies (1996).

To sum up, the younger children's profile of scores differed from the older groups insofar as the former performed higher for body knowledge than for visual–spatial capacity, whereas the latter groups performed equally well in the two domains. This finding fits the sequence of cerebral maturation, showing that parietal maturation precedes prefrontal maturation (Chiron et al., 1992; Giedd et al., 1999).

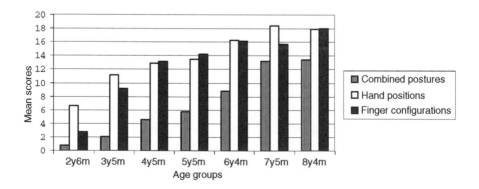

FIGURE 8.2. Scores of different types of imitation according to age.

Imitation of Meaningless Gestures by Low-Functioning Children with an Autistic Spectrum Disorder

Twenty-five children with an autistic spectrum disorder (ASD) as defined by DSM-IV (American Psychiatric Association, 1994) and the Childhood Autism Rating Scale (CARS; Schopler, Reichler, Devellis, & Daly, 1980) were presented with the same task. Their ages ranged from 4 to 17 years, with a range of developmental ages (DA) from 18 to 96 months (assessed by psychoeducational profile—revised; PEP-R). Nine children participated in the introductory play session, but they were not willing to be involved in the imitation session. The influence of DA on the willingness to imitate meaningless gestures was significant: The children who rejected the imitation session all presented the lowest evaluations of DA (less than 27 months, as assessed by PEP-R). A minimal DA is thus required to imitate meaningless gestures on request.

The 16 children with ASD who took part in the imitation task were divided into two subgroups according to their DA (Group 1, DA < 42 months, $n = 7$; Group 2, DA > 42 months, $n = 9$). We chose 42 months as a developmental landmark that was likely to reveal a different developmental profile in children with autism than in the typically developing children: A lower performance in hand positions would indicate specific deficits similar to those found by Goldenberg in patients with apraxia, who give very poor performance in hand positions and high performance in finger configurations (Goldenberg, 1996).

Data analyses show a significant difference between the two developmental groups of children with autism for global scores as well as for scores concerning each type of gesture. Below 42 months of DA, children with ASD showed similar difficulties when they had to imitate hand positions and finger configurations. No child with ASD in this group imitated any combined posture. Children with ASD above 42 months of DA obtained relatively good scores when imitating hand positions and finger configurations, but scored lower in combined gestures.

Comparison between Typically Developing Children and Children with an Autistic Spectrum Disorder

The two groups of children with ASD of DA less or greater than 42 months were compared with two groups of typically developing children matched on DA. The main result concerned imitation of hand positions in children with ASD younger than 42 months: Their scores were significantly lower than those of the typical children of the same DA. We did not find such a difference for the group with ASD older than 42 months compared with the

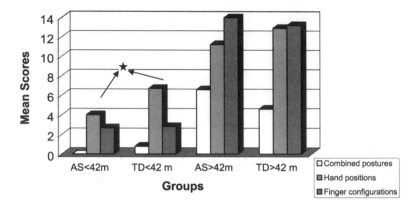

FIGURE 8.3. Scores of different types of imitation according to age (</> 42 months) and population. AS, autistic spectrum; TD, typical development.

elder group of typical children. Other scores did not differ between clinical and typical matched groups (see Figure 8.3).

Taken together, our results suggest that the basic bodily knowledge displayed by typical 30-month-olds may not be available for some low-functioning children with ASD, thus generating, in a cascading effect, paucity of motor experiences, limited capacity of intermodal transfer, and slow development of self-agency. For children with autism with a DA above 42 months, however, no evidence of a deficit in body knowledge appeared. Although larger groups are needed to support this claim further, our finding suggests that the hypothesis of an impairment of praxis in children with ASD should be restricted to subgroups of these children, and is not demonstrated to be universal across the autistic spectrum. Rogers and colleagues' comprehensive exploration of imitation performance in toddlers with autism led them recently to come to similar conclusions when they wrote:

> A very thorough examination of motor functioning in this study did not yield evidence supportive of an autism-specific difficulty with motor coordination or generalized motor planning or motor execution. . . . This suggests that a mechanism other than a *generalized* dyspraxia lies behind the motor imitation difficulty in autism. (Rogers, Hepburn, Stackhouse, & Wehner, 2003, p. 776; italics in original)

A question that comes to mind is to what extent the "motor imitation difficulty" pointed out by Rogers and colleagues (2003) may be due to a deficit in shared motor representations and social resonance. This question is of major importance for future imitation intervention programs. The use of robots that model imitation or imitate, as does Robota, a little robotic doll designed by Aude Billard (Dautenhahn & Billard, 2002), may help to disambiguate the influence of impaired social resonance on the difficulty shown by some children with autism to imitate on request. Another important option is to adopt a functionalist stance and to consider that imitation should primarily be evaluated (and stimulated) when embedded in a context that gives meaning and purpose to this adaptive behavior.

SPONTANEOUS IMITATION EMBEDDED IN A MEANINGFUL CONTEXT

In everyday life, imitations are certainly not as accurate as those required in experimental conditions such as those previously described. In contrast, the spontaneous use of imitation reveals components of an imitative system that cannot be observed when a "do like me" methodology is involved. The constraint of such methodology obviously explains the amazingly long-standing neglect of the other facet of imitation, namely the detection and understanding of being imitated. The motives that lead infants to imitate in their everyday lives appear to our focus of observation only when we focus on self-driven imitation. Long ago, one of us made a claim that comes only now to be largely echoed in the international community of psychologists: Imitation is of frequent use during infancy not only for learning purpose but also for communication (Nadel, 1986). This claim was not a trivial statement concerning the social nature of imitation: Learning also requires socially embedded conditions. Rather, the claim concerned the specific features of a communicative system and focused on the two main components of communication: turn taking and synchrony of action and reenactment. Learning via imitation exploits a basic human attraction toward novelty and allows the individual to acquire cultural knowledge (Tomasello, 1998). Communicating via imitation is another main adaptive function of imitation that exploits an innate capacity for social resonance and provides the preverbal child a format for social exchanges: Temporal synchrony of action and reenactment and approximate morphological similarity in postural signatures are sufficient indices for the imitators to demonstrate their attraction toward their models and for the "imitatees" to notice that they are being imitated

Preverbal infants use synchronic imitation extensively for communicative purposes (Nadel, 1986; Nadel-Brulfert & Baudonnière, 1982; Nadel, Guérini, Pézé, & Rivet, 1999). This was shown in a series of our experiments in which triads (or dyads) of preverbal children met in a setting richly arranged with three (or two) sets of 10 identical objects. In this setting, there was no adult present. There was no task assigned. Nothing was said to the young children, except that they could play with the objects. The meetings were filmed with a hidden camera. The objects were classic toys such as dolls or inflated balloons and attractive pieces of clothing such as cowboy hats, sunglasses, and umbrellas chosen so as to afford postures. The toddlers could choose to play solitarily or together, with different or similar items. We chose to present identical sets of objects because the contemporary literature had started to show that objects are important mediators of nonverbal communication (Bates, Benigni, Bretherton, Camaioni, & Volterra, 1979). We reasoned that similar objects would mediate similar actions and lead to similar here-and-now experiences, thus enhancing the positive emotional feeling of sharing. Neuroimaging studies give us new explanations. Perception of objects generates motor representations of possible actions. Positron emission tomography (PET) studies have found similar brain activation for perception of objects and of actions related to these objects (Grèzes & Decety, 2002). Perception of similar objects could thus activate similar motor representations, leading to shared motor representations that facilitate imitations. Our initial guess was revealed to be a good one. Results are clear (Nadel, 1986; Mertan, Nadel, & Leveau, 1993; Nadel-Brulfert & Baudonnière, 1982) and can be replicated at any time by everyone: After 18 months and up to 42 months, children prefer identical objects (they choose identical objects 75% of the time in triads and 83% in dyads) and use them to perform identical actions. Actions are mainly familiar uses of objects that are part of the children's motor repertoire. They can also be nonaffordant uses, such as holding a chair on one's head.

Of course, imitating the other's action is not enough to communicate. The striking point is that young children take advantage of the two facets of imitation to take communicative turns: They alternately imitate their partner's actions and propose actions to be imitated. As a consequence, we found a highly significant relationship between the number of times the children were imitators and the number of times they were imitated (Nadel, 1986; Nadel-Brulfert & Baudonnière, 1982). Not only do the children take turns, but they also synchronize their tempo: When needed, the model waits while the imitator hurries in order to maintain synchrony. The result is that imitator and model are mostly doing the same thing at the same time, as Figure 8.4 shows.

To sum up, spontaneous imitation, when combined with recognition of being imitated, functions as a communicative system that allows children to take turns and to synchronize their behavior with that of their partners. Ecologically valid settings that support meaningful use of imitation reveal the important role of the capacity to detect being imitated in the development of a nonverbal but powerful communicative language. Such use of imitation cannot be observed when we elicit imitation in a classic "like-me" context. Inspired by these findings, we have created a three-step design allowing us to

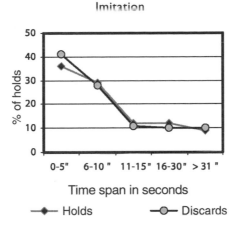

FIGURE 8.4. Temporal delay between holds and discards of identical objects. This figure illustrates how short the delay is between initiating the hold or the discard of an object and the subsequent imitation displayed by the partner(s). As the objects are attractive items, this suggests that the importance of being alike is stronger than the interest in owning objects. The analysis concerns 31,875 seconds of meeting (time unit: 1 second).

explore and to compare the capacities of children with autism for spontaneous imitation, recognition of being imitated, and induced imitation.

A TOOL TO COMPARE IMITATION AND IMITATION RECOGNITION

As seen, induced imitation and self-driven imitation require some common mechanisms, but each of the two kinds of imitation also involves specific underlying processes. It is thus not plausible that we can derive a good evaluation of children's capacity to initiate imitation from their capacity to perform induced imitation.

We propose that performance in induced imitation contexts mainly informs us about the learning function of imitation, whereas performance in spontaneous imitation contexts informs us about the availability of a communicative use of imitation. Our tool can help document how the two functions are intermeshed and exactly what role recognition of being imitated plays in the development of imitation as a communicative system. Spontaneous imitation requires the child to monitor synchrony, and when combined with recognition of being imitated, it leads to turn taking, as we have seen in the preceding section. This is really a relevant point for intervention. Usually interventions focus on an effort to make the children imitate or on an effort to imitate the children so as to attract their attention. The idea here is to alternate imitating the child and proposing attractive actions likely to be imitated. Most of the children will soon start taking the turns that are offered, because they know exactly what to do next: either imitating the other or modeling an action to be imitated by the other. It will be the beginning of social communication via imitation. Once the principle of turn taking is understood as such, it can be applied to other formats of communication than imitation.

Setting for the Three-Step Procedure

The setting used is the double setting already designed for the meeting of typically developing children. The three-step procedure starts with an evaluation of the capacity to initiate imitation. The experimenter develops attractive actions with an item of the double set of objects without directing any request toward the child. The actions are simple familiar actions (for instance, stirring a spoon in a cup) or actions that require planning for the combination of two or three simple subgoals (for instance, taking an umbrella, opening it, and holding it above the head); actions can be also nonaffordant simple actions (for instance, stirring sunglasses in a cup) or complex actions (for instance, taking the bear toy, putting it in the umbrella, and tossing it). Moreover, three meaningless gestures are displayed by the experimenter, one from each category of gestures in Goldenberg's task, selected according to the developmental study described in the first section of this chapter. The second step consists of imitating everything the child does, including as many of the various aspects as possible: postures, actions with the identical objects, vocalizations (if any). The criteria for awareness of being imitated are: staring at the imitator, smiling, close proximity, and kisses or affectionate social gestures. Criteria for understanding of being imitated as the intentional initiative of the imitator are tests for control of the imitator's intent: stopping action, changing goal, changing tempo, and initiating funny actions while looking at the imitator.

The third step consists of asking the children to "do like me" while demonstrating attractive actions of the same kinds as those displayed at the first step of the procedure. Again we repeat each action once, and again we propose three meaningless gestures, one from each category of gestures in Goldenberg's task, reflecting the same developmental level as in the evaluation of spontaneous imitation.

The analysis of findings is still in progress. Three clinical centers are participating in the data collection. Sixty-five children with autism, diagnosed using DSM-IV (American Psychiatric Association, 1996) and CARS (Schopler et al., 1980), have now been included in the study. So far we have computed the results for 36 of these children. They range from 3 to 7 years of age, and their DAS, as evaluated by PEP-R (Schopler, Reichler, & Rochen-Renner, 1988), the revised Brunet–Lézine scale (Brunet & Lézine, 1996), or the Kaufman Assessment Battery for Children (K-ABC, Kaufman

& Kaufman, 1983), varied from 6 months to 65 months. All children with autism were able to spontaneously imitate at least simple familiar actions as 6- to 9-months-old typical infants do. When the DA of the children with autism was the criterion, instead of the chronological age (CA), the developmental path of spontaneous imitation appeared to parallel the developmental path of typical young children during the first 2 years of life (Nadel, Revel, Andry, & Gaussier, 2004). A highly significant correlation was found between DA and scores of spontaneous imitations. Concerning elicited imitation, however, the picture was mixed: Some children who were good spontaneous imitators did not imitate when requested to do so and left the room, some had an equal score in the two conditions, and others who did not imitate spontaneously performed quite well when imitation was requested. Although not as informative as expected, these first results at least deliver the important message that elicited imitation reveals only part of the child's capacity to imitate. As suggested by Tony Charman, in his comments on the chapter, these results raise the issue of matching an individual child's profile of strengths and weaknesses to an intervention approach. An intervention based on imitation would benefit from a precise evaluation of what kind of imitation the child performs better and what kind of information the imitation conveys regarding object–action relationships, or the role of prompt in the child's performance, or the capacity to select means to achieve goals.

Remarkably, children with autism displayed a selective use of spontaneous imitation: None of them spontaneously imitated the meaningless gestures that the adult displayed besides goal-directed actions. These gestures did not convey any conventional or symbolic meaning. They were just neglected as nonsense in a meaningful context, although some of them were imitated on request a few minutes later. Such a selective use of imitation indicates that children with autism do not display unintended and automatic imitation similar to echopraxia found in frontal patients (Lhermitte, Pillon, & Seradou, 1986).

CONCLUDING COMMENTS

Imitation is not a unitary phenomenon. We have focused on an analysis of the many aspects of immediate imitation, without any regard to deferred imitation. This is not to say that deferred imitation is of no interest and that it should not be a part of intervention programs. But limiting our study to immediate imitation already underlines the many aspects involved and the different mechanisms that may be in play according to the function and the content concerned: body knowledge, visual–spatial analysis, motor planning, motor synchronization, awareness of other's tempo, awareness of other's intent.

Elicited imitation and spontaneous imitation require the involvement of different executive capacities. When "do like me" methodologies are used, imitation requires the child to overcome the executive difficulty of reproducing an observed action without a personal purpose. Alternatively, when imitation is done at will, the child must select among all available models the one that actually meets his or her motives, thus requiring the executive capacity to inhibit the imitation of the other possible models.

Imitation has two main adaptive functions: learning and communication. We have stressed the idea that only ecological contexts can afford the observation of everyday functional uses of imitation. For instance, the role of recognition of being imitated in early communication cannot even be suspected when free interaction is not part of the social context.

A distinction that may be relevant in imitation interventions concerns the role played by imitation training: Is the training aimed at increasing imitative capacities in order to fulfill a learning function, or is it a way to improve communication skills? What might enhance intervention effects would be to stimulate imitation in its two functions. Knowing that the intermeshing of the learning and of the communicative use of imitation has cascading effects on the development of the motor repertoire, thus speeding up the improvement of both learning and gestural communication skills.

Moreover, such improvements are not limited to the domain of imitation skills: They spread largely over more general domains, such as visual attention to the other's actions (Dawson & Adams, 1984; Tiegerman & Primavera, 1984), motor memory, and shared motor representations. When induced imitation is trained, the capacity to respond to external requests is stimulated. We suggest that the stimulation of imitation and recognition of being imitated can be used as a remediation to enhance autonomous actions and to favor the development of an awareness of self- and other agency. When imitating and being imitated, children with autism relate self-actions to others' actions. The good news is that imitation and recognition of being imitated develop when children are offered repeated opportunities to practice (Field, Field, Sanders, & Nadel, 2001). Children then start to use turn taking and to share tempos while imitating; in a word, they start to communicate. Just try it—it works!

REFERENCES

American Psychiatric Association. (1994). *Diagnostic and statitsical manual of mental disorders* (4th ed.). Washington, DC: Author.
Bates, E., Benigni, I., Bretherton, I., Camaioni, L., & Volterra, V. (1979). *The emergence of symbols*. New York: Academic Press.
Bergès, M., & Lézine, I. (1972). *Test d'imitation de gestes* (2nd ed.). Paris: Masson.

Brunet, O., & Lézine, I. (1996). *Le développement psychologique de la première enfance* (rev. version). Issy-Les-Moulineaux, France: Editions Scientifiques de Psychologie.

Charman, T., & Baron-Cohen, S. (1994). Another look at imitation in autism. *Development and Psychopathology, 6*, 404–413.

Chiron, C., Raynaud, C., Maziére, B., Zilbovicius, M., Laflamme, L., Masure, M. C., et al. (1992). Changes in regional cerebral blood flow during brain maturation in children and adolescents. *Journal of Nuclear Medicine, 33*(5), 696–703.

Dautenhahn, K., & Billard, A. (2002). Games children can play with Robota, a humanoïd robotic doll. In S. Keates, P. J. Clarkson, P. M. Langdon, & P. Robinson (Eds.), *Universal access and assistive technology* (pp. 83–105). London: Springer-Verlag.

Dawson, G., & Adams, A. (1984). Imitation and social responsiveness in autistic children. *Journal of Abnormal Child Psychology, 12*, 209–226.

Decety, J., Grèzes, J., Costes, N., Perani, D., Jeannerod, M., Procyk, E., et al. (1997). Brain activity during observation of action: Influence of action content and subject's strategy. *Brain, 120*, 1763–1777.

De Renzi, E., Fabrizia, M., & Nichelli, P. (1980). Imitating gestures. *Archives of Neurology, 37*, 6–10.

Dewey, D. (1993). Error analysis of limb and oro-facial praxis in children with developmental motor deficits. *Brain and Cognition, 23*, 203–221.

Field, T., Field, T., Sanders, C., & Nadel, J. (2001). Children display more social behaviors after repeated imitation sessions. *Autism, 5*, 317–323.

Giedd, J. N., Blumenthal, J., Jeffries, N. O., Castellanos, F. X., Liu, H., Zijdenbos, A., et al. (1999). Brain development during childhood and adolescence: A longitudinal MRI study. *Nature Neuroscience, 2*, 861–863.

Goldenberg, G. (1996). Defective imitation of gestures in patients with damage in the left or right hemispheres. *Journal of Neurology, Neurosurgery, and Psychiatry, 61*, 176–180.

Goldenberg, G. (1999). Matching and imitation of hand and finger postures in patients with damage in the left or right hemispheres. *Neuropsychologia, 37*, 559–566.

Goldenberg, G., & Hagmann, S. (1997). The meaning of meaningless gestures: A study of visuo-imitative apraxia. *Neuropsychologia, 35*, 333–341.

Grèzes, J., & Decety, J. (2002). Does the perception of objects afford action? Evidence from a neuroimaging study. *Neuropsychologia, 40*, 212–222.

Heron, M., & Slaughter, V. (2002, April). *Infants' discrimination of normal and atypical human and nonhuman shapes.* Poster presented at the International Conference on Infant Studies, Toronto, Ontario, Canada.

Hill, E. (1998). A dyspraxic deficit in specific language impairment and developmental coordination disorder. *Developmental Medicine and Child Neurology, 40*, 388–395.

Kaufman, A. S., & Kaufman, N. L. (1983). *Batterie pour l'examen psychologique de l'enfant (K-ABC). Manuel d'administration et de cotation.* Paris: Editions du Centre de Psychologie Appliquée.

Kools, J. A., & Tweedie, D. (1975). Development of praxis in children. *Perceptual and Motor Skills, 40*, 11–19.

Lhermitte, F., Pillon, B., & Seradou, M. (1986). Human autonomy and the frontal lobes: Part I. Imitation and utilization behavior: A neuropsychological study of 75 patients. *Annals of Neurology, 19*, 326–334.

Mertan, B., Nadel, J., & Leveau, H. (1993). The effect of adult presence on communicative behaviour among toddlers. In J. Nadel & L. Camaioni (Eds.), *New perspectives in communicative development* (pp. 190–201). London: Routledge.

Nadel, J. (1986). *Imitation et communication entre jeunes enfants.* Paris: Presses Universitaires de France.

Nadel, J. (2002). Imitation and imitation recognition: Their functional role in preverbal infants and nonverbal children with autism. In A. Meltzoff & W. Prinz (Eds.), *The imitative mind: Development, evolution and brain bases* (pp. 42–62). Cambridge, MA: Cambridge University Press.

Nadel, J. (2006). Does imitation matter to children with autism? In S. J. Rogers & J. H. G. Williams (Eds.), *Imitation and the social mind: Typical development and autism.* New York: Guilford Press.

Nadel, J., Guérini, C., Pezé, A., & Rivet, C. (1999). The evolving nature of imitation as a format for communication. In J. Nadel & G. Butterworth (Eds.), *Imitation in infancy* (pp. 209–234). Cambridge, UK: Cambridge University Press.

Nadel, J., & Pézé, A. (1993). What makes immediate imitation communicative in toddlers and autistic children? In J. Nadel & L. Camaioni (Eds.), *New perspectives in communicative development* (pp. 139–156). London: Routledge.

Nadel, J., Revel, A., Andry, P., & Gaussier, P. (2004). Toward communication: First developmental steps of imitation in infants, children with autism, and robots. *Studies of Interaction, 5*, 45–75.

Nadel-Brulfert, J., & Baudonnière, P. M. (1982). The social function of reciprocal imitation in 2–year-old peers. *International Journal of Behavioral Development, 5*, 95–109.

O'Hare, A. (1999). Development of an instrument to measure manual praxis. *Developmental Medicine and Child Neurology, 41*, 597–607.

Rogers, S. (1999). An examination of the imitation deficit in autism. In J. Nadel & G. Butterworth (Eds.), *Imitation in infancy* (pp. 254–283). Cambridge, UK: Cambridge University Press.

Rogers, S., Bennetto, L., McEvoy, R., & Pennington, B. (1996). Imitation and pantomime in high-functioning adolescents with autism spectrum disorders. *Child Development, 67*, 2060–2073.

Rogers, S., Hepburn, S., Stackhouse, T., & Wehner, E. (2003). Imitation performance in toddlers with autism and those with other developmental disorders. *Journal of Child Psychology and Psychiatry, 44*, 763–781.

Schopler, E., & Reichler, R. (1979). *Individualized assessment and treatment for autistic and developmentally disabled children: Vol. 1. Psychoeducational profile* (2nd ed.). Austin, TX: PRO-ED.

Schopler, E., Reichler, R., Devellis, R., & Daly, K. (1980). Toward objective classification of childhood autism: Childhood Autism Rating Scale (CARS). *Journal of Autism and Developmental Disorders, 10*, 91–103.

Schopler, E., Reichler, R., & Rochen-Renner, B. (1988). *The Childhood Autism Rating Scale (CARS).* Austin, TX: Western Psychological Services.

Smith, I., & Bryson, S. (1994). Imitation and action in autism: A critical review. *Psychological Bulletin, 116*, 259–273.

Smith, I., & Bryson, S. (1998). Gesture imitation in autism: Nonsymbolic postures and sequences. *Cognitive Neuropsychology, 15*, 747–770.

Stone, W., Ousley, O., & Littleford, C. (1997). Motor imitation in young children with autism: What's the object? *Journal of Abnormal Child Psychology, 25*, 475–485.

Sunderland, A., & Sluman, S. M. (2000). Ideomotor apraxia, visuomotor control and the explicit representation of posture. *Neuropsychologia, 38*, 923–934.

Tiegerman, E., & Primavera, L. (1984). Imitating the autistic child: Facilitating communicative gaze behavior. *Journal of Autism and Developmental Disorders, 14*, 27–38.

Tomasello, M. (1998). Emulation learning and cultural learning. *Behavioral and Brain Sciences, 21*, 703–704.

Uzgiris, I., & Hunt, J. McV. (1975). *Assessment in infancy: Ordinal scales of psychological development*. Urbana: University of Illinois Press.

9

Augmentative and Alternative Communication Systems for Children with Autism

PATRICIA HOWLIN

ALTERNATIVE COMMUNICATION SYSTEMS FOR CHILDREN WITH AUTISM

The term *alternative communication* can be interpreted in a variety of different ways, but the Committee on Augmentative Communication of the American Speech-Language-Hearing Association (ASHA; 1991) has defined alternative and augmentative communication (AAC) systems as follows: "An integrated group of components, including the symbols, aids, strategies and techniques used by individuals to enhance communication. The system serves to supplement any gestural, spoken and/or written communication abilities" (pp. 9–10).

Symbols are defined as "a visual, auditory and/or tactile representation of conventional concepts (e.g., gestures, photographs, manual signs, picto-ideographs, printed words, objects or Braille)." An *aid* is "a physical object or device used to transmit or receive messages (e.g., a communication book, board, charts, mechanical or electronic device, or computer)." *Strat-*

egy is "a specific way of using AAC aids, symbols, and/or techniques more effectively for enhanced communication." *Technique* refers to the method of transmitting messages (signing, pointing, etc.), and a *multimodal system* is one that "utilizes the individual's full communication capabilities, including any residual speech or vocalizations, gestures, signs, and aided communication."

The need for a range of augmentative strategies to enhance the communication skills of children with autism is evident given the severity and pervasiveness of their speech and language deficits. Communication difficulties are often the first symptoms to give rise to parental concerns (Howlin & Moore, 1997) and are among the main reasons that parents seek diagnostic help. Follow-up studies indicate that the development of language is an important prognostic indicator and that, unless some useful language is established by the age of around 6 years, the likelihood of children subsequently acquiring spoken language is very small (Lord & Bailey, 2002). Statistics suggest that around 25% of individuals with autism remain without functional speech (Lord & Bailey, 2002), and the risk of severe and persisting language impairment is particularly high among children with nonverbal IQs below 50. Impaired communication is also one of the three principal diagnostic criteria for autism (American Psychiatric Association, 1994; World Health Organization, 1993). Many children fail entirely to develop spoken language, and there is rarely any spontaneous attempt to compensate for this lack of speech via alternative means such as gesture or mime. In children who do develop language, onset is usually, although not invariably, delayed. When speech does emerge, it tends to be characterized by many abnormal features, such as: echolalia (both immediate and delayed); repetitive, stereotyped, and idiosyncratic utterances; pronominal reversal; neologisms; socially inappropriate use of language; impaired communicative intent; and a marked inability to initiate or sustain reciprocal conversation. Speech abnormalities are accompanied by deficits in nonverbal communication; comprehension is severely affected; and there are impairments, too, in abstract ability, imagination, and play.

The challenge for therapeutic approaches in this area is thus enormous. A truly successful program must aim not only to provide the child with more effective means of communication but also to improve understanding, both verbal and nonverbal; to increase motivation to communicate; and to enhance imaginative and abstract skills. In this chapter a variety of different approaches designed to improve the communication skills of children with autism are discussed, and the evidence in support of their effectiveness is reviewed. However, it should be noted that, unlike most of the other chapters in this book, much of the research involves children of primary school age (5 years plus) or older.

THE DISAPPOINTING RESULTS
OF EARLY VERBAL TRAINING PROGRAMS

Studies of language training with children with autism first began to appear in the United States in the mid-1960s (Baer, Wolf, & Risley, 1968; Risley & Wolf, 1967), with the emphasis being on the use of operant methods to teach imitative responses and/or the elimination of "inappropriate" speech. However, despite claims that such methods could result in the establishment of "near normal speech" (Daley, Cantrell, Cantrell, & Aman, 1972), in many cases progress was painfully slow. Lovaas (1977), for example, reported that 90,000 trials were required to teach one unfortunate child two simple word approximations; other studies reported little change after many hours of intensive treatment (Howlin, 1989). The outcome of spoken-language-training programs was particularly poor for children whose comprehension and vocal skills were most severely impaired, and it became clear that, for them, an alternative approach to intervention was required.

ALTERNATIVES TO SPEECH

Signing

Studies reporting on the use of sign language to improve the communicative competence of children with autism first began to appear in the 1970s (e.g., Bonvillian & Nelson, 1976; Fulwiler & Fouts, 1976; Konstantareas, Oxman, & Webster, 1978). It was argued that signing should be easier to acquire than speech because it bypassed the children's fundamental deficit in verbal communication. Moreover, in that signs are less transient than words, it was suggested that they should make fewer demands on verbal memory and abstract understanding. Manual signs are also far easier to prompt than vocalizations.

Initially, most signing programs were based on the formal systems, such as American Sign Language (ASL) or British Sign Language (BSL), used in deaf communities, but as it became evident that these were often too complex and abstract for individuals with additional learning and communication problems, new systems were developed. The Paget–Gorman system (Paget, Gorman, & Paget, 1976), for example, had a structure much closer to spoken English, and for some years it was widely used in schools for children with intellectual disabilities and/or autism. However, many of the signs used in Paget–Gorman are relatively abstract, competence in the use of two-handed signs is required, and the system also assumes a relatively high level of communicative intent among users. For these reasons, during the 1980s the Paget–Gorman system was largely replaced in U.K. schools for children with autism by the Makaton system (Walker, 1980).

Although based on BSL, Makaton signs were generally simpler, many requiring the use of only one hand, and the core "vocabulary" was modified, at least to some extent, to suit the needs of the individual student.

Despite the rapid spread of sign-based programs in schools and units for children with autism, evaluative research was limited. Most studies were lacking in experimental rigor, controlled trials were virtually nonexistent, and reported outcomes were variable. In an early review, Kiernan (1983) noted the methodological limitations of most studies. Small sample size was also a major problem, one of the few exceptions being the study by Layton (1988) that included 60 participants and random assignment to groups. Kiernan (1983) also commented on the heterogeneity of the participants and the programs involved. Although most participants were described as being severely or profoundly retarded, data on cognitive abilities were generally sparse. The age range of participants spanned preschool to adolescence, and initial language levels ranged from mute to simple speech. Intervention programs lasted from 17 days to more than 3 years, and outcome varied from 2 to 400 signs. In around half the studies reviewed, children subsequently developed some spoken language; in the other half, they did not. Almost two decades later, Goldstein (2002) was able to identify only 10 studies involving signed communication for children with autism that met basic experimental requirements, and even among these few studies, the findings were variable. Moreover, most outcome research focused on the *number* of signs acquired, rather than on the impact on children's pragmatic competence. When this was assessed, the results were not impressive. Many individuals used only a small proportion of the learned signs spontaneously (Duker & van Lent, 1991), and Attwood, Frith, and Hermelin (1988) found that the ability to sign did not necessarily improve social communication. Thus the spontaneous signing of children with autism tended to be stereotyped and repetitive and used mainly to achieve immediate needs; signs were rarely used for the purposes of social interaction or to share experiences. Bonvillian and Blackburn (1991) noted that the extent and complexity of spontaneous signing following training was closely associated with pretreatment levels of cognitive, fine motor, social, and receptive language skills. The children with autism who were most impaired in these areas acquired only very limited working sign vocabularies.

Lack of empirical data on the effectiveness of sign language programs for children with autism did not deter specialist schools from adopting such systems as their primary communication programs. Even as late as 1990, Grove and Walker (1990, p. 15) claimed (though without supporting statistics) that "The Makaton system is one of the most widely used systems of augmentative communications in the United Kingdom." However, although there is some *suggestive* evidence that sign teaching may be more effective in increasing communication in children with autism than the teaching of spoken language (Goldstein, 2002), the overall findings are far from conclusive. With hindsight, this is hardly surprising, given that it is now well established that children with autism typically have difficulties with motor movements (Hauck & Dewey, 2001; Manjiviona & Prior, 1995; Rapin, 1996), with motor planning and sequencing (Hughes, 1996; Minshew, Goldstein, & Siegel, 1997), and, crucially, in many different aspects of imitation (Charman et al., 1997; Nadel, Guerini, Peze, & Rivet, 1999; Stone, Ousley, & Littleford, 1997; Rogers, Hepburn, Stackhouse, & Wehner, 2003; Williams, Whiten, & Singh, 2004). Recent research also suggests that successful sign acquisition may be related not only to children's motor ability (Seal & Bonvillian, 1997) but also to their functioning in other domains, including symbolic processing and social skills (Bonvillian & Blackburn, 1991) and executive function (Seal & Bonvillian, 1997). Perhaps rather than advocating specific signing systems, such as Makaton, for this highly heterogeneous group of children, research efforts might have done better to focus on identifying the particular profiles of children who seem to benefit most from signing, or on exploring particular areas of skill or deficit that seem to be associated with successful acquisition.

Symbol and Picture Communication Systems

The failure of signing programs to increase the communicative competence of many children with autism led to a gradual shift, during the 1970s and 1980s, toward increasingly concrete methods of training. There is considerable research evidence demonstrating that visual abilities are relatively intact in autism, and in the educational field, visual teaching methods had already proved effective in enhancing general skill acquisition (cf. the TEACCH program; Schopler, Mesibov, & Hearsey, 1995). Thus it was only a matter of time before visual strategies began to be used to increase communication skills as well. A variety of symbol systems have been developed over recent years (see Beukelman & Mirenda, 1998, for details), but Rebus (Clark, Davis, & Woodcock, 1974) and Bliss symbols (Bliss, 1965) were among the first to be used with people with learning disabilities. Rebus is a pictographic system with cartoon-type illustrations that can mostly, though not invariably, be identified without difficulty (e.g., a sketch of a car for *car*). Rebus symbols have been used in communication programs for individuals with a variety of disabilities, although only a few studies report their use with people with autism (Reichle & Brown, 1986). Blissymbolics (Bliss, 1965) have also been widely adopted as an augmentative communication system. However, these symbols are highly stylized, non-iconic characters (e.g., ↑ for *tree*), and a number of research studies have indicated that of all the representational systems in common use Blissymbols are the least transparent, the most difficult to learn, and the hardest to retain (Beukleman & Mirenda, 1998). In both Rebus and Bliss systems, the written label is placed beneath the symbol, as much for the benefit of the child's audience as for the child him- or herself. As with studies of signing, well-controlled experimental research in this area is limited, but there is some evidence that iconic symbols tend to be acquired more easily than non-iconic symbols (Konstantareas, 1996). From a practical point of view, pictures and pictographs also seem to have a number of potential advantages over signs or abstract symbols: They make fewer demands on memory or cognitive skills, they are (at least in principle) always available, they require only minimum motor ability, and they are easily understood by observers and are easy to prompt. However, they are a relatively slow and inflexible means of communication (competent language speakers use between 150 and 250 words per minute; symbols and pictographs are typically used at a rate of 2–8 words per minute), turn taking is restricted, and symbolic or picture systems make it difficult to convey syntactic or semantic relations with ease. Successful acquisition of symbol systems also tends to be very unpredictable, with some individuals developing relatively large "vocabularies" and others making limited progress (Abrahamsen, Romski, & Sevcik, 1989). Konstantareas (1987) and Kiernan (1983) also reported specific problems in teaching symbols to children with autism. They found that unprompted, spontaneous use was rare, that pictographs tended to be used for requests rather than providing information or initiating social contact, and that generalization to unfamiliar people or situations was often poor. Despite such caveats and the general lack of any experimental evidence for their effectiveness, pictographs or other pictorial systems became widely used in schools for children with autism. The Makaton signing system was also later extended to include picture symbols, but although the resulting combination of signs and symbols was claimed to "teach total communication to people with a wide range of disabilities" (Grove & Walker, 1990, p. 25), no evidence exists in support of this claim.

Improvements in computer technology in recent years have greatly increased the potential for picture and symbol systems to be used by individuals with a wide range of different abilities and across many different settings. Problems of access and transportability can be readily overcome by the use of personalized communication boards kept in each of the settings in which the child spends time. Portable and handheld computers have also increased the ease with which pictorial systems can be used, because large, individualized lexicons can be stored in a relatively small space. Commercially available programs (e.g., Lightwriter or Boardmaker) also make it possible for teachers and parents to construct an extensive picture vocabulary with minimal time and effort.

There have been no large-scale comparative studies of the effectiveness of symbols versus signs by children with autism, and the results of research with other groups are conflicting. Foreman and Crews (1998) reported that signing resulted in more frequent communication than symbol use in children with Down syndrome. In contrast, Udwin and Yule (1990, 1991a) found no significant differences between the use of Bliss symbols and Makaton signs in 40 language-impaired children with cerebral palsy. Although some progress was made by children in both groups, acquisition was generally very slow, and "utterance length" rarely exceeded a single sign or symbol. Udwin and Yule (1991b) also note that exposure to both systems was limited and that, despite schools' claims that they were using these systems extensively, the average time *per week* spent in teaching was only 100 minutes for Bliss and 63.5 minutes for Makaton. Hardly enough to expect a major improvement in communication! Grove and Dockrell (2000) also found that nonverbal children using Makaton rarely progressed beyond Mean Length of Utterance (MLU) Stage 1 in terms of semantic and lexical development. Like Udwin and Yule (1990), these authors comment on the limited use of signing by the children's parents, teachers, and peers, an issue also highlighted by Konstantareas (1996) in a more recent review of communication training programs for children with autism.

The Picture Exchange Communication System

Unlike most alternative/augmentative systems, which have been developed for children with learning and communication problems more generally, the Picture Exchange Communication System (PECS) was specifically designed for children within the autistic spectrum (Bondy & Frost, 1994a). It is also one of the few communication programs to have focused particularly (though not exclusively) on preschool children. PECS is a systematic approach to communication training using standardized sets of pictographs, communication books and communication boards, and a highly prescriptive teaching manual. Training is divided into the following six levels, which should be followed in strict sequence:

1. *Requesting*—prompted exchange of picture by child to "communicative partner" in order to obtain desired object
2. *Increasing distance* between child and communicative partner; fading of prompts
3. *Picture discrimination*—choosing appropriate picture from a selection of pictures in communication book/board
4. *Using phrases*—child combines pictures indicating set phrases (e.g., "I want") with picture of desired object
5. *Responding to questions*—appropriate pictures (+ verbalization) used in response to question "What do you want?"

6. *Commenting*—pictures (+ verbalization) used to respond to questions such as "What do you see/hear?" "What is it?" and so forth

There have been enthusiastic claims for the effectiveness of PECS by Bondy and Frost (1994a, 1994b, 1994c). PECS is described as "a rapidly acquired, self-initiated functional communication system" that parallels typical language development, so that children with a mental age of 10–12 months can learn the initial phases (Bondy & Frost, 2001, p. 725). Over half (59%) of children age 5 or younger were said to have developed independent speech and to use this as their sole mode of communication after having been taught PECS; a further 30% developed speech in conjunction with PECS—a total success rate of 89% (Bondy & Frost, 1994a). Independent evaluations, however, are limited. In a single-case, multiple-baseline study, Kravits, Kamps, Kemmerer, and Potucek (2002) reported increases in spontaneous communication (verbal and PECS) in settings in which PECS was implemented, together with some restricted generalization to other settings. Charlop-Christy, Carpenter, Le, Le Blanc, and Kellet (2002) recorded increases in PECS usage, speech, social communication, and joint attention in 3 children following a PECS program. A concomitant decrease occurred in problem behaviors. Ganz and Simpson (2004) also report improvements in use and level of PECS and spoken vocabulary in 3 young, PECS-trained children. In a larger scale study involving 31 preschool children, Schwartz, Garfinkle, and Bauer (1998) found that after an average of 14 months (range 3–28 months) the children were using PECS in a functional manner to communicate with peers and adults. Eighteen children were followed up for a further year. Their use of PECS generalized to untrained snack- and playtime sessions, and 44% demonstrated marked increases in spoken language. Magiati and Howlin (2003) monitored the progress of 34 children (average chronological age 7.8 years; average Vineland communication age 1.5 years) attending specialist schools for children with autism in which teachers received training and ongoing consultation sessions in the use of PECS. Compared with baseline levels, the children made significant progress in the frequency with which they used PECS; the extent of their PECS vocabulary also increased, as did overall PECS level. Children who were using some speech when intervention began made similar progress to those who had no language. However, verbal communication skills changed little, in either the initially verbal or nonverbal children. As Schwartz et al. (1998) and Magiati and Howlin (2003) make clear, these were *not* experimental studies, and they lack control groups or independent, blind assessments. Rather, they confirm that PECS can be readily acquired by children with autism and that levels of PECS usage increase following training.

The impact on verbal communication skills, the extent of generalization to other settings, and the comparative effectiveness of PECS compared with other teaching methods still require experimental validation. Nevertheless, Chambers and Rehfeldt (2003) suggest that PECS may be acquired more rapidly than other systems, such as signs, because it offers distinct discriminative stimuli that prompt the correct response. Thus the correct use of PECS, at least in the early phases, is predominantly a *recognition* task; in contrast, the correct use of signs is a *recall* task that clearly makes more demands on cognitive functioning. The fact that only a single topographical response (pointing to or giving a picture or object) is required, rather than the multiple and varied responses needed in signing, is also likely to enhance PECS usage.

Other Forms of Picture Communication

Despite the apparent value of PECS for many children, there is no evidence that the specific materials involved are optimal and/or necessary or that the prescribed stages of training are essential for progress. Certainly, there are no data to indicate that commercially produced (and hence relatively expensive) equipment is the only option. "Homemade" charts with photographs indicating different activities throughout the day or what food will be on offer at mealtimes can be very successful in increasing understanding or in enabling individuals with autism to indicate their own choices more effectively (cf. the procedures developed by the TEACCH program; Schopler et al., 1995). Children can easily be provided with their own personal set of photographs or pictures to enable them to indicate basic needs or wishes (e.g., to leave the building, have a drink, go to the bathroom, etc.). Picture systems have been used to increase children's tolerance of new activities and to reduce the disruption that may occur if their routines need to be changed (Krantz, MacDuff, & McClannahan, 1993). Keen, Sigafoos, and Woodyatt (2001) also demonstrate how prelinguistic behaviors, such as pointing or reaching, can be gradually shaped until children are able to use photographs to indicate the same needs.

Whatever the exact system chosen, in order to be of any real value the materials must be readily accessible to both the child and those living and working with him or her. Communication boards allow the display of a relatively large number of pictures, words, or symbols (cf. Calculator & Luchko, 1983), but although useful within the classroom setting, they can be unwieldy in other settings. For greater ease of use, important or frequently used pictures or photos might be attached to a key ring on a belt, kept in a waist bag, or hung on a neck chain of the type used for company identity badges—anything that is age appropriate. Digitally produced photographs allow multiple copies of varying sizes to be made with ease, thereby providing identical pictures for adults and children, as well as for a central display. Whatever materials are used, it is essential to ensure that these are adequately protected, preferably laminated, and that they are updated and replaced as necessary. Worn, out-of-date pictures that are no longer of relevance to the child will be of little use.

Not all individuals with autism learn to use such materials with great frequency or spontaneity, and their use tends to be particularly limited among those who are older and/or severely intellectually impaired. However, even within this group, consistent prompting can help gradually to establish the link between the picture and the related activity or object, thereby offering caregivers or teachers a more effective means of communicating with that individual. Picture cards also have the advantage, particularly in new, large, or busy settings, of being readily understood by strangers, whereas signs or more complex symbols can be used or interpreted only by individuals who are familiar with that system. This is important because no system is likely to be effective unless it is consistently reinforced in a wide range of settings.

Social Stories

Pictures have also been used to increase social skills and social understanding among children with autism. The "Social Stories" approach, developed by Gray (1995), uses sequences of simple line drawings to help children with autism as young as 3 years of age to "explain" why they have experienced specific social problems, why other people react as they do, and how behavior might be modified in the future. There are now several positive accounts of this approach (cf. Bledsoe, Smith-Myles, & Simpson, 2003; Gray & Garand, 1993; Hagiwara & Myles, 1999; Lorimer, Simpson, Myles, & Gantz, 2002; Myles & Simpson, 2001; Norris & Datillo, 1999; Swaggart et al., 1995), but group sizes tend to be very small, and experimental controls are generally absent. Although Thiemann and Goldstein (2001), using a multiple-baseline design, were able to demonstrate changes in social behavior in 5 students with intellectual disabilities, their study combined social stories with other strategies, including video feedback, and hence experimental evidence of the *specific* effectiveness of social stories remains limited.

Written Communication

Most communication systems for children with autism utilize modalities that are assumed to be "simpler" than speech. However, there have been some reports of the value of using written language with individuals with autism, even including those with severe intellectual and language impairments. La Vigna (1977), for example, used fading procedures to teach 3 severely handicapped adolescents with autism to recognize and respond to written words. However, mastery of just three words required up to 1,642 trials. Success is more likely when working with cognitively more able children. Howlin and Rutter (1987) describe how shaping procedures (progressing from pictures plus words to words alone) proved effective for a 4-year-old child with autism who, although entirely nonverbal, had a performance IQ of over 120. Within 2 months he learned to respond to written labels, and by the end of 12 months he could respond appropriately to more than 100 written instructions. Comprehension of spoken commands also showed a small improvement, and although he has never learned to speak, he eventually progressed to using a computerized "communicator." Training in the use of symbols such as Bliss can also be a transitional stage in the development of written skills (McNaughton, 1995).

Written scripts have also been employed to increase social functioning and group activities in late elementary school-age and middle school-age children. Krantz and colleagues (1993) used written scripts to teach 9- to 12-year-old children how to initiate conversations with peers. As conversational initiations increased, scripted statements and questions were gradually faded, and the children began to use unscripted initiations. Similar, though simplified, strategies have been used successfully with preschool children who had only minimal reading skills, and McClannahan and Krantz (1999) cite a number of studies using this approach. Hunt, Alwell, Goetz, and Sailor (1990) also report on the use of communication books to develop conversational skills.

It may be that for certain children, particularly those who, although nonspeaking, are of at least average nonverbal IQ, the teaching of written language may be a very effective alternative to speech. However, again, there are no well-controlled or large-scale studies of this approach, and hence no conclusions can be drawn about its potential effectiveness.

Finally, it is also worth bearing in mind that written communication may assist older individuals who are able to talk but for some reason are reluctant to do so. Howlin (2004) reports the case of a patient who had developed speech late in his childhood. He had never been a fluent speaker, and during a period of severe depression he ceased speaking almost completely. This muteness continued even after his depression finally responded to treatment. Rather than insisting that he try to talk, his parents and daycare staff encouraged him to communicate in writing. This he was willing to do, and eventually he began to use speech spontaneously once more.

Facilitated Communication

One system that relies strongly on written language is Facilitated Communication, which became prominent during the early 1990s. In this system, a facilitator supports the client's hand, wrist, or arm while he or she uses a keyboard or letter board to spell out words, phrases, or sentences. Its use with people with autism was based on the theory that many of their difficulties result from a physical inability to express themselves rather than from more fundamental social or communication deficits. The technique was claimed to prove that individuals with autism who had previously been considered to be severely intellectually impaired were actually of superior intelligence. Facilitators were encouraged to assume that the client possessed unrecognized literacy skills and that the provision of physical support could lead to "communication unbound" (Biklen, 1993). Facilitated Communication has now been the focus of at least 50 studies involving several hundred participants (see reviews by Bebko, Perry, & Bryson, 1996; Green, 1994; Jacobsen, Mulick, & Schwartz, 1995; Mostert, 2001; Simpson & Myles, 1995). These have shown virtually no evidence of independent communication. On the contrary, all well-controlled investigations have consistently indicated that responses are almost invariably under the control of the facilitator, not the client. Moreover, so extensive have been the concerns arising from the use of this technique (including many unsupported claims of sexual abuse) that, in 1994, the American Psychological Association adopted the resolution that "Facilitated Communication is a controversial and unproved procedure with no scientifically demonstrated support for its efficacy." Similarly, the American Academy of Pediatrics Committee on Children with Disabilities (1998) concluded that "there are good scientific data showing (FC) to be ineffective. Moreover . . . the potential for harm does exist, particularly if unsubstantiated accusations of abuse occur using FC" (p. 432). However, although the method is now widely discredited among researchers, it still has its proponents, as various websites testify, and it continues to be used within some schools despite the damage it may cause to families ("Facilitated Communication," 2000).

Computerized Systems

Developments in computer hardware and software in recent years have helped to improve the functioning of children with autism in many areas, including attention and performance in classroom activities (Jordan & Powell, 1990a, 1990b; Moore & Calvert, 2000; Pleinis & Romanczyk, 1985) and interactions with teachers (Tjus, Heimann, & Nelson, 2001); social problem solving and social skills (Bernard-Opitz, Sriram, & Nakhoda-Sapuan, 2001; Panyan, 1984); literacy (Heimann, Nelson, Tjus, & Gillberg, 1995; Nelson, Heimann, & Tjus, 1997; Tjus, Heimann, & Nelson, 1998; Williams, Wright, Callaghan, & Coughlan, 2002); and emotion recognition (Silver & Oaks, 2001; Baron-Cohen, 2002).

The rapid growth of computerized communicative aids also has great potential for nonverbal individuals with autism. Sets of progressively more complex keyboards make it possible for children to proceed gradually from single-symbol boards (e.g., a large colored square or circle that emits a sound when pressed) to multisymbol displays depicting a wide variety of stimuli that can be personally tailored to the individual's own environment, needs, or interests. The development of improved speech output software has also resulted in computers becoming a far more effective means of communication. Colby (1973) was one of the first to demonstrate the potential of computers in enhancing the communication skills of nonverbal children with autism. Computer games were used to teach the children to associate letters on the keyboard with words or phrases, accompanied by animated displays. Following training 13 children were reported to have developed speech. Heimann et al. (1995) and Tjus et al. (1998) have reported increases in spoken language skills among school-age children exposed to similar but more sophisticated computerized strategies. Bernard-Opitz, Sriram, and Sapuan (1999) assessed the use of the IBM Speech Viewer system (which provides visual reinforcement on the production of sounds) with 10 nonverbal children with autism and found a significant increase in vocal imitations compared with training by teachers or parents. Moore and Calvert (2000) reported significantly greater increases in receptive vocabulary acquisition among children exposed to computer-based training programs than among those trained directly by teachers. Hetzroni and Tannous (2004), in a study of five elementary school-age pupils with autism, found that the use of specially designed computer software to encourage play, eating, and hygiene activities resulted in the children using fewer echolalic and irrelevant utterances and more communicative speech. These improvements also generalized to the natural classroom environment. Bosseler and Massaro (2003) have described the use of "Baldi," a three-dimensional computer-animated tutor. This character has far more naturalistic speech patterns than is typically the case for computers, together with interactive visual displays. Vocabulary is individually tailored and based on items from the child's everyday environment and activities. Using a within-subject design, the researchers demonstrated how, following training, their sample of 6 school-age children with autism (IQ range < 35–94) learned and retained significant numbers of new words; they also showed generalization to untrained stimuli and settings. Although, as in most studies of its kind, sample size was small, Bosseler and Massaro (2003) believe that this program has great potential for developing the receptive and expressive skills of children with autism. The fact that the "tutor" can also mimic naturalistic teeth, tongue, and palate movements may also, it is believed, help to improve any existing articulation difficulties.

Although most of the programs described here have involved children of elementary school age or older, rapid progress in the development of computerized systems clearly offers many potential advantages to preschool children with autism. As Bosseler and Massaro (2003) note, computers can be permanently available, they are unfailingly patient, they do not become angry, tired, or bored, and they offer a one-on-one learning environment. There is also evidence that the attitudes of listeners/observers toward people with disabilities are more favorable when more complex augmentative systems, such as computers, are used. Gorenflo and Gorenflo (1991), for example, found that, at least in an experimental setting, an adult using voice-assisted computerized technology to communicate was rated more positively and viewed as less impaired than one using an alphabet board.

Functional Communication Training

Although *facilitated* communication is now discredited, this should not be confused with programs that focus on *functional* communication training. This approach derives primarily from studies of "challenging behavior" particularly in nonverbal and severely intellectually impaired individuals with autism. Functional analysis of so-called challenging behaviors frequently indicated that many such behaviors, far from being *inappropriate,* may be the only way in which someone with very limited communication skills can rapidly, effectively, and predictably gain control over his or her environment (Durand & Carr, 1991). Indeed, analysis of the function of these responses often indicates that so-called maladaptive behaviors may be extremely *adaptive* if an individual is unable to express his or her needs, feelings, or emotions in any other way. Head banging, throwing the TV across the room, or pulling someone's hair are all likely to result in rapid and usually predictable responses from others. Unwanted demands may cease or boredom be relieved, and certainly attention will be received. Over the past decade, many different studies have demonstrated the effectiveness of teaching students to use "assistative" communication devices to replace these undesirable responses. These strategies can range from a simple hand movement to buzzers, red "stop" or green "go" signs, simplified computer keyboards, or microswitches that trigger prerecorded audio messages (Wacker et al., 1990). These devices enable individuals to express their need for assistance, to obtain attention or desired objects, or to escape unwanted situations in a more acceptable manner. In addition, there is strong evidence that these strategies, as well as increasing communicative competence, frequently result in a decrease in disruptive, aggressive, stereotyped, and self-injurious behaviors (see Durand & Merges, 2001, for a review).

Although the majority of studies involving functional analysis and functional communication training have been conducted within experimental settings, there have been some attempts to adapt this methodology to more naturalistic environments. For example, Schuler, Peck, Willard, and

Theimer (1989) developed a relatively simple measure to assess both children's communicative forms and their communicative functions (see Figure 9.1) This strategy can be used by teachers and others to determine how a child communicates and what he or she is communicating about. The use of such a matrix helps to demonstrate how, even if children are nonverbal and apparently noncommunicating, many of their behaviors (including screaming, self-injury, crying, grabbing, etc.) do have an important communicative role. Once these functions are identified, then the child may be taught alternative *forms* of communication.

Developed along similar lines, but in a slightly different format, is the interview protocol devised by Finnerty and Quill (1991). This categorizes

Communication profile	Cries	Screams	Self-injures	Just looks	Moves to person	Pulls other's hand	Grabs/reaches	Does/gets it by self	Goes away	Makes sound	Looks at person/object	Gives object	Points/simple gesture	Uses pictures/symbols	Uses signs (e.g., Makaton)	Echoes	Uses single words	Uses phrases/sentences	No indication of needs
What does x usually do if she/he wants:																			
Adult attention																			
Help with dressing, washing, etc.																			
To play a game/have a story																			
To go outside																			
To go shopping, etc.																			
Object out of reach																			
Favorite food/drink																			
Music/TV/video																			
Games, books, etc.																			
Other special object																			
What happens if:																			
Usual routine is stopped																			
Favorite object removed/lost																			
Ongoing activity stopped																			
Wants to show you something																			
Wants a break																			
Dislikes something																			
Made to go somewhere/ do something she/he doesn't want																			

FIGURE 9.1. Establishing a communication profile. Example derived from Schuler, Peck, Willard, and Theimer (1989).

verbal and nonverbal behaviors into 23 communicative functions, and sample scenarios are provided to guide the interview. The authors suggest that their schedule can be used to summarize the child's skills in several different areas, including the range of communicative means and of communicative functions, the ability to use more than one means to convey each function, the ability to repair strategies, and the ability to identify different communicative styles with different people or in different situations (Quill, 1995).

Watson, Lord, Schaffer, and Schopler (1987) have also described the approach used within the TEACCH program to analyze spontaneous language usage. This identifies the *form* of communication used (motor acts, speech vocalizations, and gestures), the *target* of the interaction (peer, teacher, other adult, etc.), and the *function* of the interaction. Functions include: getting attention, use as part of a social routine, requesting, commenting, refusing/rejecting, giving information, seeking information, expressing feelings, and social interaction. Using this system with children with autism, Stone and Caro-Martinez (1990) found that the first three functions—getting attention, use as part of a social routine, and requesting—together accounted for approximately two-thirds of children's communicative acts. The final four (seeking information, expressing feelings, and interacting socially) accounted for only around 10%.

Once the child's current communicative modes and functions are identified, the information gathered can be used to plan ways in which alternative and more acceptable responses might be established. Moreover, by helping parents or teachers to appreciate that certain behaviors may be a function of poor *communication* skills, rather than being "deliberate" acts of aggression or provocation, this approach can also have a very positive effect on other people's attitudes and their responses toward the child.

Multiple Communication Systems

Although many different types of alternative communication programs appear to result in short-term gains, evidence of longer term effects on individuals' communicative competence is limited. Several studies indicate that generalization to untrained settings is often poor; spontaneous generative use is limited, and maintenance often requires constant and consistent adult prompting (Schlosser, Belfiore, Nigam, Blischak, & Hetzroni, 1995; Udwin & Yule, 1990). In order to reduce problems of this kind, it has been argued that multimodal systems using a combination of speech and AAC methods or two AAC strategies in tandem might prove more effective. Goldstein (2002), for example, in a review of interventions involving signing, suggests that a *combination* of signs and speech may help to enhance vocabulary, because signs offer an additional symbolic system for representing objects and actions. Foreman and Crews (1998), working with children with

Down syndrome, also found that a multimodal system using symbols and signing together was more effective than either strategy in isolation. However, studies involving children with autism have produced more equivocal results. Several early reports claimed positive effects for multimodal training programs (Benaroya, Wesley, Ogilvie, Klein, & Meaney, 1977; Gaines, Leaper, Monahan, & Weickgenant, 1988; Layton, 1988), but whereas some small-scale control studies suggest that multimodal training is superior to training in a single modality (Barrera & Sulzer-Azaroff, 1983; Brady & Smouse, 1978; Konstantareas & Lelbovitz, 1981; Sisson & Barrett, 1984), others have failed to find differential effects (Remington & Clarke, 1983, 1993), and still others have found that different children respond to different methods (Carr & Dores, 1981; Yoder & Layton, 1988). Surprisingly, there have been few recent studies exploring these unresolved issues, and because most existing research is based on very small groups or single-case reports, there is no conclusive evidence for the effectiveness of single versus multimodal training or for particular combinations of augmentative systems. Nevertheless, in a recent review, Goldstein (2002) concludes that presenting signs or symbols, as well as speech, may help to "jump start" early vocabulary learning in that such systems are both less transient and easier to prompt than words alone.

CHOOSING AN APPROPRIATE SYSTEM

Communicative Forms

With so many systems to choose from, how can teachers, therapists, or parents go about selecting the most effective program for the child in their care? Light and colleagues (Light, Roberts, Dimarco, & Greiner, 1998; Light, McNaughton, & Parnes, 1994) have developed a detailed protocol for assessing clients' communication skills that can then be used as the basis for designing an appropriate AAC program. A much simpler system, proposed by Layton and Watson (1995), analyzes the different skills required for using signs, pictures, or written words and indicates which systems are most likely to succeed with different clients (see Table 9.1). However, there have been no attempts to test the validity of such systems, and in view of the fact that alternative communication strategies of various kinds are now widely used in schools for children with autism, it is disturbing that so little research has been conducted concerning the characteristics of children who seem to respond best to particular systems. There is anecdotal evidence that systems using pictures or photographs make the fewest demands on cognitive, linguistic, or memory skills and are thus more likely to succeed with children who have greatest deficits in these areas; but experimental data in support of such hypotheses remain lacking.

TABLE 9.1. Assessment for Choosing Alternative Communication Strategies

	Signing	Pictures/Pictographs	Writing
Characteristics of AAC system			
Easily shaped	xx	xxx	x
Portability	xxx	xx	xxx
Permanence	–	xxx	xxx
Speed	x	x	xx
Phrases possible	xx	xx	xxx
Iconicity	–/x	xxx	–
Reciprocity	x	x	xx
Demands on others' understanding	xxx	x	x
Child skills required			
Motor skills	xxx	x	xx
High cooperation	x	x	xx

Note. Example from Watson and Layton (1995). xxx, characteristic definitely applies/high level of skill required; xx, characteristic somewhat applies/moderate level of skill required; x, characteristic minimally applies/low level of skill required; –, characteristic does not apply/skill not required.

Communicative Functions

Whatever communication system is chosen, it would seem essential that this system fully reflect the child's individual interests or needs and that it is directly relevant to his or her environment. Nevertheless, in many behaviorally based interventions, the focus of training has tended to be on teaching and prompting predetermined labeling skills ("It's a cat"; "It is green" etc.), and such strategies continue to be a central component of many preschool intensive behavioral programs (cf. the stages described in Morris, Green, & Luce, 1996; see Table 9.2).

However, a number of studies indicate that communication training is much more likely to succeed if the system taught builds on children's existing and spontaneous attempts to communicate, thereby providing them with greater control over the environment. Studies of language acquisition in normal infants have shown that one of the primary goals of early communication is the manipulation of the immediate environment. Labeling and naming of objects for the purpose of sharing experiences do occur, but instrumental and regulatory utterances ("wanna," "gimme," "more," "no," etc.) tend to be among the most frequently used. Some years ago, Wetherby (1986) was able to demonstrate marked differences in the communicative functions displayed by typically developing preschool children and by those

TABLE 9.2. **Stages in Behavioral Language Program**

- Identify body parts/objects ("Show/Give me"; "What's this?").
- Identify pictures ("Show/Give me"; "What's this?").
- Perform actions ("Show me drinking, hugging").
- Request desired objects ("I want . . . ").
- Answer social questions ("What's your name?"; "How old are you?").
- Use verb labels ("What are you/is he doing?").
- Label familiar people ("Who is this?").
- Describe function of objects ("What do you do with pencil, cup?").

Note. Data from Morris, Green, and Luce (1996).

with autism. The children with autism rarely spontaneously used labels or descriptive comments, as the typically developing children did, but they frequently indicated their need for particular objects or expressed a wish to terminate activities. Rather than attempting to teach children to express concepts that are of little practical value to them, training is likely to be more successful if it takes account of their already existing "communicative profiles." Schuler et al. (1989), for example, analyzed the communicative functions expressed by two young children with autism prior to intervention (i.e., whether they made requests for objects, action, affection, etc., and whether these were communicated by looks, cries, aggression, vocalizations, etc.). Once it was clear how and why the children spontaneously tried to communicate, signs were successfully taught to replace existing strategies. Durand and Carr (1991) analyzed the "communicative intent" of self-injurious behaviors, and having established the "messages" conveyed by these actions ("want out," "want help," "too difficult," etc.), they then taught the children the signs to convey, more appropriately, the same functions. Durand and Carr (1991) and Prizant and Schuler (1987) have adopted similar approaches in the modification of echolalic and stereotyped speech. Instead of merely dismissing such utterances as "inappropriate" and therefore needing to be extinguished, they analyzed their communicative functions. They then successfully taught equivalent but appropriate verbal responses to replace them.

By means of this functional analysis of existing communication strategies, the complexity of the newly taught task for the child is much reduced. Instead of having to learn to use both new forms *and* new functions, the child is taught to "map" an alternative and more socially acceptable mode of communication onto an existing and spontaneously used communicative function. By ensuring that the new system results in the rapid elicitation of a desired response, the need for any extrinsic reinforcers is also reduced.

ENHANCING MOTIVATION TO COMMUNICATE

Improving the child's motivation to use the chosen system is crucial for successful and spontaneous usage. Motivational theories of learning suggest that the learning of new tasks in a series will be dependent on earlier successes in the same series. Thus, if communication skills are taught in the context of other, regularly occurring chains of behavior, they are more likely to become part of the habit chain and more likely to be strengthened. This finding highlights the importance of making communication training an integral part of more generalized teaching programs, rather than relying on teaching in isolation. Studies by Koegel and Koegel (1995) indicate that acquisition and generalization of communication skills by children with autism are more likely to be established if training is intrinsically linked to the teaching of other daily living skills. Many other authors have stressed the need for environmental restructuring if newly acquired communication skills are to be used spontaneously and effectively. There is little point, for example, in teaching a child to use the symbol or sign for an object he wants if that object is readily accessible without any additional effort. Changing environmental contingencies (i.e., placing toys, food, etc., out of immediate reach) so that the child needs to make greater use of taught strategies has obvious advantages. It increases the occurrence of stimulus-specific reinforcement and, by providing the child with greater control over the environment, makes it more likely that the newly acquired skills will be used on future occasions.

A number of studies also illustrate how deliberate disruption of the child's habitual routines can be used to increase communication. McClenny, Roberts, and Layton (1992) found that children communicated more frequently during sessions when they were exposed to "infringements" of previously well-established joint-action routines. These included making a desired object inaccessible (placing it in a locked box or on a high shelf); violating object function (using a spoon too large to fit in a jar of yogurt or one with holes in it to serve liquid; attempting to scoop out peanut butter with a broken plastic knife), or mislabeling objects or actions (e.g., calling a cup an "elephant"). Withholding objects resulted in the highest frequency of communicative attempts, and violations of object function were more effective than mislabeling objects. Similar strategies are described by Quill (1995), who provides examples of a variety of "unexpected" events used to elicit communication—for example, switching the contents or labels of well-known containers; demonstrating a wind-up toy but then handing the child a broken one; or handing out a container of juice but not providing any cups. Hawkins (1995) suggests making changes to daily routines, such as removing an item (e.g., soap) required to complete a regular behavior (e.g., hand washing), or delaying access to a particular item (e.g., offering one glove but not the other). Howlin (1998) also describes how gentle but systematic intrusion into the child's ritualistic activities can be used to encourage communication. These more "naturalistic" strategies clearly have many advantages over techniques that rely on artificial settings, methods, and materials. The resulting improvements in communication may also help to reduce problem behaviors. Koegel and colleagues (Koegel, Koegel, & Surratt, 1992) suggest that because such naturalistic reinforcement procedures are so effective, motivation to cooperate with the communication programs is enhanced, and hence children will be less likely to resort to disruptive behaviors. Certainly, as long as there is close cooperation and consistency among the adults in the child's environment, this approach seems more likely to ensure generalization and maintenance of communication skills. However, initially, any intrusions into the child's activities should be introduced gradually and with care in order to avoid unnecessary distress, and only minimal communicative attempts should be required. Otherwise anger and confusion, rather than reciprocal interaction, are likely to result.

LIMITATIONS OF EXISTING RESEARCH

A recent review (Law, Garrett, & Nye, 2004) of speech and language therapies for communication-impaired children concluded that, although there was evidence of improvement in children with phonological and expressive problems, the effect on those with more severe communication difficulties was limited. Evidence for a positive impact of nonverbal forms of communication training is even weaker, as is apparent from this chapter. Particular systems seem to leap to prominence and then to disappear from the literature almost without trace. Thus most reports of signing appeared in the 1970s; research on the use of symbols and of simultaneous communication methods systems emerged, and then largely disappeared again, in the 1980s, and in the 1990s picture communication systems came into prominence. There have been few systematic attempts to compare the relative effectiveness of different types of communication strategies, and although most published reports indicate improvements in the specific area of skill trained (increased use of signs, symbols, pictures, etc.), there is no evidence that any one program is superior to others in terms of producing higher rates of spontaneous and generative communication or in wider generalization. The few studies that have attempted to address these questions have been small scale, often single case; reports of treatment effectiveness are frequently anecdotal, control groups are rare, and randomized control trials are virtually nonexistent. Moreover, when particular methods have been shown to have some positive effects in experimental environments, generalization to more naturalistic settings or maintenance over longer periods has rarely been demonstrated.

Crucially, too, there is no reliable evidence concerning which systems work best with which children. Most of the programs described herein have involved children of primary school age or older, or interventions have included very heterogeneous age groups (sometimes mixing young children and adults; Goldstein, 2002). Mental age is rarely considered at all. Thus on the basis of present data there is no way of establishing the relative effectiveness of different approaches with preschool children. Uncontrolled studies indicate that PECS is likely to be effective in this younger age group, but whether it is more or less successful than other strategies remains to be demonstrated.

A further, unanswered question concerns *when* alternative communication systems should be introduced. Many of the programs described herein were implemented years after the stage at which typically developing children begin to speak. Studies of second-language acquisition (and alternative communication systems might well be regarded as a "second language") generally indicate that peak proficiency, in terms of phonology, semantics, and syntax, depends, for most people, on exposure in infancy or very early childhood. Proficiency, especially in the more complex grammatical aspects of language, tends to decline once children reach 4–6 years of age (Newport, 2002). For children with additional learning and communication problems, delays in introducing appropriate communication strategies are likely to have an even greater impact. On the basis of information from normal linguistic development, it would seem crucial that intervention begin as early as possible. Parents and preschool teachers sometimes express fears that the implementation of a nonverbal system may further delay or even prevent the emergence of speech. In fact, although evidence is limited, reviews of this area indicate that augmentative systems may actually encourage previously nonverbal children to speak. Thus, as soon as it is apparent that a child is significantly delayed in speech (i.e., no words or word approximations by 24 months), it would seem important to introduce an augmentative system without delay. In the absence of empirical data on the optimal system to use, it is probably wisest to introduce a system that builds on the child's existing skills. For example, a simple sign system may work with a child who imitates or uses gesture readily; a system such as PECS may suit a child who is interested in pictures or who spontaneously uses objects to indicate needs; and a computerized system may work well with those children with autism who show good computer skills.

A final and related question concerns the extent of exposure to specialist language programs that is required for the acquisition of fluent communication. Not only are communication programs for children with specific language difficulties generally introduced very late, but they also tend to be implemented for only very short periods each day (Grove & Dockrell, 2000; Konstantareas, 1996; Udwin & Yule, 1990). Early access to appropriate interventions and *constant* exposure to the chosen system are likely to be crucial for fluency of communication and generalization and maintenance.

CONCLUSIONS

Although the choice of appropriate communication programs for children with autism should be based on empirical evidence, current interventions are often based more on the whim of the moment. The complexity of children's communication deficits is rarely taken into account when assigning them to specific treatment programs, and little attention has been paid to the need to match the child's profile of strengths and difficulties to the components of different interventions. Furthermore, the range of alternative strategies employed has remained relatively limited. Thus, despite the increasing sophistication of computerized communication systems developed for use by individuals with severe physical disabilities (Beukelman & Mirenda, 1998), there has been little systematic evaluation of the use of these methods for children with autism.

The age at which augmentative programs should be introduced for optimal progress also remains unknown, although long-term outcome is almost certain to be affected by the age at which intervention begins. Delaying the introduction of alternative means of communication until the primary school years or later, as is the case in many of the studies reviewed here, is likely to result in limited acquisition, restricted fluency, and impaired generalization.

Finally, it is also apparent that whatever alternative systems are chosen for use with *children,* the use of these methods by their parents, teachers, and peers often remains extremely limited. Typically developing children learn to speak because they are surrounded by speech from the very moment they are born. To expect children with profound language impairments to develop effective communication skills using a system that they are exposed to intermittently and perhaps for only a few hours or less each day is hardly realistic. There is an urgent need to improve not only experimental work in this area but also attitudes and practices.

REFERENCES

Abrahamsen, A. A., Romski, M. A., & Sevcik, R. A. (1989). Concomitants of success in acquiring an augmentative communication system: Changes in attention, communication, and sociability. *American Journal on Mental Retardation, 5,* 475–496.

American Academy of Pediatrics Committee on Children with Disabilities. (1998). Auditory integration training and facilitated communication for autism. *Pediatrics, 102,* 431–433.

American Psychiatric Association. (1994). *Diagnostic and statistical manual of mental disorders* (4th ed.). Washington, DC: Author.

American Speech-Language-Hearing Association. (1991). *Report: Augmentative and alternative communication, 33*(Suppl. 5), 9–12.

Attwood, T., Frith, U., & Hermelin, B. (1988). The understanding and use of interpersonal gestures by autistic and Down's syndrome children. *Journal of Autism and Developmental Disorders, 18,* 241–257.

Baer, D. M., Wolf., M. M., & Risley, T. R. (1968). Some current dimensions of applied behavior analysis. *Journal of Applied Behavior Analysis, 1,* 91–97.

Baron-Cohen, S. (2002). *Mind reading: The interactive guide to emotions.* Cambridge, UK: University of Cambridge.

Barrera, R. D., & Sulzer-Azaroff, B. (1983). An alternating treatment comparison of oral and total communication training programs with echolalic autistic children. *Journal of Applied Behavior Analysis, 16,* 379–394.

Bebko, J. M., Perry, A., & Bryson, S. (1996). Multiple method validation study of facilitated communication: II. Individual differences and subgroup results. *Journal of Autism and Developmental Disorders, 26,* 19–42.

Benaroya, S., Wesley, S., Ogilvie, H., Klein, L. S., & Meaney, M. (1977). Sign language and multisensory input training of children with communication and related developmental disorders. *Journal of Autism and Childhood Schizophrenia, 7,* 23–31.

Bernard-Opitz, V., Sriram, N., & Nakhoda-Sapuan, S. (2001). Enhancing social problem solving in children with autism and normal children through computer-assisted instruction. *Journal of Autism and Developmental Disorders, 31,* 377–384.

Bernard-Opitz, V., Sriram, N., & Sapuan, S. (1999). Enhancing vocal limitations in children with autism using the IBM Speech Viewer. *Autism: International Journal of Research and Practice, 3,* 131–147.

Beukelman, D. R., & Mirenda, P. (1998) *Augmentative and alternative communication: Management of severe communication disorders in children and adults* (2nd ed.). Baltimore: Brookes.

Biklen, D. (1993). *Communication unbound: How facilitated communication is challenging traditional views of autism and ability/disability.* New York: Teachers College Press.

Bledsoe, R., Smith Myles, B., & Simpson, R. L. (2003). Use of a social story intervention to improve mealtime skills of an adolescent with Asperger syndrome. *Autism: International Journal of Research and Practice, 7,* 289–295.

Bliss, C. (1965). *Semantography.* Sydney, Australia: Semantography.

Bondy, A., & Frost, L. (2001). The Picture Exchange Communication System. *Behavior Modification, 25,* 725–744.

Bondy, A. S., & Frost, L. A. (1994a). PECS: *The Picture Exchange Communication System training manual.* Cherry Hill, NJ: Pyramid Educational Consultants.

Bondy, A. S., & Frost, L. A. (1994b). The Delaware Autistic Program. In S. L. Harris & J. S. Handleman (Eds.), *Preschool education programs for children with autism* (pp. 37–54). Austin, TX: PRO-ED.

Bondy, A. S., & Frost, L. A. (1994c). The Picture Exchange Communication System. *Focus on Autistic Behavior, 9,* 1–19.

Bonvillian, J. D., & Blackburn, D. (1991). Manual communication and autism: Factors relating to sign language acquisition. In P. Siple & S. D. Fischer (Eds.), *Issues in sign language research* (pp. 187–209). Chicago: University of Chicago Press.

Bonvillian, J. D., & Nelson, K. E. (1976). Sign language acquisition in a mute autistic boy. *Journal of Speech and Hearing Disorders, 41,* 339–347.

Bosseler, A., & Massaro, D. W. (2003). Development and evaluation of a computer-animated tutor for vocabulary and language learning in children with autism. *Journal of Autism and Developmental Disorders, 33,* 653–672.

Brady, D., & Smouse, A. (1978). A simultaneous comparison of three methods for language training with an autistic child: An experimental single case analysis. *Journal of Autism and Childhood Schizophrenia, 8,* 271–279.

Calculator, S., & Luchko, C. (1983). Evaluating the effectiveness of a communication board training program. *Journal of Speech and Hearing Disorders, 48,* 185–191.

Carr, E. G., & Dores, P. A. (1981). Patterns of language acquisition following simultaneous communication with autistic children. *Analysis and Intervention in Developmental Disabilities, 1,* 347–361.

Chambers, M., & Rehfeldt, R. A. (2003). Assessing the acquisition and generalization of two mand forms with adults with severe developmental disabilities. *Research in Developmental Disabilities, 24,* 265–280.

Charlop-Christy, M. H., Carpenter, M., Le, L., LeBlanc, L. A., & Kellett, K. (2002). Using the Picture Exchange Communication System (PECS) with children with autism: Assessment of PECS acquisition, speech, social-communicative behavior, and problem behavior. *Journal of Applied Behavior Analysis, 35,* 213–231.

Charman, T., Swettenham, J., Baron-Cohen, S., Cox, A., Baird, G., & Drew, A. (1997). Infants with autism: An investigation of empathy, pretend play, joint attention and imitation. *Developmental Psychology, 33,* 781–789.

Clark, C., Davis, C., & Woodcock, R. (1974). *Standard rebus glossary.* Circle Pines, MN: American Guidance Service.

Colby, K. M. (1973). The rationale for computer-based treatment of language difficulties in non-speaking autistic children. *Journal of Autism and Childhood Schizophrenia, 3,* 254–260.

Daley, D., Cantrell, R., Cantrell, M., & Aman, L. (1972). Structuring speech therapy contingencies with an oral apraxic child. *Journal of Speech and Hearing Disorders, 37,* 22–32.

Duker, P. C., & van Lent, C. (1991). Inducing variability in communicative gestures used by severely retarded individuals. *Journal of Applied Behavior Analysis, 24,* 379–386.

Durand, B. M., & Carr, E. G. (1991). Functional communication training to reduce challenging behavior: Maintenance and application in new settings. *Journal of Applied Behavior Analysis, 24,* 251–254.

Durand, V. M., & Merges, E. (2001). Functional communication training: A contemporary behavior analytic intervention for problem behavior. *Focus on Autism and Other Developmental Disorders, 16,* 110–119.

Facilitated communication is not reliable as evidence. (2000, July 26). *Law report, London Times.*

Finnerty, J., & Quill, K. (1991). *The communication analyzer*. Lexington, MA: Educational Software Research.

Foreman, P., & Crews, G. (1998). Using augmentative communication with infants and young children with Down syndrome. *Down Syndrome Research and Practice, 5,* 16–25.

Fulwiler, R. L., & Fouts, R. S. (1976). Acquisition of American Sign Language by a non-communicating autistic child. *Journal of Autism and Childhood Schizophrenia, 6,* 43–51.

Gaines, R., Leaper, C., Monahan, C., & Weickgenant, A. (1988). Language learning and retention in young language disordered children. *Journal of Autism and Developmental Disorders, 18,* 281–296.

Ganz, J. B., & Simpson, R. L. (2004). Effects on communicative requesting and social development of the Picture Exchange Communication System in children with characteristics of autism. *Journal of Autism and Developmental Disorders, 34* 395 409.

Goldstein, H. (2002). Communication intervention for children with autism: A review of treatment efficacy. *Journal of Autism and Developmental Disorders, 32,* 373–396.

Gorenflo, C. W., & Gorenflo, D. W. (1991). The effects of information and augmentative communication technique on attitudes toward nonspeaking individuals. *Journal of Speech and Hearing Research, 34,* 19–26.

Gray, C. A. (1995). Teaching children with autism to "read" social situations. In K. A. Quill (Ed.), *Teaching children with autism: Strategies to enhance communication and socialization* (pp. 219–242). New York. Delmar.

Gray, C. A., & Garand, J. D. (1993). Social stories: Improving responses of students with autism with accurate social information. *Focus on Autistic Behavior, 8,* 1–10.

Green, G. (1994). The quality of the evidence. In H. C. Shane (Ed.), *Facilitated communication: The clinical and social phenomenon* (pp. 157–226). San Diego, CA: Singular.

Grove, N., & Dockrell, J. (2000). Multisign combinations by children with intellectual impairments: An analysis of language skills. *Journal of Speech, Language, and Hearing Research, 43,* 309–323.

Grove, N., & Walker, M. (1990). The Makaton Vocabulary: Using manual signs and graphic symbols to develop interpersonal communication. *Augmentative and Alternative Communication, 6,* 15–28.

Hagiwara, T., & Myles, B. S. (1999). A multimedia social story intervention: Teaching skills to children with autism. *Focus on Autism and Other Developmental Disabilities, 14,* 82–95.

Hauck, J. A., & Dewey, D. (2001). Hand preference and motor functioning in children with autism. *Journal of Autism and Developmental Disorders, 31,* 265–278.

Hawkins, D. (1995). Spontaneous language use. In R. L. Koegel & L. K. Koegel (Eds.), *Teaching children with autism* (pp. 43–52). Baltimore: Brookes.

Heimann, M., Nelson, K., Tjus, T., & Gillberg, C. (1995). Increasing reading and communication skills in children with autism through an interactive multimedia computer program. *Journal of Autism and Developmental Disorders, 25,* 459–480.

Hetzroni, O. E., & Tannous, J. (2004). Effects of a computer-based intervention program on the communicative functions of children with autism. *Journal of Autism and Developmental Disorders, 34,* 95–113.

Howlin, P. (1989). Changing approaches to communication training with autistic children. *British Journal of Disorders of Communication, 24,* 151–168.

Howlin, P. (1998). *Children with autism and Asperger syndrome.* Chichester, UK: Wiley.

Howlin, P. (2004). *Autism and Asperger syndrome: Preparing for adulthood.* London: Routledge.

Howlin, P., & Moore, A. (1997). Diagnosis in autism: A survey of over 1200 parents. *Autism: International Journal of Research and Practice, 1,* 135–162.

Howlin, P., & Rutter, M. (1987). The consequences of language delay for other aspects of development. In W. Yule & M. Rutter (Eds.), *Language development and disorders* (pp. 271–94). Oxford, UK: MacKeith Press.

Hughes, C. (1996). Planning problems in autism at the level of motor control. *Journal of Autism and Developmental Disorders, 26,* 99–109.

Hunt, P., Alwell, M., Goetz, L., & Sailor, W. (1990). Generalized effects of conversation skill training. *Journal of the Association for Persons with Severe Handicaps, 15,* 250–260.

Jacobson, J. W., Mulick, J. A., & Schwartz, A. A. (1995). A history of facilitated communication: Science, pseudoscience, and anti-science. *American Psychologist, 50,* 750–765.

Jordan, R., & Powell, S. (1990a). Teaching autistic children to think more effectively. *Communication, 24,* 20–22.

Jordan, R., & Powell, S. (1990b). Improving thinking in autistic children using computer presented activities. *Communication, 24,* 23–25.

Keen, D., Sigafoos, J., & Woodyatt, G. (2001). Replacing prelinguistic behaviors with functional communication. *Journal of Autism and Developmental Disorders, 31,* 385–398.

Kiernan, C. (1983). The use of nonvocal communication techniques with autistic individuals. *Journal of Child Psychology and Psychiatry, 24,* 339–375.

Koegel, R. L., & Koegel, L. K. (1995). *Teaching children with autism: Strategies for initiating positive interactions and improving learning opportunities.* Baltimore: Brookes.

Koegel, R. L., Koegel, L. K., & Surratt, A. V. (1992). Language intervention and disruptive behavior in pre-school children with autism. *Journal of Autism and Developmental Disorders, 22,* 141–153.

Konstantareas, M. (1987). Autistic children exposed to simultaneous communication training: A follow-up. *Journal of Autism and Developmental Disorders, 17,* 115–132.

Konstantareas, M. (1996). Communication training approaches in autistic disorder. In J. H. Beitchman, N. J. Cohen, M. Konstantareas, & R. Tannock (Eds.), *Language, learning, and behavior disorders* (pp. 467–487). Cambridge, UK: Cambridge University Press.

Konstantareas, M. M., & Lelbovitz, S. F. (1981). Early communication acquisition by autistic children: Signing and mouthing versus signing and speaking. *Sign Language Studies, 31,* 135–154.

Konstantareas, M., Oxman, J., & Webster, C. (1978). Iconicity: Effects on the acquisition of sign language by autistic and other severely dysfunctional children. In P. Siple (Ed.), *Understanding language through sign language research* (pp. 213–237). New York: Academic Press.

Krantz, P. J., MacDuff, M. T., & McClannahan, L. E. (1993). Programming participation in family activities for children with autism: Parents' use of photographic activity schedules. *Journal of Applied Behavior Analysis, 26,* 137–138.

Kravits, T. E., Kamps, D. M., Kemmerer, K., & Potucek, J. (2002). Brief report: Increasing communication skills for an elementary-aged student with autism using the Picture Exchange Communication System. *Journal of Autism and Developmental Disorders, 32,* 225–230.

LaVigna, G. W. (1977). Communication training in mute autistic adolescents using the written word. *Journal of Autism and Childhood Schizophrenia, 7,* 135–149.

Law, J., Garrett, Z., & Nye, C. (2004). Speech and language therapy interventions for children with primary speech and language delay or disorder (Cochrane Review). In *The Cochrane Library* (Issue 3). Chichester, UK: Wiley.

Layton, T. L. (1988). Language training with autistic children using four different models of presentation. *Journal of Communication Disorders, 21,* 333–350.

Layton, T. L., & Watson, L. R. (1995). Enhancing communication in non-verbal children with autism. In K. Quill (Ed.), *Teaching children with autism: Strategies to enhance communication and socialization,* (pp. 73–104). New York: Delmar.

Light, J., McNaughton, D., & Parnes, P. (1994). *A protocol for the assessment of the communication interaction skills of nonspeaking severely handicapped adults and their facilitators.* Toronto, Ontario, Canada: Augmentative Communication Service, Hugh MacMillan Medical Centre.

Light, J. C., Roberts, B., Dimarco, R., & Greiner, N. (1998). Augmentative and alternative communication to support receptive and expressive communication for people with autism. *Journal of Communication Disorders, 31,* 153–180.

Lord, C., & Bailey, A. (2002). Autism spectrum disorders. In M. Rutter & E. Taylor (Eds.), *Child and adolescent psychiatry* (4th ed., pp. 636–663). Oxford, UK: Blackwell.

Lorimer, P. A., Simpson, R., Myles, B. S., & Ganz, J. (2002). The use of social stories as a preventative behavioral intervention in a home setting with a child with autism. *Journal of Positive Behavioral Interventions, 4,* 53–60.

Lovaas, O. (1977). *The autistic child: Language development through behavior modification.* New York: Wiley.

Magiati, I., & Howlin, P. (2003). A pilot evaluation study of the Picture Exchange Communication System (PECS) for children with autistic spectrum disorders. *Autism: International Journal of Research and Practice, 7,* 297–320.

Manjiviona, J., & Prior, M. (1995). Comparison of Asperger syndrome and high functioning autistic children on a test of motor impairment. *Journal of Autism and Developmental Disorders, 25,* 23–40.

McClannahan, L. E., & Krantz, P. J. (1999). *Activity schedules for children with autism: Teaching independent behavior.* Bethesda, MD: Woodbine.

McClenny, C., Roberts, J., & Layton, T. (1992). Unexpected events and their effect on children's language. *Child Language Teaching and Therapy, 8,* 229–264.

McNaughton, S. (1995). Responding to "What is your latest thinking on Bliss?" *Communicating Together, 12,* 22–23.

Minshew, N. J., Goldstein, G., & Siegel, D. J. (1997). Neuropsychologic functioning in autism: Profile of a complex information processing disorder. *Journal of International Neuropsychological Society, 3,* 303–316.

Moore, M., & Calvert, S. (2000). Brief report: Vocabulary acquisition for children with autism: Teacher or computer instruction. *Journal of Autism and Developmental Disorders, 30,* 359–362.

Morris, C., Green, G., & Luce, S. C. (Eds.). (1996). *Behavioral interventions for young children with autism: A manual for parents and professionals.* Austin, TX: PRO-ED.

Mostert, M. P. (2001). Facilitated communication since 1995: A review of published studies. *Journal of Autism and Developmental Disorders, 31,* 287–313.

Myles, B. S., & Simpson, R. (2001) Effective practices for students with Asperger syndrome. *Focus on Exceptional Children, 34,* 1–14.

Nadel, J., Guerini, C., Peze, A., & Rivet, C. (1999). The evolving nature of imitation as a format for communication. In J. Nadel & G. Butterworth (Eds.), *Imitation in infancy* (pp. 209–234). Cambridge, UK: Cambridge University Press.

Nelson, K. E., Heimann, M., & Tjus, T. (1997). Theoretical and applied insights from multimedia facilitation of communication skills in children with autism, deaf children and children with other disabilities. In L. B. Adamson & M. A. Romski (Eds.), *Communication and language acquisition: Discoveries from atypical development* (pp. 295–325). Baltimore: Brookes.

Newport, E. L. (2002). Critical periods in language development. In L. Nadel (Ed.), *Cognitive science* (pp. 737–740). London: Macmillan.

Norris, C., & Dattilo, J. (1999). Evaluating effects of a social story intervention on a young girl with autism. *Focus on Autism and Other Developmental Disabilities, 14,* 180–186.

Paget, R., Gorman, P., & Paget, G. (1976). *The Paget–Gorman Sign System* (6th ed.). London: Association for Experiments in Deaf Education.

Panyan, M. V. (1984). Computer technology for autistic students. *Journal of Autism and Developmental Disorders, 14,* 375–382.

Pleinis, A., & Romanczyk, R. G. (1985). Analyses of performance, behavior and predictors for severely disturbed children: A comparison of adult vs, computer instruction. *Analysis and Intervention in Developmental Disabilities, 5,* 345–356.

Prizant, B., & Schuler, A. (1987). Facilitating communication: Language approaches. In D. Cohen & A. Donnellan (Eds.), *Handbook of autism and pervasive developmental disorders* (pp. 316–332). New York: Wiley.

Quill, K. (1995). Enhancing children's social-communicative interactions. In K. Quill (Ed.), *Teaching children with autism: Strategies to enhance communication and socialization* (pp. 163–192). New York: Delmar.

Rapin, I. (1996). *Preschool children with inadequate communication: Developmental language disorder.* London: MacKeith Press.

Reichle, J., & Brown, L. (1986). Teaching the use of a multipage direct selection communication board to an adult with autism. *Journal of the Association for Persons with Severe Handicaps, 11,* 68–73.

Remington, B., & Clarke, S. (1983). Acquisition of expressive signing by autistic children: An evaluation of the relative effects of simultaneous communication and sign-alone training. *Journal of Applied Behavior Analysis, 16,* 315–328.

Remington, B., & Clarke, S. (1993). Simultaneous communication and speech comprehension: Part I. Comparison of two methods of teaching expressive signing and speech comprehension skills. *Augmentative and Alternative Communication, 9*, 36–48.

Risley, T., & Wolf, M. (1967). Establishing functional speech in echolalic children. *Behaviour Research and Therapy, 5*, 73–88.

Rogers, S. J., Hepburn, S. L., Stackhouse, T., & Wehner, E. (2003). Imitation performance in toddlers with autism and those with other developmental disorders. *Journal of Child Psychology and Psychiatry, 44*, 763–781.

Schlosser, R. W., Belfiore, P. J., Nigam, R., Blischak, D., & Hetzroni, O. (1995). The effects of speech output technology on the learning of graphic symbols. *Journal of Applied Behavior Analysis, 28*, 537–549.

Schopler, E., Mesibov, G. B., & Hearsey, K. (1995). Structured teaching in the TEACCH system. In E. Schopler & G. B. Mesibov (Eds.), *Learning and cognition in autism* (pp. 243–268). New York: Plenum Press.

Schuler, A. L., Peck, C. A., Willard, C., & Theimer, K. (1989). Assessment of communicative means and functions through interview: Assessing the communicative capabilities of individuals with limited language. *Seminars in Speech and Language, 10*, 51–61.

Schwartz, I. S., Garfinkle, A. N., & Bauer, J. (1998). The Picture Exchange Communication System: Communicative outcomes for young children with disabilities. *Topics in Early Childhood Special Education, 18*, 144–159.

Seal, B. C., & Bonvillian, J. D. (1997). Sign language and motor functioning in students with autistic disorders. *Journal of Autism and Developmental Disorders, 27*, 437–466.

Silver, M., & Oakes, P. (2001). Evaluation of a new computer intervention to teach people with autism or Asperger syndrome to recognize and predict emotions in others. *Autism: International Journal of Research and Practice, 5*, 299–316.

Simpson, R. L., & Myles, B. S. (1995). Facilitated communication and children with disabilities: An enigma in search of a perspective. *Focus on Exceptional Children, 27*, 1–16.

Sisson, L. A., & Barrett, R. P. (1984). An alternating-treatments comparison of oral and total communication training with minimally verbal retarded children. *Journal of Applied Behavior Analysis, 17*, 559–566.

Stone, W. L., & Caro-Martinez, L. M. (1990). Naturalistic observations of spontaneous communication in autistic children. *Journal of Autism and Developmental Disorders, 20*, 437–453.

Stone, W. L., Ousley, O. Y., & Littleford, C. D. (1997). Motor imitation in young children with autism: What's the object? *Journal of Abnormal Child Psychology, 25*, 475–485.

Swaggart, B. L., Gagnon, E., Bock, S. J., Earles, T. L., Quinn, C., Myles, B. S., et al. (1995). Using social stories to teach social and behavioral skills to children with autism. *Focus on Autistic Behavior, 10*, 1–16.

Thiemann, K. S., & Goldstein, H. (2001). Social stories, written text clues, and video feedback: Effects on social communication of children with autism. *Journal of Applied Behavior Analysis, 34*, 425–446.

Tjus, T., Heimann, M., & Nelson, K. E. (1998). Gains in literacy through the use of a specially developed multimedia research strategy: Positive findings from 13 children with autism. *Autism: International Journal of Research and Practice, 2,* 139–156.

Tjus, T., Heimann, M., & Nelson, K. E. (2001). Interaction patterns between children and their teachers when using a specific multi-media and communication strategy: Observations from children with autism and mixed intellectual disabilities. *Autism: International Journal of Research and Practice, 5,* 175–187.

Udwin, O., & Yule, W. (1990). Augmentative communication systems taught to cerebral palsied children: A longitudinal study: I. The acquisition of signs and symbols, and syntactic aspects of their use over time. *British Journal of Disorders of Communication, 25,* 295–309.

Udwin, O., & Yule, W. (1991a). Augmentative communication systems taught to cerebral palsied children: A longitudinal study: II. Pragmatic features of sign and symbol use. *British Journal of Disorders of Communication, 26,* 137–148.

Udwin, O., & Yule, W. (1991b). Augmentative communication systems taught to cerebral palsied children: A longitudinal study: III. Teaching practices and exposure to sign and symbol use in schools and homes. *British Journal of Disorders of Communication, 26,* 149–162.

Wacker, D., Steege, M., Northup, J., Sasso, G., Berg, W., Reimers, T., et al. (1990). A component analysis of functional communication training across three topographies of severe behavior problems. *Journal of Applied Behavior Analysis, 23,* 417–429.

Walker, M. (1980). *Makaton vocabulary* (rev. ed.). Surrey, UK: The Makaton Vocabulary Development Project.

Watson, L. R., Lord, C., Schaffer, B., & Schopler, E. (1989). *Teaching spontaneous communication to autistic and developmentally handicapped children.* New York: Irvington.

Wetherby, A. M. (1986). Ontogeny of communicative functions in autism. *Journal of Autism and Developmental Disorders, 16,* 295–316.

Williams, C., Wright, B., Callaghan, G., & Coughlan, B. (2002). Do children with autism learn to read more readily by computer assisted instruction or traditional book methods? *Autism: International Journal of Research and Practice, 6,* 71–91.

Williams, J. H. G., Whiten, A., & Singh, B. (2004). A systematic review of action imitation in autistic spectrum disorder. *Journal of Autism and Developmental Disorders, 34,* 285–299.

World Health Organization. (1993). *The ICD-10 classification of mental and behavioral disorders: Diagnostic criteria for research.* Geneva, Switzerland: Author.

Yoder, P. J., & Layton, T. L. (1988). Speech following sign language training in autistic children with minimal verbal language. *Journal of Autism and Developmental Disorders, 18,* 217–230.

PART IV

Developmental and Neurobiological Issues

This section provides a conceptual and empirical framework that outlines developmental and neuroscientific approaches to early social-communicative development, drawing on research with typically developing infants, children with developmental delay, and children with ASD.

Walden and Hurley, in Chapter 10, provide a conceptual framework for understanding the myriad influences on early social-communicative development. As well as summarizing work with children, they draw on comparative studies illustrating the effects of environmental factors and experience on gene expression and neurological development. The chapter outlines the typical and atypical developmental pathways of joint attention, emotional responsivity, and imitation abilities. Parallel and divergent research trends in the literature on typical and atypical development are discussed, with an eye toward integrating these different approaches. This framework is important in reminding us that the future is not a "given" for children with ASD and that their experiences from early in life will, in part, determine the progress that they make and competencies that they develop. Such empirically based theoretical principles should both motivate and underpin intervention approaches.

Mundy and Thorp, in Chapter 11, examine the empirical evidence relevant to establishing the neural basis of early social-communicative behavior in autism, with a particular focus on joint attention. The chapter emphasizes the fact that ASD is a multisystem, multiprocess neurodevelopmental disorder that must be understood at both the behavioral and brain levels. Results from neuroimaging, electrophysiological, and neuropsychological studies are reviewed, providing strong evidence that initiating joint attention and responding to joint attention are subserved by different cortical systems. The authors discuss clinical implications of these findings in terms of understanding how children with ASD learn and offer a framework for developing neuroscientifically based early interventions that target both types of joint-attention skills.

10

A Developmental Approach to Understanding Atypical Development

TEDRA A. WALDEN
JENNIFER J. HURLEY

Development is complex. Each individual child develops as a unique melding of biological and social forces, which interact throughout life to create an individual path of development. To ignore the complexity of the developmental process or to focus on one or a few aspects of development misrepresents each individual.

Current developmental accounts hold that it is not possible to find a single underlying cause for typical or atypical development in children. Rather, maintaining or changing direction on a path depends on interactions among many factors (Cicchetti & Sroufe, 2000). We can no longer ask what is *the* cause for a child's developmental path, but instead must ask how *combinations* of factors act in concert to maintain or change a particular path of development (Cicchetti & Sroufe, 2000).

Developmental psychopathology provides a general orientation to understanding how disorders arise and are maintained. This approach acknowledges the complexity of human behavior and the need to integrate individual and contextual processes in a dynamic ecological model (Sameroff, 1992; Sameroff & Seifer, 1990). For example, Sroufe and Rutter (1984) described the approach as "the study of the origins and course of individual patterns of behavioral adaptation" (p. 18). Cicchetti and Toth (1995) argued that it is important to evaluate the dynamic transaction with the "inner" constitutional and "outer" environmental characteristics that may lead to outcomes that either inhibit or exacerbate early deviations or maintain or disrupt early adaptation.

Cicchetti and Sroufe (2000) referred to developmental psychopathology as a "big tent" under which many disciplines of study can combine efforts to facilitate progress. Consideration of perspectives from multiple disciplines will help us to understand the processes of development in general and is imperative for gaining a greater understanding of developmental processes in atypically developing children (Dykens, 2003). Dawson et al. (2002) have advocated "an integration of concepts" approach to understanding development in children with autism.

In this chapter we discuss some important coactions among different factors that affect development. We highlight the effects of experience on developing systems because experiences can be targets of intervention and change. We then discuss three early social-communicative behaviors—joint attention, emotional communication, and imitation—for typically developing children and those with autism and note the importance of each as a foundation for later development, especially language and communication skills.

CAUSALITY AND COACTIONAL RELATIONS AMONG AGENTS OF DEVELOPMENT

Gottlieb and Halpern (2002) characterized the interactions among different agents of development, such as environment, behavior, neural structure, and genetic activity, as "bidirectional traffic." The factors act together, with the direction of influence moving back and forth and with development occurring as a product of the relation among the factors (coaction). What accounts for development, then, is this coaction—not the individual factors. In this section we discuss evidence that experience interacts with other factors in development. We consider some effects that may go unnoticed because most members of the species have functionally equivalent experiences in the normal rearing environment. However, appreciating the impact of experiences can focus attention on possible opportunities for interventions for children with atypical development.

Effects of Experience on Species-Typical Behavior

Outcomes, even those said to be "innate," develop through a complex interplay of genetic propensities and sensitivities with environmental and social factors, some of which may be subtle (making them easy to overlook). To say that a characteristic is "innate" or "genetic" does not explain how it develops; we must still explain how genetic factors express themselves as physical or behavioral characteristics.

An example of work focusing on social factors that influence "innate" characteristics is that of Gottlieb and colleagues, who have studied the development of attachment behaviors (preference for one individual, usually the mother) in young birds. They proposed that, rather than complex or even simple behaviors being encoded directly in the genes, what are encoded are sensitivities to particular kinds of stimulation or experiences. As described next, their work shows that normally occurring experiences (which occur for most members of a species) can be the basis for developing important behaviors that are "typical" of the species (e.g., recognizing one's own species; Dmitrieva & Gottlieb, 1994; Gottlieb, 1985; Gottlieb, 1998).

Gottlieb studied the ability of mallard ducklings to recognize the call of their species, a behavior long considered to be "innate." The behavior is important for individual survival (because it influences caregiving) and necessary for the continuance of the species (because it guides mating with members of one's own species). Gottlieb (1991) reported a series of experimental studies showing that recognizing the call of one's species was neither "genetically determined" nor "innate." Rather, the *experience* of hearing sounds during a time of increased sensitivity created a familiarity with and preference for that sound. Experiences involving hearing maternal calls while inside the egg, the calls of young siblings, or even self-produced vocalizations (prior to hatching) were all effective in producing the preference. Exposure to calls of another species produced a preference for that call instead of those of one's own species. Furthermore, experiences prior to hatching and after hatching were both effective. It was difficult to reverse the preference once it was established; that is, sensitivity to the auditory experiences was limited. Thus the development of preferences for one's own species, a behavior that was previously thought to be "genetically determined," depends on social experiences.

In subsequent work, Randell and Gottlieb (1992) found that excessive stimulation (i.e., constant movement) made the developing organism unresponsive to other types of stimulation, even that to which it would typically be highly responsive (e.g., calls). They exposed duck embryos to the call of their species while the young received various levels of water-bed stimulation. The ducklings that experienced constant movement did not learn to recognize the call, whereas those with minimal or alternating stimulation did.

These studies show that behaviors of typically developing members of a species can result from the interplay of genetic sensitivities with experiences. These experiences may occur under normal rearing conditions, but they can be altered (and sometimes without noticing or appreciating what has changed). This idea has enormous implications for early intervention with children with atypical development because it suggests that early intervention might be effective in maintaining or redirecting children's behavior to a more normal course.

Effects of Experience on Gene Expression

The effects of genes used to be viewed as deterministic and invariant, but we now understand that genes do not have constant effects. We have learned that, despite the fact that every cell in the body has exactly the same genotype, each has a different developmental history and different characteristics. This differentiation is an environmental effect stemming from different experiences of each cell (Sameroff, 1992). Genes vary in their effects across development, and they are responsive to context. Structural genes are activated and inactivated by operator and regulator genes, which respond to the environment in which the gene functions. Thus to think of genetic effects as "determined" misrepresents their complexity. Furthermore, genes create their effects by producing particular strings of protein, and there are many steps between proteins and behavioral characteristics.

An example of the impact of experience on gene expression is a study of serotonin concentration and behaviors in monkeys (Bennett et al., 2002). In rhesus monkeys, the transporter gene 5-HTT is responsible for serotonin release into the system. Genetic variation in serotonin expression has been associated with depression, aggression-related personality traits, and anxiety (e.g., Veenstra-VanderWeele, Anderson, & Cook, 2000). Some, but not all, monkeys with a short allele for 5-HTT have lower levels of serotonin and display aggressive, risky behavior (e.g., making longer leaps between trees). Bennett and colleagues (2002) randomly assigned monkeys with short and long alleles to be raised by either their mothers or their peers. Only monkeys who were raised by peers *and* had short alleles showed lower concentrations of serotonin and risky, aggressive behaviors, whereas monkeys with both short and long alleles who were raised by mothers had typical levels of serotonin and typical behavior. Experience, in this case rearing condition, interacted with the genetic constellation of these monkeys to result in different developmental outcomes. Thus genes did not "determine" atypical development, but the coaction between environment and genes acted together to influence development.

Another coactional relation between environment and genetics may apply to children with atypical development. When children display behaviors or have particular physical characteristics (e.g., stereotypies), they may evoke a certain type of response from others. These are called evocative genotype–phenotype interactions (Scarr & McCartney, 1983). The development of children with a genetically identifiable syndrome may be mediated by the social responses of others. Evocative effects of genotype on environment may operate for children with particular syndromes or etiological causes for their mental retardation (Dykens, 1995).

For example, an evocative effect may account for social responses to children with Down syndrome, who have a craniofacial appearance that is perceived as youthful. Fidler and Hodapp (1999) showed photographs of children with Down syndrome and children with 5p-syndrome (associated with mental retardation) to adult raters, who perceived children with Down syndrome as being more "baby faced" and more immature (e.g., more naive, kind, and cuddly). A youthful appearance may be endearing to adults and elicit positive social behaviors and behaviors that might typically be directed toward younger children. In support of this hypothesis, Fidler (2003) found that parents of children with Down syndrome spoke to their children with a distinctly different style than did parents of children with other etiologies of mental retardation. Their speech had characteristics associated with infant-directed speech or "motherese" (i.e. higher pitch and greater pitch variability). Thus, genetic factors may produce differences in the environment experienced by the children, which contributes to their development.

The role of the social environment in mediating the impact of genetic factors is suggested in a series of studies of social referencing with typical children and those with Down syndrome by Walden and colleagues. Typically, by 12 months of age, children who are confronted with events that are novel or ambiguous (e.g., new foods or toys) refer to the reactions of other people to help evaluate the event and know how to respond. Walden, Knieps, and Baxter (1991) reported that preschool children with Down syndrome were less likely than typically developing mental-age (MA) matched peers to regulate their behavior to novel events based on social referencing of their mothers' emotional reactions to the events. Also, parents of children with Down syndrome had trouble timing their social referencing messages to be contingent on their children's social looks at them. That is, parents were instructed not to communicate until the child had initiated a social look toward the parent; however, parents of children with Down syndrome gave many "false alarms," or uncued messages. This was important because Down syndrome children with more contingent parents (who waited for the children to initiate an interaction before giving emotional messages) behaved like typically developing children, basing their behavior on parents' emotional messages. However, children with Down syndrome with less contingent parents did not. Thus, parents of children with Down syndrome developed a response bias, failing to wait for their children to initiate communication, behavior that was associated with poor social referencing.

In a follow-up study, Walden (1996) evaluated differences in social signals (social looks) produced by typically developing children and by those with Down syndrome. Adults watched video segments of unfamiliar children and their parents during social referencing episodes. The participants judged whether each child looked at the parent or not in each segment and rated their level of confidence in making each judgment. These judgments were evaluated for accuracy by comparing them with those of trained coders who used frame-by-frame coding in slow motion. The social looks of the typically developing children were easier to judge correctly, and judges were more confident of their evaluations of them than they were of their evaluations of the looks produced by children with Down syndrome. The judges "missed" many of the looks from children with Down syndrome when they occurred. Even when the participants did judge correctly for the children with Down syndrome that a social look had occurred, they were less confident about their decisions than about those for typically developing children. Interestingly, the difficulty and lack of confidence extended to parents of children with Down syndrome, parents of children with typical development, and nonparents with no experience with small children—thus they could not be said to be the result of parenting experiences.

These studies suggest that hard-to-interpret social signals of children with Down syndrome pose a challenge for parents (and others) during social interactions. Noncontingent responding makes it harder for children to interpret the meaning of social messages, and social referencing suffers. The genetic syndrome sets the stage for atypical social interactions that impair the development of children with Down syndrome.

Social signals of young children with Down syndrome are more difficult to interpret, so these children may elicit less responsive and contingent behaviors in general. Having responsive caretakers who interpret and respond to signals appropriately is a critical component of social and cognitive development (Lamb & Easterbrooks, 1981). Furthermore, because the social looks of children with Down syndrome did not elicit appropriate responses from their parents, this behavior might be expected to decline in frequency and appropriateness in the future, creating further social difficulties. In this way, experiences can interact with genetic factors to produce a phenotype such as Down syndrome.

The preceding studies illustrate ways in which genetic propensities interact with experiences to produce atypical experiences leading to undesirable outcomes. These experiences could be the focus of interventions designed to compensate for deficits or to build on strengths in order to interrupt a cascade of effects. That is, early intervention might help to maintain or redirect behavior to a more normal course.

Effects of Experience on Neurological Structure

We now understand that experience can affect neural development at structural and functional levels. In addition, neural structure influences experience. Thus an understanding of development requires combining knowledge of neurobiological processes and behavioral development to understand how typical and atypical development diverge and how the interaction between neural structure and environment can deflect or maintain an individual on a path of typical or atypical development (Cicchetti & Cannon, 1999).

An example of an effect of experience on neural structure is that reported by Wu and Kass (2002). They examined the neural structures of squirrel and galago monkeys who had accidentally lost limbs when they were under the age of 2 months. When the monkeys were 4–8 years of age, their brains were examined to assess the plasticity of neural restructuring after limb loss. The monkeys' bodies were injected with dye in different locations. The dye traveled to and stained the corresponding terminations of sensory afferents in the spinal cord and brainstem. Stains in areas of the brain corresponding to the intact limb were larger than those in areas corresponding to the amputated limb. The afferents from areas surrounding the stump after amputation encroached on portions of the brain and spinal cord that would have been responsive to the arm or leg before amputation. Wu and Kass (2002) explain the size differences and encroachment as due to brain development that occurs in response to either stimulation or lack of stimulation. This study shows that the brain can undergo structural changes as a result of experience.

Effects of Experience on Children with Atypical Development

Given that brain structure and functioning, as well as experience, influence the developmental path, understanding the relations among these factors has significance for early intervention. Cicchetti (2002) described the coacting relations among neural, genetic, and experiential agents as "scaffolding" and described three types of scaffolding that affect the process of neural development. *Gene-driven processes* occur when genes influence brain development. For example, genes guide the migration of neurons (Rakic, 1988). *Experience-expectant processes* occur during sensitive periods or when the brain is primed for information or experiences needed for typical development (Cicchetti, 2002). For example, during early visual development, there is an overproduction of synapses, which decrease when not used. Visual deprivation during this sensitive period produces lasting damage to the visual cortex, even when typical visual experiences are later restored (described in Greenough, Black, & Wallace, 1987). Similarly, Rema, Armstrong-James, & Ebner (2003) exposed rats to sensory deprivation and evaluated the effect of later stimulation on neural cortical cell responses. Rats who had experienced early sensory deprivation were impaired in responding to stimulation, even when later sensory experiences were provided. *Experience-dependent* effects are not restricted by temporal periods but occur throughout the lifetime when the brain is affected by new experiences (Cicchetti, 2002). An experience-dependent effect can be seen in recent research evaluating the effects of different environments on brain development in rats (e.g., Jones, Klintsova, Kilman, Sirevaag, & Greenough, 1997; Rema & Ebner, 1999; Turner & Greenough, 1985).

Rema and Ebner (1999) evaluated the effects of enriched rearing on young rats with prenatal alcohol exposure (PAE). Rats who received enriched rearing were provided with ladders, platforms, a variety of toys, and other rats for social stimulation. Environmental stimulation increased brain plasticity, that is, experience-dependent neural change, in rats with PAE when compared with rats with PAE who did not receive stimulation. Specifically, for rats with PAE, enriched rearing accelerated neuronal responsiveness, increased the magnitude of responses, and accelerated the rate of a type of response modification that indicates cortical plasticity. The stimulated rats with PAE never demonstrated the levels of responsiveness as rats without PAE, but they did improve. By providing environmental stimulation, the responsiveness and plasticity of cortical neurons were increased.

Turner and Greenough (1985) and Jones and colleagues (1997) demonstrated that experience-dependent effects occur in adult animals. Rats who were provided with complex and standard laboratory cages were compared; increased cortical volume and thickness and a higher number of synapses per neuron were found in rats provided with the complex environment (Turner & Greenough, 1985). Jones and colleagues (1997) found a greater number of multiple synaptic contacts among individual dendrites and axons in rats with the complex environment. These studies demonstrate that neural structures are influenced by experiences provided by the environment.

Experience-dependent aspects of cortical development have implications for special education and intervention efforts. Interventions that capitalize on the plasticity of the brain and focus on providing children with autism with experiences designed to influence the brain are promising. By studying the impact of intervention efforts on the neural functions of children with autism, we will develop a better understanding of the plasticity of neural functions and structures and how these are linked to behavioral changes (Dawson et al., 2002). For example, Field and colleagues (Escalona, Field, Singer-Strunck, Cullen, & Hartshorn, 2001; Field, 1995) have shown that pressure massage improves the behavioral functioning of infants and children with a wide range of disorders (including autism) and that associated changes in catecholamines (epinephrine, norepinephrine, cortisol) and food-absorption hormones (gastrin, insulin) stimulated by increased vagal activity are likely to contribute to the effects. They speculate that increased parasympathetic activity, or slowed and organized physiological state, may cause both the physiological and behavioral changes.

Behavioral interventions (i.e., interventions designed to alter the environment or experiences of a person to result in a change in behavior) have been developed to influence language (Leonard, 1998), social (McConnell, 2002), and other developmental outcomes of children. Camarata and Yoder (2002) suggest using neural imaging techniques to identify associated neural changes. Few intervention studies use such techniques, possibly due to difficulties using neural imaging with young children. Bruer (2002) warns that unless we observe specific behavioral correlates of brain changes, we do not know the significance of brain changes for changes in behavior. Thus we need to better specify the links between particular behaviors and neural characteristics. However, more specific measures are needed to assess the core behavioral phenotype of autism in order to discover which genes and regions of the brain are linked to specific behaviors.

Summary

We have characterized development as involving many interacting forces, with changes in one process or structure having implications for changes in others. This view of development argues against the notion that we will identify a single, isolated cause of autism. There are undoubtedly multiple "causes" for the autism phenotype. This fact may partly explain why individuals with autism vary. Causes will be identified at different levels of analysis and in different areas of function and structure, and experiences will play a role in each causal process. Each of these causes offers opportunities for intervention, particularly at times of transition and reorganization, such as the onset of language or entry to school.

VIEWING ATYPICAL AND TYPICAL DEVELOPMENT TOGETHER

Developmental psychopathology views development through a multidisciplinary lens (Cicchetti, 2002) and argues that one must have an understanding of typical processes to understand atypical development (e.g.,

Achenbach, 1990; Cicchetti & Sroufe, 2000). The same processes often account for both typical and atypical development. There has been a long history of evaluating the development of children with mental retardation relative to typically developing children (e.g., Hodapp, Burack, & Zigler, 1998; Zigler & Hodapp, 1986), and this is true for autism, as well.

Although deficits in social and communicative skills are a defining feature of autism, research suggests that young children with autism show a specific pattern of strengths and weaknesses, rather than overall deficits. Three behaviors—joint attention, emotional communication, and imitation—have been considered to be fundamentally different in young children with autism and also to be the foundation for later social behavior and communication, including language (Mundy & Crowson, 1997). In this section, the typical development of joint attention, emotional communication, and imitation are described, followed by a description of these skills in children with autism. The link between the early development of these critical skills and later language and communication skills is discussed.

One must be cautious not to confuse between-group differences with causes of development. If a variable differs among children with different syndromes, it does not mean that difference is the cause of the outcome. Furthermore, we cannot assume that causal influences go only in one direction. For example, we argued earlier that neural structure affects the types of experiences a child can have and that a child's experiences affect the structure and functioning of the brain.

Joint Attention in Typically Developing Children

Joint attention is the ability to coordinate one's attention with that of a partner in reference to an event or object (Carpenter, Nagell, & Tomasello, 1998). It has been described as a triadic exchange because it involves two communication partners and an event or object (Bakeman & Adamson, 1986). Joint attention involves sharing an internal experience (attention) and can be achieved in two ways: A child can follow (respond to) a communicative partner's focus, or the child can initiate an attempt to recruit the partner's attention. Initiating joint attention reflects a child's ability to elicit and direct a partner's attention, whereas responding to joint attention reflects the ability to follow a partner's attention-specifying cues.

Behaviors involved in joint-attention acts emerge during the first year of life. Many 6-month-old infants shift gaze to follow their mother's visual focus (Butterworth & Jarrett, 1991; Morales, Mundy, & Rojas, 1998). However, they cannot do so if she looks behind them or if her visual focus is outside their visual field (Morales et al., 1998). Children begin to follow pointing gestures between 9 and 12 months (Butterworth & Jarrett, 1991; Deak, Flom, & Pick, 2000) and improve during the second year of life.

Children alternate eye gaze between an object and a communicative partner at 10–15 months of age (Ninio & Bruner, 1978). During the first year of life, children increase in responding to gaze-only cues from adults (Striano & Rochat, 1999). By the middle of the second year, children can follow points, verbal directives (e.g., "Look at the banana!"), and gaze direction (Deak et al., 2000). Over the course of the second year, children increasingly monitor social partners and respond to their attentional shifts (Walden, Deak, & Yale, 2005).

Joint attention can also be thought of in terms of function: (1) *imperative* acts, in which the child uses joint attention to meet a need, such as requesting assistance, and (2) *declarative* acts, in which the child shares an experience or awareness of an event or object (Mundy Sigman, & Kasari, 1993). Late in the first year of life, infants begin to initiate joint attention, first for the purpose of requesting a desired object (imperative) and later to share an experience (declarative) with a communicative partner. Children initiate joint attention for requesting with their mothers increasingly during the second year. By 13 months, more than half of all children point to requested objects (Bretherton, McNew, & Beeghley-Smith, 1987; Carpenter et al., 1998).

Declarative joint attention is observed beginning around 10 months of age (Ninio & Bruner, 1978). Some researchers (e.g., Tomasello, 1995) believe that this type of attention signals that children perceive other people as intentional agents because they understand that others have internal states such as attention, interest, desires, and intentions and that these internal states can be shared and/or acted on. Infants show objects around 10 or 11 months of age (Carpenter et al., 1998), and pointing and gazing have been reported at around the same time (Bretherton et al., 1987), with declarative pointing observed shortly after (Carpenter et al., 1998). Franco, Fabia, and Butterworth (1996) reported a developmental sequence in coordinating declarative pointing and eye gaze. At around 12 months, children point to an object and then look at the adult; at around 14 months, they point at the object and look at the adult simultaneously; and at 16 months, they check to see if the adult is looking at them before pointing to the object.

The development of joint-attention skills has been linked to later language development (Mundy & Gomes, 1998; Tomasello & Todd, 1983). Morales and colleagues (1998) found that infants' ability to follow their mothers' directional gaze at 6 months of age was positively correlated with vocabulary at 12, 18, 21, and 24 months. Morales et al. (2000) found a positive association between children's early ability to respond to joint attention bids and later vocabulary development.

The ability to engage in joint attention is thought to be critical for language learning. Following cues to others' attention helps children filter and select information so they can focus on important aspects of the situation at hand. During joint-attention episodes, an object or event of interest can be identified by the infant as the referent of the verbal label provided by another person, thereby facilitating language learning (Tomasello, 1988; Tomasello & Farrar, 1986). Thus joint attention enables children to link spoken words with the objects and events to which they refer, that is, to map words onto their referents. Without the ability to share attention, children have difficulty processing social input in ways that facilitate acquiring language.

Joint Attention in Children with Autism

Deficits in joint attention are strong indicators of autism and distinguish young children with autism from those with other disorders (Mundy & Crowson, 1997; Mundy, Sigman, Ungerer, & Sherman, 1986). Young children with autism perform more poorly on joint-attention tasks than MA-matched peers with developmental delays (Mundy et al., 1986; Mundy, Sigman, & Kasari, 1990; Mundy, Sigman, & Kasari, 1994). Findings that children with autism perform significantly worse on joint-attention tasks than children with other types of delays support the position that deficits in joint-attention skills are a distinctive feature of autism.

Deficits in joint-attention skills for children with autism may be more severe for declarative acts. Charman (1998) reported that young children with autism are more likely to use joint-attention bids to meet a need (an imperative act) than to communicate about an object or event of interest (a declarative act). Mundy and colleagues (1986) found that the rate of eye contact with a conversational partner was higher in children with autism when it was used to obtain a preferred object that was out of reach (a requesting function) than for sharing an experience (a declarative function).

Joint attention is positively related to later language in children with and without autism. Studies have linked early joint attention with later language in children with pervasive developmental delay (Charman et al., 2003) and autism (Charman et al., 2003; Mundy et al., 1990; Sigman & Ruskin, 1999). Preschoolers' nonverbal joint-attention bids with a commenting function, but not those with a requesting function, have been positively associated with language scores 1 year later (Mundy et al., 1990). Similarly, Charman and colleagues (2003) found that nonverbal "comments" at 20 months (gaze switches between an adult and a mechanical toy that had stopped working) were related to receptive, but not expressive, language at 42 months.

Stone and Yoder (2001) suggested three reasons that declarative joint attention (comments) may be related to later language: (1) when children engage in joint attention, it signals to caregivers that they want language input (e.g., Lock, Young, Service, & Chandler, 1990); (2) when a child engages in joint attention, it may elicit language input from adults (e.g., Franco et al., 1996); and (3) children who engage in more joint attention may have more interest in sharing experiences (e.g., Mundy, 1995). These suggestions focus on the role of the child in shaping his or her experience in that children with autism may elicit different language-relevant behaviors from those around them.

Joint attention is important for making sense of and detecting order in the world, as well as for language development. Word learning can occur without visual joint attention (as in blind children, who perhaps use more tactile approaches); however, joint attention aids in mapping words to objects and events. Children with autism are prone to mapping errors when faced with ambiguous labels; that is, they do not link words with objects the speaker is talking about (Baron-Cohen, Baldwin, & Crowson, 1997). Thus deficits in joint attention are important in their own right and also because they may interfere with development of other skills.

Emotional Communication in Typically Developing Children

The ability of young children to interpret and respond to affective signals of caregivers and the ability to communicate these to partners is critical for typical social and communicative development (Walden & Knieps, 1996). Emotional communication involves the transmission of emotional information and emotional responses. Two early ways in which emotional communication occurs are affect sharing and social referencing.

Beginning early in the first year of life, affect sharing involves establishing coordinated emotional states during mother–child interactions (Field, 1994; Lundy, Field, & Pickens, 1996). Positive affect predominates in most interactions, but some high-risk dyads (e.g., depressed mothers and their infants) may establish patterns of negative affect (Lundy et al., 1996; Field, 1994). Furthermore, disrupting the flow of interaction is upsetting for typically developing infants, as is illustrated by findings from the "still-face" procedure (Tronick, 2003; Weinberg & Tronick, 1996). Later in the first year of life, infants look at a conversational partner to share positive affect, sometimes including an object that the infant "shows" the partner (Carpenter et al., 1998).

By the end of the first year of life, typically developing infants begin to engage in social referencing with their parents and others. This occurs when infants are interested in others' emotional reactions to objects and events, particularly if the events are unfamiliar or arousing. Infants spontaneously reference others and are sensitive to their emotional messages. That is, when others have negative reactions, the infants themselves are more negative and avoidant than they are when others have positive reactions to objects and events (Sorce, Emde, Campos, & Klinnert, 1985; Walden & Ogan, 1988).

The expression of emotion and language acquisition have been linked. Bloom and Capatides (1987) examined the relation between infants' affect and the emergence of language between 9 months and 2 years of age. They found that children's language achievements (first word spoken and spurt in vocabulary size) were negatively correlated with frequent or intense positive or negative emotional expressions and that the more time the child spent in a neutral affective state, the earlier was the onset of language. Bloom and Capatides (1987) suggested that language learning is facilitated when children adopt a "reflective stance," a neutral, alert state that supports cognitive activity needed for language acquisition. Because emotion and cognition draw on the same attentional resources, children who are more emotional are less able to achieve a reflective stance and are less able to process environmental cues necessary for language learning. Bloom and Tinker (2001) found that young children's rate of emotional expression decreased during times of planning or effort before the emergence of new skills (e.g., first words and sentences) and increased once they were more proficient in using new language skills.

Baldwin (2000) discussed the role of attention to others' affect in language acquisition. She argued that when infants hear an unfamiliar word, they pay attention to cues such as emotional expressions and use these cues to understand the new word. Tomasello, Strosberg, and Akhtar (1996) reported two experiments in which 18-month-old infants used adults' emotional cues to identify target objects associated with verbal labels when adult gaze was not helpful. Saylor and Troseth (2005) found that 2½-year-old children used information about an experimenter's preferences for one of two toys to help them learn novel labels for the toys. By 3½ years the children did so even when their own preferences conflicted with those of the experimenter. Thus language learning is powered by skill in making inferences about the affective states of others.

Emotional communication is a fundamental process underlying relationships, sociability, and even turn-taking skills. Understanding that others have emotions, that emotions can be acted on, that they influence social interactions, and that they provide valuable information about how to interpret and cope with events are significant achievements for infants (Walden & Knieps, 1996). These achievements are linked with cognitive, language, and social development.

Emotional Communication in Children with Autism

In studies of children with autism, two aspects of early emotional development have received attention: (1) affect during joint-attention tasks (Kasari,

Sigman, Mundy, & Yirmiya, 1990; Mundy, Kasari, & Sigman, 1992) and (2) monitoring and response to others' emotions (Bacon, Fein, Morris, Waterhouse, & Allen, 1998; Charman et al., 1997; Sigman, Kasari, Kwon, & Yirmiya, 1992).

Adamson and Bakeman (1984) proposed that affect sharing is likely to occur during instances of joint attention. Similarly, Mundy and colleagues (1992) argued that affect helps distinguish between imperative (requesting) and declarative (commenting) joint attention because declarative joint attention bids are more likely to be accompanied by positive affect. They found positive affect in over 50% of episodes of declarative joint attention, as compared with 36% of imperative episodes. Kasari and colleagues (1990) found that for typically developing children, positive affect sharing during instances of declarative joint attention was higher than during requesting. However, young children with autism had low levels of positive affect during both requesting and sharing. These findings suggest that joint attention should be viewed not only as the coordination of attention between communicative partners but also as a context in which an affective experience can be communicated, shared, or compared. Thus joint-attention deficits in children with autism are not limited only to reduced shared attention with communicative partners but also to fewer instances of positive affect sharing.

Sigman and colleagues (1992) investigated responses of young children with autism to the negative affect of others and compared the responses with those of children who were typically developing and at the same developmental level and those of children who were the same chronological age (CA) and developmental level. In a series of vignettes, adults expressed mock distress, pain, and discomfort. Children with autism looked at the adults less often and less quickly than children in the other two groups. Rather, children with autism spent more time looking at and playing with a toy than other children, even after the adult feigned injury. The children with autism appeared to be less concerned about the distress of the adults than the other children.

Bacon and colleagues (1998) also evaluated the attention of children to others' affective displays. Children with autism were divided into high- and low-functioning groups based on nonverbal IQ and were compared with children with language impairments, mental retardation, and typical development. Children participated in one episode with an ambiguous stimulus (an unusual loud sound) and two in which adults feigned distress about losing a pen or bumping a body part. Children with autism who were lower functioning looked at or referenced the adult less than the other children; the difference was accounted for by the children's level of language functioning. Higher functioning children with autism performed similarly to the other children. However, both high- and low-functioning children with autism spent less time looking at the faces of the adults following the uncertain stimulus; that is, they did less social referencing.

Important aspects of emotional development typically occur during the first year of life. Yet during this time, children with autism show less interest in others' emotions and are less responsive to emotion in a social context. They also share less positive affect during joint-attention contexts in which typically developing children spontaneously show and share positive reactions with others. These behaviors contribute to the development of interpersonal understanding and serve as a foundation for social behavior, language, and many cognitive skills. Failing to take advantage of opportunities to coordinate one's view of the world with that of others may contribute to later aberrations in social and emotional behavior.

Imitation in Typically Developing Children

Imitation is an important guide for behavior in a wide range of species (Prinz & Meltzoff, 2002). Imitation involves a network of behaviors: (1) an act is demonstrated by a model and observed by an observer, (2) the observer uses perceptions of the action to develop an action plan, (3) the observer engages in the motor output to perform the action (Meltzoff, 2002; Prinz, 2002). Imitation of caregivers is one of the earliest reciprocal interactions, and it is a vehicle through which infants gain a shared understanding of others (Meltzoff & Moore, 1983b).

The ability to imitate others is a critical skill for young children, enabling them to learn and master new behaviors (Meltzoff & Moore, 1983a). A child's cognitive and social development are fostered through imitation. Also, imitation helps the infant to understand that he or she is an individual who is separate from others, though related (Meltzoff & Gopnik, 1993). Furthermore, imitation is linked with understanding others' intentions. Thus imitation is an important early skill that facilitates development.

Nadel (2002) proposed that imitation is one semantic foundation for language development because it is an effective tool for thought in preverbal children, allowing them to represent events, roles, goals, and actions. Imitation is based on an intermodal representational system that unites the child's own body transformations and those of others (Meltzoff & Moore, 1983b). The ability to represent actions intermodally has been suggested to be the start of psychological development (Meltzoff & Moore, 1983a).

Nadel (2002) argued that preverbal children communicate during imitative episodes in that they share topics and apply rules. For example, when children engage in imitation, there are two roles, the imitated and the imitator, and children switch roles and take turns. Nadel (2002) evaluated peer imitation in infant dyads and triads and found that most children imitated peers by 18 months of age. Children used imitation to initiate and respond to social interactions. That is, imitation, imitation monitoring, and recognition of being imitated serve communicative functions before the development of spoken language.

Infants as young as 2 to 3 weeks imitate facial expressions, and 6-month-old infants imitate a hand movement (Meltzoff & Moore, 1977). With age, the ability to imitate others changes and expands. For example, older children are able to imitate actions that are more complex (McCabe & Uzgiris, 1983), and older children more frequently imitate novel actions than do younger infants (Masur & Ritz, 1984).

Snow (1989) examined rates of different types of imitation in 14- and 20-month-old infants and found that object-mediated imitation (manipulation of an object) was more frequent than gestural imitation. Higher rates of gestural imitation were correlated with higher language ability (e.g., number of nouns and verbs produced, total productive vocabulary, and production/comprehension ratios), whereas higher rates of object-mediated imitation were negatively correlated with language ability. Early vocal imitation was related to higher language abilities.

Imitation in Children with Autism

Several studies have found that imitation is deficient in young children with autism. Stone, Ousley, and Littleford (1997) found that young children with autism performed more poorly on imitation tasks than typically developing children and children with developmental delays, despite controlling for MA, cognitive development, and expressive language ability. Rogers, Hepburn, Stackhouse, and Wehner (2003) found that children with autism performed more poorly on a battery of imitation tasks than children with developmental disorders or typical development and that imitation was correlated with autism severity. Stone and colleagues (1997) further found that although children with autism improved between 2 and 3 years of age, they continued to have poorer motor imitation skills than developmentally matched controls.

Imitation impairments in children with autism vary with the type of imitation task performed (Rogers et al., 2003). For example, Stone and colleagues (1997) evaluated two types of imitation in young children with autism: body imitation (e.g., opening and closing a fist) and object-related imitation (e.g., pushing a car across a table). Imitation involving body movement was more impaired. Rogers and colleagues (2003) found that imitation of oral motor behaviors (e.g., blowing a cotton ball across a table) and of object-related behaviors were poorer in children with autism than in children with developmental disabilities and with typical development.

Early imitation abilities have been linked to later language performance in children with autism. Consistent with Snow's (1989) study with typically developing children (described earlier), body imitation at age 2 years has been positively related to expressive vocabulary at 2 and 3 years of age in children with autism; however, there appears to be no association between object imitation skills and later language abilities (Stone et al., 1997). In addition, Stone and Yoder (2001) found a positive association between the performance of children with autism on the Motor Imitation Scale at age 2 and expressive language at age 4.

Charman and colleagues (2003) found that better imitation skills at 20 months were associated with better receptive language at 42 months for children with pervasive developmental delay (PDD) and autism. Imitation and later expressive language were not significantly related in this small sample. Carpenter, Nagell, and Tomasello (1998) found a positive correlation between imitative learning of arbitrary actions and referential language in children with autism. They suggested that because imitation is a *relative* strength for children with autism (though not as good as for typically developing children) compared with other early social-communicative behaviors such as joint attention, imitation skills should be considered as one route to language acquisition for children with autism. That is, an alternative route to language that capitalizes on the relative strengths of children with autism may be possible.

Cognitive achievements that have been said to underlie imitation include the ability to make attributions about the model's intentions, to plan and act out imitative behaviors, and to establish turn taking and role switching. These skills involve interpersonal understanding. Baldwin (2000) suggested that poor interpersonal understanding is one reason that children with autism show delays in language acquisition: Deficits in interpersonal understanding impair their ability to separate relevant from irrelevant linguistic input and to map words to objects.

Imitation appears to be a transitory system used by preverbal infants to communicate and may be one mechanism of early language development. When young children master language, the communicative function of imitation diminishes, and the rate of imitative episodes declines (Nadel, 2002). The role of imitation in preverbal social interactions and the association between early imitative skills and later language (Carpenter, Pennington, & Rogers, 2002; Charman et al., 2003; Stone et al., 1997; Stone & Yoder, 2001) underscore the importance of this early social-communicative skill.

Summary

Autism is a disorder defined by a pattern of strengths and weaknesses, especially in social and communicative behaviors. Although children with autism have deficits in joint attention, emotional communication, and imitation, these deficits are not absolute or pervasive. Imitation, although deficient, may be an area of relative strength for children with autism (Carpenter et al., 2002). Reports that imitation is associated with later language for children with autism indicate that regardless of whether there is an average difference between typically developing and children with autism, imitation and later language are related for both groups.

The relative strength in imitation skills for children with autism suggests that interventions might feature imitation strategies. Hodapp and Ricci (2002) proposed that interventions for different etiologies might "play to children's strengths." For example, children with fragile-X and Prader–Willi syndromes show relative strength in simultaneous processing (e.g., identifying incomplete drawings) and deficits in sequential processing (e.g., imitating series of movements; Dykens, Hodapp, & Leckman, 1994; Hodapp et al., 1992); teaching approaches can be used that facilitate learning in children with simultaneous processing styles. Similarly, Garfinkle and Schwartz (2002) capitalized on the relative strength of imitation skills in children with autism by using peer imitation to build play skills.

UNDERSTANDING AUTISM

Understanding the development of autism is difficult, for it is a complex disorder, and variability among children with autism is striking. Autism is linked to genes, but the links are complicated. Experience matters, for all genes are expressed in a context. Individuals can never be understood apart from the context in which they develop, whether they are developing typically or atypically. Characteristics of individuals also influence their experiences (e.g., Scarr & McCartney, 1983). In addition, individuals construct understandings and giving meaning to the world (Cicchetti, 2002). The individual's active role in contributing to outcomes is central in development. A multidisciplinary approach to autism that considers multiple agents of development is necessary.

Mundy and Crowson (1997) proposed a model in which frontal neu rological processes and experience interact in the development of joint-attention skills in children with autism. In this "cybernetic" model of autism, initial insult to the frontal lobe leaves a child unable to process the early social experiences needed for further neurological shaping. As a result, the initial frontal lobe problem, the *initial pathological process,* leads to disturbances in the child's early social communication. Neural development is impaired because the brain does not receive input to further shape neurological connections, a *secondary neurological disturbance.* This results in a dysfunctional "environmental-induced neurological shaping process." Children with autism may miss important periods of *neurological* shaping due to aberrant *social* interactions and thus maintain an aberrant path, the phenotype associated with autism. Note that causes (and interventions) and effects can be in *different domains* (e.g., social effects on brain structure).

Timing an intervention is important, as interventions vary in their effectiveness depending on internal and external factors, as well as on the developmental level of the individual (e.g., sensitive periods in experience-expectant processes). Both theory and data suggest that it may be difficult for neural structure to continue on a typical developmental path following early deprivation. Thus early interventions to provide experiences necessary for cortical growth are critical. Times of reorganization or transition may be particularly efficient and effective points at which to intervene. Dynamic-systems theorists (echoing ideas from Piaget and others) claim that when systems are far from equilibrium, as they are during times of transition, elements are reorganized and eventually linked into stable orderly arrangements (self-organization). Developmental transitions are opportunities to influence a system before it stabilizes and becomes self-perpetuating (Lewis, 2000).

Longitudinal studies with children who are at a higher risk for developing autism have the potential to help identify early markers for autism. One approach is to study the development of younger siblings of children with autism, because siblings are at increased risk for autism (Jorde et al., 1991). Such studies may identify early behaviors associated with autism before it is diagnosed, and they can describe patterns of growth in children with different outcomes. Furthermore, such studies may help us to understand whether there is a "broader phenotype" of autism, that is, shared characteristics of autism (or more subtle forms of those characteristics) among relatives who do not have autism. In this way, we can better understand the early developmental trajectories of children at risk for autism.

This chapter has highlighted some fundamental puzzles of autism: What are the links between brain and behavior? Why is there variability among individuals with autism? Can experiences alter the developmental course? When we understand the links between brain and behavior, can predict variability among individuals and across situations, and can identify what experiences shape development in particular ways, we will have a better understanding not only of autism but of typical development as well.

ACKNOWLEDGMENTS

Support for Jennifer J. Hurley was provided by Grant No. T32-HD07226 from the National Institute of Child Health and Human Development. Thanks to Paul Yoder, Georgene Troseth, and Bob Hodapp for suggestions on an earlier draft.

REFERENCES

Achenbach, T. M. (1990). Conceptualization of developmental psychopathology. In M. Lewis & S. M. Miller (Eds.), *Handbook of developmental psychopathology* (pp. 3–13). New York: Plenum Press.

Adamson, L., & Bakeman, R. (1984). Coordinating attention to people and objects in mother–infant and peer–infant interaction. *Child Development, 55,* 1278–1289.

Bacon, A. L., Fein, D., Morris, R., Waterhouse, L., & Allen, D. (1998). The responses of autistic children to the distress of others. *Journal of Autism and Developmental Disorders, 28*(2), 129–141.

Bakeman, R., & Adamson, L. (1986). Infants' conventionalized acts: Gestures and words with mothers and peers. *Infant Behavior and Development, 9,* 215–230.

Baldwin, D. A. (2000). Interpersonal understanding fuels knowledge acquisition. *Current Directions in Psychological Science, 9*(2), 40–45.

Baron-Cohen, S., Baldwin, D. A., & Crowson, M. (1997). Do children with autism use the speaker's direction of gaze (SDG) strategy to crack the code of language? *Child Development, 68,* 48–57.

Bennett, A. J., Lesch, K. P., Heils, A., Long, J., Lorenz, J., Shoaf, S. E., et al. (2002). Early experience and serotonin transporter gene variation interact to influence primate CNS function. *Molecular Psychiatry, 7,* 118–122.

Bloom, L., & Capatides, J. B. (1987). Expression of affect and the emergence of language. *Child Development, 58,* 1513–1522.

Bloom, L., & Tinker, E. (2001). The intentionality model and language acquisition. *Monographs of the Society for Research in Child Development, 66*(4, Serial No. 267).

Bretherton, I., McNew, S., & Beeghley-Smith, M. (1987). Early person knowledge as expressed in gestural and verbal communication: When do infants acquire a "theory of mind"? In J. Oates & S. Sheldon (Eds.), *Cognitive development in infancy* (pp. 219–246). Hillsdale, NJ: Erlbaum.

Bruer, J. T. (2002). Avoiding the pediatrician's error: How neuroscientists can help educators (and themselves). *Nature Neuroscience Supplement, 5,* 1031–1033.

Butterworth, G. E., & Jarrett, N. L. M. (1991). What minds have in common is space: Spatial mechanisms serving joint visual attention in infancy. *British Journal of Developmental Psychology, 9,* 55–72.

Camarata, S., & Yoder, P. (2002). Language transactions during development and intervention: Theoretical implications for developmental neuroscience. *International Journal of Developmental Neuroscience, 20,* 459–465.

Carpenter, M., Nagell, K., & Tomasello, M. (1998). Social cognition, joint attention, and communicative competence from 9 to 15 months of age. *Monographs for the Society for Research in Child Development, 63*(4, Serial No. 231).

Carpenter, M., Pennington, B. F., & Rogers, S. J. (2002). Interrelations among social-cognitive skills in young children with autism. *Journal of Autism and Developmental Disorders, 32*(2), 91–106.

Charman, T. (1998). Specifying the nature and course of joint attention impairment in autism in the preschool years: Implications for diagnosis and intervention. *Autism: The International Journal of Research and Practice, 2*(1), 61–79.

Charman, T., Baron-Cohen, S., Swettenham, J., Baird, G., Drew, A., & Cox, A. (2003). Predicting language outcome in infants with autism and pervasive developmental disorder. *International Journal of Language and Communication Disorders, 38*(3) 265–285.

Charman, T., Swettenham, J., Baron-Cohen, S., Cox, A., Baird, G., & Drew, A. (1997). Infants with autism: An investigation of empathy, pretend play joint attention, and imitation. *Developmental Psychology, 33*, 781–789.

Cicchetti, D. (2002). The impact of social experience on neurobiological systems: Illustration from a constructivist view of child maltreatment. *Cognitive Development, 17*, 1407–1428.

Cicchetti, D., & Cannon, T. D. (1999). Neurodevelopmental processes in the ontogenesis and epigenesis of psychopathology. *Development and Psychopathology, 11*, 375–393.

Cicchetti, D., & Sroufe, L. A. (2000). The past as prologue to the future: The times, they've been a-changin' [Editorial]. *Development and Psychopathology, 12*, 255–264.

Cicchetti, D., & Toth, S. L. (1995). Developmental psychopathology and disorders of affect. In D. Cicchetti & D. J. Cohen (Eds.), *Developmental psychopathology: Vol. 2. Risk, disorder and adaptation* (pp. 369–420). New York: Wiley.

Dawson, G., Webb, S., Schellenberg, G. D., Dager, S., Friedman, S., Aylward, E., et al. (2002). Defining the broader phenotype of autism: Genetic, brain, and behavioral perspectives. *Development and Psychopathology, 14*, 581–611.

Deak, G., Flom, R., & Pick, A. (2000). Effects of gesture and target on 12- and 18-month olds' joint visual attention to objects in front of or behind them. *Developmental Psychology, 36*, 511–523.

Dmitrieva, L. P., & Gottlieb, G. (1994). Influences of auditory experience on the development of brain stem auditory-evoked potentials in mallard duck embryos and hatchlings. *Behavioral and Neural Biology, 61*(1), 19–28.

Dykens, E. M. (1995). Measuring behavioral phenotypes: Provocations from the "New Genetics." *American Journal on Mental Retardation, 99*(5), 522–532.

Dykens, E. M. (2003). Anxiety, fears, and phobias in persons with Williams syndrome. *Developmental Neuropsychology, 23*(1&2), 291–316.

Dykens, E. M., Hodapp, R. M., & Leckman, J. F. (1994). *Behavior and development in fragile X syndrome*. Newbury Park, CA: Sage.

Escalona, A., Field, T., Singer-Strunck, R., Cullen, C., & Hartshorn, K. (2001). Brief report: Improvements in the behavior of children with autism following massage therapy. *Journal of Autism and Developmental Disorders, 31*, 513–516.

Fidler, D. J. (2003). Parental vocalizations and perceived immaturity in Down syndrome. *American Journal on Mental Retardation, 108*(6), 425–434.

Fidler, D. J., & Hodapp, R. M. (1999). Craniofacial maturity and perceived personality in children with Down syndrome. *American Journal on Mental Retardation, 104*(5), 410–421.

Field, T. (1994). The effects of mother's physical and emotional unavailability on emotion regulation. *Monographs of the Society for Research in Child Development, 59*(2–3), 208–227.

Field, T. (1995). Massage therapy for infants and children. *Developmental and Behavioral Pediatrics, 16*, 105–111.

Franco, F., Fabia, F., & Butterworth, G. (1996). Pointing and social awareness: Declaring and requesting in the second year. *Journal of Child Language, 23*, 307–306.

Garfinkle, A. N., & Schwartz, I. S. (2002). Peer imitation: Increasing social interactions in children with autism and other developmental disabilities in inclusive preschool classrooms. *Topics in Early Childhood Special Education, 22*, 26–38.

Gottlieb, G. (1985). Social interaction with siblings is necessary for visual imprinting of species-specific maternal preferences in ducklings. *Journal of Comparative Psychology, 99*(4), 371–379.

Gottlieb, G. (1991). Experiential canalization of behavioral development: Results. *Developmental Psychology, 27*(1), 35–39.

Gottlieb, G. (1998). Normally occurring environmental and behavioral influences on gene activity: From central dogma to probabilistic epigenesis. *Psychological Review, 105*(4), 792–802.

Gottlieb, G., & Halpern, C. T. (2002). A relational view of causality in normal and abnormal development. *Development and Psychopathology, 14*, 421–435.

Greenough, W. T., Black, J. E., & Wallace, C. S. (1987). Experience and brain development. *Child Development, 58*, 539–559.

Hodapp, R. M., Burack, J. A., & Zigler, E. (1998). Developmental approaches to mental retardation: A short introduction. In J. A. Burack, R. M. Hodapp, & E. Zigler (Eds.), *Handbook of mental retardation and development* (pp. 3–19). New York: Cambridge University Press.

Hodapp, R. M., Leckman, J. F., Dykens, E. M., Sparrow, S. S., Zelinsky, D., & Ort, S. I. (1992). K-ABC profiles in children with fragile X syndrome, Down syndrome, and non-specific mental retardation. *American Journal on Mental Retardation, 97*, 39–46.

Hodapp, R. M., & Ricci, L. A. (2002). Behavioral phenotypes and educational practice: The unrealized connection. In G. O'Brien & O. Udwin (Eds.), *Behavioral phenotypes in clinical practice* (pp. 137–151). London: Mac Keith Press.

Jones, T. A., Klintsova, A. Y., Kilman, V. L., Sirevaag, A. M., & Greenough, W. T. (1997). Induction of multiple synapses by experience in the visual cortex of adult rats. *Neurobiology of Learning and Memory, 68*, 13–20.

Jorde, L. B., Hasstedt, S. J., Ritvo, E. R., Mason-Brothers, A., Freeman, B. J., Pingree, S., et al. (1991). Complex segregation analysis of autism. *American Journal of Human Genetics, 49*, 932–938.

Kasari, C., Sigman, M., Mundy, P., & Yirmiya, N. (1990). Affective sharing in the context of joint attention interaction of normal, autistic, and mentally retarded children. *Journal of Autism and Developmental Disorders, 20*(1), 87–101.

Lamb, M. E., & Easterbrooks, M. A. (1981). Individual differences in parental sensitivity: Origins, components, and consequences. In M. E. Lamb & L. R. Sherrod (Eds.), *Infant social cognition: Empirical and theoretical considerations* (pp. 127–153). Hillsdale, NJ: Erlbaum.

Leonard, L. (1998). *Specific language impairment*. Cambridge, MA: MIT Press.

Lewis, M. (2000). The promise of dynamic systems approaches for an integrated account of human development. *Child Development, 71*, 36–43.

Lock, J., Young, A., Service, B., & Chandler, P. (1990). Some observations on the origin of the pointing gesture. In B. Volterra & C. J. Erting (Eds.), *From gesture to language in hearing and deaf children* (pp. 42–55). Berlin, Germany: Springer-Verlag.

Lundy, B., Field, T., & Pickens, J. (1996). Newborns of mothers with depressive symptoms are less expressive. *Infant Behavior and Development, 19*(4), 419–424.

Masur, E. F., & Ritz, E. (1984). Patterns of gestural, vocal, and verbal imitation performance in infancy. *Merrill–Palmer Quarterly, 30,* 369–392.

McCabe, M., & Uzgiris, I. C. (1983). Effects of model and action on imitation in infancy. *Merrill–Palmer Quarterly, 29,* 69–82.

McConnell, S. R. (2002). Interventions to facilitate social interaction for young children with autism: Review of available research and recommendations for educational intervention and future research. *Journal of Autism and Developmental Disorders, 32*(5), 351–372.

Meltzoff, A., & Gopnik, A. (1993). The role of imitation in understanding persons and developing a theory of mind. In S. Baron-Cohen, H. Tager-Flusberg, & D. J. Cohen (Eds.), *Understanding other minds: Perspectives from autism* (pp. 335–366). Oxford, UK: Oxford University Press.

Meltzoff, A. N. (2002). Elements of a developmental theory of imitation. In A. N. Meltzoff & W. Prinz (Eds.), *The imitative mind: Development, evolution and brain bases* (pp. 19–41). Cambridge, UK: Cambridge University Press.

Meltzoff, A. N., & Moore, M. K. (1977). Imitation of facial and manual gestures by human neonates. *Science, 198,* 75–78.

Meltzoff, A., & Moore, M. K. (1983a). The origins of imitation in infancy: Paradigm, phenomena, and theories. In L. P. Lipsitt & C. Rovee-Collier (Eds.), *Advances in infancy research* (Vol. 2, pp. 265–301). Norwood, NJ: Ablex.

Meltzoff, A., & Moore, M. K. (1983b). Newborn infants imitate adult facial gestures. *Child Development, 54,* 702–709.

Morales, M., Mundy, P., Delgado, C. E. F., Yale, M., Messinger, D., Neal, R., et al. (2000). Responding to joint attention across the 6– through 24–month age period and early language acquisition. *Journal of Applied Developmental Psychology, 21*(3), 283–298.

Morales, M., Mundy, P., & Rojas, J. (1998). Following the direction of gaze and language development in 6–month-olds. *Infant Behavior and Development, 21*(2), 373–377.

Mundy, P. (1995). Joint attention and social-emotional approach behavior in children with autism. *Development and Psychopathology, 7,* 63–82.

Mundy, P., & Crowson, M. (1997). Joint attention and early social communication: Implications for research on intervention with autism. *Journal of Autism and Developmental Disorders, 27*(6), 653–676.

Mundy, P., & Gomes, A. (1998). Individual differences in joint attention skill development in the second year. *Infant Behavior and Development, 21,* 469–482.

Mundy, P., Kasari, C., & Sigman, M. (1992). Nonverbal communication, affective sharing, and intersubjectivity. *Infant Behavior and Development, 15,* 377–381.

Mundy, P., Sigman, M., & Kasari, C. (1990). A longitudinal study of joint attention and language development in autistic children. *Journal of Autism and Developmental Disorders, 20,* 115–128.

Mundy, P., Sigman, M., & Kasari, C. (1993). The theory of mind and joint attention in autism. In S. Baron-Cohen, H. Tager-Flusberg, & D. Cohen (Eds.), *Understanding other minds: Perspectives from autism* (pp. 181–203). Oxford, UK: Oxford University Press.

Mundy, P., Sigman, M., & Kasari, C. (1994). Joint attention, developmental level, and symptom presentation in young children with autism. *Development and Psychopathology, 6,* 389–401.

Mundy, P., Sigman, M., Ungerer, J., & Sherman, T. (1986). Defining the social deficits of autism: The contribution of nonverbal communication measures. *Journal of Child Psychology and Psychiatry, 27,* 657–669.

Nadel, J. (2002). Imitation and imitation recognition: Functional use in preverbal infants and nonverbal children with autism. In A. N. Meltzoff & W. Prinz (Eds.), *The imitative mind: Development, evolution and brain bases* (pp. 42–62). Cambridge, UK: Cambridge University Press.

Ninio, A., & Bruner, J. (1978). The achievement and antecedents of labelling. *Journal of Child Language, 5,* 1–15.

Prinz, W. (2002). Experimental approaches to imitation. In A. N. Meltzoff & W. Prinz (Eds.), *The imitative mind: Development, evolution and brain bases* (pp. 143–162). Cambridge, UK: Cambridge University Press.

Prinz, W., & Meltzoff, A. N. (2002). An introduction to the imitative mind and brain. In A. N. Meltzoff & W. Prinz (Eds.), *The imitative mind: Development, evolution and brain bases* (pp. 1–15). Cambridge, UK: Cambridge University Press.

Rakic, P. (1988). Specification of cerebral cortex areas. *Science, 241,* 170–176.

Randell, P. L., & Gottlieb, G. (1992). Developmental intersensory interference: Augmented prenatal sensory experience interferes with auditory learning in duck embryos. *Developmental Psychology, 28*(5), 795–803.

Rema, V., Armstrong-James, M., & Ebner, F. F. (2003). Experience-dependent plasticity is impaired in adult rat barrel cortex after whiskers are unused in early postnatal life. *Journal of Neuroscience, 23*(1), 358–366.

Rema, V., & Ebner, F. F. (1999). Effects of enriched environment rearing on impairments in cortical excitability and plasticity after prenatal alcohol exposure. *Journal of Neuroscience, 15,* 10993–11006.

Rogers, S. J., Hepburn, S. L., Stackhouse, T., & Wehner, E. (2003). Imitation performance in toddlers with autism and those with other developmental disorders. *Journal of Child Psychology and Psychiatry, 44*(5), 763–781.

Sameroff, A. J. (1992). Principles of development and psychopathology. In A. J. Sameroff & E. Robert (Eds.), *Relationship disturbance in early childhood: A developmental approach* (pp. 17–32). New York: Basic Books.

Sameroff, A. J., & Seifer, R. (1990). Early contributors to developmental risk. In J. E. Rolf & A. S. Masten (Eds.), *Risk and protective factors in the development of psychopathology* (pp. 52–66). New York: Cambridge University Press.

Saylor, M. M., & Troseth, G. L. (2005). *Preschoolers use information about speakers' desires to learn new words.* Unpublished manuscript, Vanderbilt University.

Scarr, S., & McCartney, K. (1983). How people make their own environments: A theory of genotype environment effects. *Child Development, 54,* 424–435.

Sigman, M. D., Kasari, C., Kwon, J., & Yirmiya, N. (1992). Responses to the negative emotions of others by autistic, mentally retarded and normal children. *Child Development, 63,* 786–807.

Sigman, M., & Ruskin, E. (1999). Continuity and change in the social competence of children with autism, Down syndrome and developmental delays. *Monographs of the Society for Research in Child Development, 64,* 1–114.

Snow, C. E. (1989). Imitativeness: A trait or a skill? In G. E. Speidel & K. E. Nelson (Eds.), *The many faces of imitation in language learning* (pp. 73–90). New York: Springer-Verlag.

Sorce, J., Emde, R., Campos, J., & Klinnert, M. (1985). Maternal emotional signaling: Its effect on the visual cliff behavior of 1–year-olds. *Developmental Psychology, 21,* 195–200.

Sroufe, L. A., & Rutter, M. (1984). The domain of developmental psychopathology. *Child Development, 55,* 17–29.

Stone, W. L., Ousley, O. Y., & Littleford, C. D. (1997). Motor imitation in young children with autism: What's the object? *Journal of Abnormal Child Psychology, 25*(6), 475–485.

Stone, W. L., & Yoder, P. J. (2001). Predicting spoken language level in children with autism spectrum disorders. *Sage, 5*(4), 341–361.

Striano, T., & Rochat, P. (1999). Developmental link between dyadic and triadic social competence in infancy. *British Journal of Developmental Psychology, 17,* 551–562.

Tomasello, M. (1988). The role of joint attention in early language development. *Language Sciences, 11,* 69–88.

Tomasello, M. (1995). Joint attention as social cognition. In C. Moore & P. Dunham (Eds.), *Joint attention: Its origins and role in development* (pp. 85–101). Oxford, UK: Oxford University Press.

Tomasello, M., & Farrar, M. J. (1986). Joint attention and early language. *Child Development, 57*(6), 1454–1463.

Tomasello, M., Strosberg, R., & Akhtar, N. (1996). Eighteen-month-old children learn words in non-ostensive contexts. *Journal of Child Language, 23*(1), 157–176.

Tomasello, M., & Todd, J. (1983). Joint attention and early lexical acquisition style. *First Language, 4,* 197–212.

Tronick, E. Z. (2003). Emotions and emotional communication in infants. In J. Raphael-Leff (Ed.), *Parent–infant psychodynamics: Wild things, mirrors and ghosts* (pp. 35–53). London, UK: Whurr.

Turner, A. M., & Greenough, W. T. (1985). Differential rearing effects on rat visual cortex synapses: I. Synaptic and neuronal density and synapses per neuron. *Brain Research, 329,* 195–203.

Veenstra-VanderWeele, J., Anderson, G. M., & Cook, E. H., (2000). Pharmacogenetics and the serotonin system: Initial studies and future directions. *European Journal of Pharmacy, 410,* 165–181.

Walden, T. A. (1996). Social responsivity: Judging signals of young children with and without developmental delays. *Child Development, 67,* 2074–2085.

Walden, T. A., Deak, G. O., & Yale, M. (2005). *Eliciting and directing one-year-old infants' attention: Effects of verbal and nonverbal cues.* Unpublished manuscript, Vanderbilt University.

Walden, T. A., & Knieps, L. (1996). Reading and responding to social signals. In M. Lewis & M. W. Sullivan (Eds.), *Emotional development in atypical children* (pp. 29–42). Hillsdale, NJ: Erlbaum.

Walden, T. A., Knieps, L. J., & Baxter, A. (1991). Contingent provision of social referential information by parents of children with and without developmental delays. *American Journal on Mental Retardation, 96*(2), 177–187.

Walden, T., & Ogan, T. (1988). The development of social referencing. *Child Development, 59*, 1230–1240.

Weinberg, K. M., & Tronick, E. Z. (1996). Infant affective reactions to the resumption of maternal interaction after the still-face. *Child Development, 67*, 905–914.

Wu, C. W. H., Kass, J. H. (2002). The effects of long-standing limb loss on anatomical reorganization of somatosensory afferents in the brainstem and spinal cord. *Somatosensory and Motor Research, 19*(2), 153–163.

Zigler, E., & Hodapp, R. (1986). *Understanding mental retardation.* New York: Cambridge University Press.

11

The Neural Basis of Early Joint-Attention Behavior

PETER MUNDY
DANIELLE THORP

Social impairments, along with problems with communication and repetitive behaviors, constitute a pathognomonic symptom cluster of autism (American Psychiatric Association, 2000). Therefore, an important goal of research on autism is to describe the neural systems involved in these social impairments. Identifying these systems will likely have important clinical implications, such as advancing the development of neuroimaging methods that assist in early detection, as well as guiding and evaluating pharmacological and behavioral treatments. Several complementary approaches have recently emerged in the literature with respect to this goal (Mundy, 2003). One approach has been to identify anomalies in the neural functions and/or neural morphometrics of people with autism. Then researchers have attempted to relate these anomalies to the social-behavior impairments of autism. Work on orienting difficulties and related cerebellar cell abnormalities in autism provides a seminal example of this approach (Carper & Courchesne, 2000; Courchesne et al., 1994; Townsend et al., 2001).

Another approach begins with the current understanding of brain systems involved in a variety of social-perceptual processes, such as face perception and recognition (Elgar & Campbell, 2001), the perception of emotional or motivation-related information (Watanabe, 1999; LeDoux, 1989), and the perception of the direction of gaze of a social partner (Kawashima et al., 1999). Comparative and human imaging studies suggest that social perception may be supported by a complex ventromedial "social brain" circuit involving the orbitofrontal cortex, the temporal cortical areas including the superior temporal sulcus (STS), as well as superior temporal gyrus (STG) and subcortical areas such as the amygdala (Adolphs, 2001; Brothers, 1990). Behavioral deficits in social perception have long been recognized in autism (e.g., Hobson, 1993; Sigman, Kasari, Kwon, & Yirmiya, 1992). Therefore, a major goal of this second approach is to examine the hypothesis that deficits in ventral "social brain" systems give rise to fundamental impairments in the social perception and social behavior of children with autism (e.g., Baron-Cohen et al., 1999; Critchley et al., 2000).

A third expedient approach is to begin with the fundamental symptoms of the disorder and attempt to understand the neural substrates of these pathognomonic features of the syndrome. For example, one criterion in DSM-IV for autism is "a lack of spontaneously seeking to share experience with others" (American Psychiatric Association, 2000, p. 75). This symptom may be assessed with measures of impairments in joint-attention behaviors such as showing or pointing (Mundy & Crowson, 1997). So several research groups have begun to explore the neural and neuropsychological foundations of the development of joint attention (Dawson et al., 2002; Griffith, Pennington, Wehner, & Rogers, 1999; Mundy, Card, & Fox, 2000). In addition to its content and face validity, this approach is important because it focuses on impairments in neural processes that may be involved the *social-output systems* that mediate the spontaneous organization, generation, and expression of social attention, behavior, and cognition (Klin, Jones, Schultz, & Volkmar, 2003; Minshew, Meyer, & Goldstein, 2002; Mundy, 1995, 2003). Impairments in the flexible generation of adaptive social behaviors is a hallmark of autism, and the flexible self-initiation of social-communication behaviors is one of the ultimate goals of intervention for children affected by this syndrome (Mundy & Crowson, 1997). Therefore, this third approach holds that the study of neural output systems involved in the self-initiation of social behaviors and social attention is an important complement to the study of neural processes involved in *social-input systems* and the social-perception paradigms that are currently prominent in the social–brain approach to autism.

Research utilizing this approach suggests that the neural substrates of social-output systems may be different from those involved in social-perception systems. Thus a complex, multiprocess neural model will likely be needed to understand the social symptoms of autism. For example, children with autism display difficulty with the development of the ability to follow gaze and to respond to the joint bids of others (Leekam, Lopez, & Moore, 2001; Mundy, Sigman, & Kasari, 1994), and this ability domain appears to involve neural activity in the STS and parietal lobes (e.g., Mundy et al., 2000; Senju, Tojo, Yaguchi, & Hasegawa, 2005; Vaughan & Mundy, in press). Children with autism also display a robust disturbance of the tendency to initiate joint-attention bids to spontaneously share experience, and this ability domain appears to involve activity of the dorsomedial and orbitomedial frontal cortex but relatively little input from the parietal and temporal cortices. (Caplan et al., 1993; Henderson, Yoder, Yale, & McDuffie, 2002; Dawson et al., 2002; Mundy et al., 2000). Hence impairments in different cortical systems may be involved in deficits in initiating and responding to the social-communication bids of others. The cortical and subcortical regions involved in these systems are illustrated in Figure 11.1.

Understanding the neural systems that support the development of joint attention and early social-communication skills provides new perspectives and hypotheses on the nature of the social disturbance in autism. These new perspectives hopefully will lead to valuable insights that contribute to the development of early identification and diagnostic neuroimaging methods. In addition, this information may play a pivotal role in guiding effective pharmacological and behavioral interventions. Specifically, a better understanding of the neural systems involved in the symptoms of autism may lead to the development of brain–behavior measurements that enable researchers to identify the specific agents of change in an intervention package or to provide better information about which aspects of a behavior system are most likely to change in response to intervention. Better biobehavioral symptom information and assessments may also allow researchers to understand the moderators of outcome in autism and, thereby, to identify children who will benefit most from specific kinds of intervention approaches. Therefore, this chapter provides an overview of the literature on the neural substrates of symptoms related to joint-attention impairment and considers what utility this information may offer for clinical research on autism. We begin with a review of our understanding of the nature and significance of joint-attention impairments in autism.

JOINT ATTENTION AND SOCIAL IMPAIRMENT IN AUTISM

Brain–behavior studies of joint attention may be critical to an understanding of autism because the early social-communication symptoms of autism are exemplified by a robust developmental failure in this domain (Mundy & Sigman, 1989). The term *joint-attention skills* refers to the capacity of

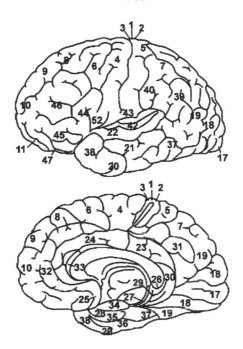

FIGURE 11.1. Lateral (top) and medial (bottom) illustrations of Brodmann's cytoarchitectonic areas of the cerebral cortex. The dorsal medial frontal cortex (DMFC) includes areas 8 and 9. The anterior cingulate is depicted as area 24. The ventral "social brain" includes the orbitofrontal cortex (area 11), the amygdala (area 22) and the superior temporal sulcus (the divisions between area 22 and 21). Adapted from Mundy (2003). Copyright 2003 by Blackwell Publishing. Adapted by permission.

individuals to coordinate attention with a social partner in relation to some object or event. In the first years of life this may only involve the social coordination of overt aspects of visual attention, such as when a toddler shows a toy to a parent. Theoretically, though, this capacity eventually becomes elaborated and integral to the social coordination of covert aspects of attention, as when social partners coordinate attention to psychological phenomena, such as ideas, intentions, or emotions (Tomasello, 1995).

Joint attention begins to emerge by at least 6 months of age (Scaife & Bruner, 1975) and takes several different behavioral forms. One behavior involves infants' ability to follow the direction of gaze, head turn, and/or pointing gesture of another person (Scaife & Bruner, 1975). This behavior may be referred to as responding to joint-attention skills (RJA; Seibert, Hogan, & Mundy, 1982; Mundy, Hogan, & Doehring, 1996). Another type of skill involves infants' use of eye contact and/or deictic gestures (e.g., pointing or showing) to spontaneously initiate coordinated attention with a social partner. The latter type of protodeclarative act (Bates, 1976) may be referred to as initiating joint-attention skills (IJA; Seibert et al., 1982; Mundy et al., 1996). These behaviors, especially IJA, appear to serve social functions. That is, the goal and reinforcement of these behaviors has been interpreted to revolve around sharing experience with others and the positive valence such early sharing has for the young child (Adamson, 1995; Bates, 1976; Mundy, 1995). Alternatively, social-attention coordination may also be used for less social but more instrumental purposes (Bates, 1976). So, for example, infants and young children may use eye contact and gestures to initiate attention coordination with another person in order to elicit aid in obtaining an object or event. This may be referred to as a protoimperative act (Bates, 1976) or initiating behavior request (IBR; Mundy et al., 1996). Figure 11.2 provides illustrations of IJA, RJA, and IBR behaviors.

Joint-attention skills are a critical milestone in early development and social learning (Bakeman & Adamson, 1984; Baldwin, 1995). Much of early language acquisition, for example, takes place in unstructured or incidental social-learning situations in which (1) parents provide learning opportunities by referring to a new object or event in the environment, but (2) infants may need to discriminate among a number of stimuli in the environment in order to focus on the correct object or event to acquire the appropriate new word association. Thus the infant is confronted with the possibility of referential mapping errors (Baldwin, 1995). To deal with this problem, infants may utilize the direction of gaze of the parent (i.e., use RJA skill) to limit the number of potential stimuli to attend to and increase the likelihood of a correct word learning experience (Baldwin, 1995). Similarly, when an infant initiates bids for joint attention, the responsive caregiver may follow the child's line of regard and take advantage of the child's focus of attention to provide a new word in a context that maximizes the opportunity to learn (cf. Tomasello, 1995). Hence joint attention may be regarded as an early developing *self-organizing facility* that is critical to much of subsequent social and cognitive development (e.g., Baldwin, 1995; Mundy & Burnette, 2005).

Children with autism, unfortunately, display robust levels of impairments in joint-attention development from at least as early as 12–18 months of age (Osterling, Dawson, & Munson, 2002; Swettenham et al., 1998). This impairment may be associated with a disruption of an early self-organizing process in social learning that contributes to the subsequent behavioral, and even neural, development of children with autism (Mundy & Crowson, 1997; Mundy & Burnette, 2005).

Interestingly, though, young children with autism display a dissociation in the development of joint-attention skills. Although children with autism display deficits in both IJA and RJA skills, they display less pro-

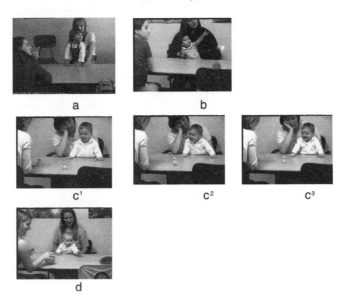

a   b

c¹   c²   c³

d

FIGURE 11.2. Illustrations from the Early Social Communication Scales (Seibert, Hogan, & Mundy, 1982; Mundy et al., 2003) of (a) responding to joint attention; (b) initiating joint attention—"pointing"; (c) initiating joint attention—"alternating gaze"; and (d) initiating behavior regulation/requests—"pointing." From Mundy and Burnette (2005). Copyright 2005 by John Wiley & Sons, Inc. Reprinted by permission.

nounced deficits in IBR or social-attention coordination for instrumental purposes (Mundy, Sigman, Ungerer, & Sherman, 1986). Moreover, young children with autism display some basic gaze-following ability by 2 years of age (Charwarska, Klin, & Volkmar, 2003), and problems in RJA may remit among older children with autism or those with higher mental ages (Mundy, Sigman, & Kasari, 1994; Leekam et al., 2001; Sigman & Ruskin, 1999). The impairment in IJA, however, remains robust even in older children (Mundy et al., 1994; Sigman & Ruskin, 1999). Indeed, research indicates that IJA, but not RJA, is related to social symptom intensity in preschool children with autism (Mundy et al., 1994). Moreover, individual differences in IJA, but not RJA, among 2- to 6-year-old children with autism significantly predict their tendency to spontaneously initiate social interaction with others 7–10 years later in life (Lord, Floody, Anderson, & Pickles, 2003; Sigman & Ruskin, 1999).

A dissociated pattern of IJA and RJA development is also observed in typical development and may occur because IJA and RJA reflect different integrations of social-cognitive and social-emotional processes (Mundy et al., 2000). IJA reflects the tendency to spontaneously initiate social-attention coordination, whereas RJA is a measure of the tendency to respond to another person's signal to shift attention. Hence, IJA may be more affected by executive and social-motivation processes involved in the generation and *self*-initiation of behavioral goals than RJA (Mundy, 1995; Mundy et al., 2000). In particular, IJA appears to involve the tendency to spontaneously initiate episodes of sharing the affective experience of an object or an event with a social partner (Mundy, Kasari, & Sigman, 1992). Indeed, a significant component of IJA disturbance in autism may be explained in terms of an attenuation of the tendency to initiate episodes of shared positive affect with a social partner (Kasari, Sigman, Mundy, & Yirmiya, 1990).

This literature has led to the instantiation of joint-attention disturbance, and especially IJA disturbance, as a central symptom of autism. For example, a "lack of spontaneous seeking to share enjoyment, interests, or achievements with other people (e.g., by a lack of showing, bringing or pointing out objects of interest)" is now one of four cardinal symptoms of the social impairment of autism in a current nosology (American Psychiatric Association, 2000, p. 75). Thus many of the current autism diagnostic and screening instruments include measures of joint attention, including the "gold standard" Autism Diagnostic Observation Schedule (ADOS; Lord et al., 1999). The ADOS even reflects the notion of a developmental dissociation in joint attention. Measures used for diagnosis with the youngest children (Module 1) include both IJA and RJA assessments. Module 2 is designed for developmentally more advanced children, and although it includes measures of both IJA and RJA, only the former is included in the diagnostic scoring.

In summary, research suggests that both IJA and RJA impairments may be important components of the early development of autism. However, with development, a dissociation appears to occur, with RJA impairments decreasing but IJA impairments remaining robust. This dissociation in development is consistent with the possibility that different neural processes are involved in the development of IJA and RJA (Mundy et al., 2000). Understanding these differences in the neurodevelopment of IJA and RJA may provide insights into the nature of autism.

THE NEURAL SUBSTRATE OF RJA

RJA is a complex behavior domain involving the perception and processing of social information, such as the direction of gaze, head orientation, and/or pointing gestures of a social partner. When studies examine the response of individuals to all of these behaviors in quasi-naturalistic situations, we refer to them as *RJA research*. However, often researchers use less naturalistic but more controlled paradigms to examine responses just to shifts in direction of gaze. Studies of this component of RJA are referred to as *gaze-following research*. Both types of research have been utilized in charting the neural correlates of RJA development.

Because RJA and gaze following involve social perception, they may be expected to be supported by a complex ventromedial "social brain" circuit. In particular, the results of several studies converge to suggest that gaze following and RJA may be mediated by part of this social brain circuit, contained primarily within the STS, STG, and adjacent parietal areas (e.g., Brodmann's area [BA] 40). These temporal and parietal areas of the brain are thought to contain neural networks that respond preferentially to faces, animate movement, and spatial orientation, including head, eye, and body orientation (e.g., Emery, 2000; Calder et al., 2002).

Wicker, Michel, Henaff, and Decety (2002) observed that neural groups in the posterior STS were activated in response to faces with direct or horizontally averted eye gaze but not to faces with downward eye gaze. Wicker et al. (2002), however, did not observe differences between direct and averted eye-gaze conditions. Alternatively, Puce, Allison, Bentin, Gore, and McCarthy (1998) reported that video of face stimuli with gaze moving horizontally from forward to averted gaze elicited greater posterior STS activation compared with faces with static forward gaze. Face matching on the basis of direction of gaze also elicited activation of neurons in the left posterior STS, whereas identity-based face matching elicited bilateral activation from the fusiform and inferior occipital gyri (Hoffman & Haxby, 2000). Similarly, George, Driver, and Dolan (2001) reported that direct-gaze stimuli elicited more fusiform activation than averted-gaze stimuli. Finally, Kingstone, Friesen, and Gazzaniga (2000) reported data in two split-brain patients that were consistent with the notion that parietal, as well as temporal, subsystems specialized for face processing and for processing of information relevant to spatial orientation combine to support the development of gaze following.

Mundy et al. (2000) have also reported observations linking RJA to parietal processes. In a study of 32 typically developing infants, these researchers examined the longitudinal relations between baseline electroencephalogram (EEG) at 14 months and RJA at 18 months as measured on the Early Social Communication Scales (ESCS; Seibert, Hogan, & Mundy, 1982; Mundy et al., 2003). The ESCS is a structured 20-minute observation instrument that provides quantitative measures of the development of RJA, IJA, and other nonverbal communication skills in children between 8 and 24 months of age. The EEG data were collected using a Lycra cap with electrodes placed bilaterally at dorsofrontal, central, temporal, parietal, and occipital sites. RJA at 18 months was predicted by 14 month EEG indexes of left-parietal activation and right-parietal deactivation. The location of the neural generators of EEG data was difficult to delineate definitively in this study. Nevertheless, the EEG data were quite consistent with previous research (Emery, 2000) that suggested that parietal areas specialized for spatial orienting and attention, along with adjacent temporal systems specialized for processing gaze, may contribute to gaze following or related RJA skill development.

The results of these human imaging, electrophysiological, and neuropsychological studies are also consistent with earlier reports from comparative research that provide experimental evidence of temporal (i.e., STS) and adjacent parietal involvement in gaze following (Emery, 2000). In two studies, presurgical monkeys demonstrated a clear ability to discriminate face stimuli on the basis of direction of gaze. After resection of the STS, however, the gaze discrimination abilities of the monkeys fell to chance (Campbell, Heywood, Cowey, Regard, & Landis, 1990; Heywood & Cowey, 1992). Eacott, Heywood, Gross, and Cowey (1993) compared two groups of monkeys, those with and without surgically induced lesions of the STS, on a task of discriminating pairs of eyes directed straight ahead or averted 5 or more degrees. The results indicated that the nonlesioned monkeys were capable of discriminating targets involving horizontal eye-gaze shifts of greater than 5 degrees, but the animals with STS lesions were not. However, Eacott et al. (1993) also reported that the lesioned animals performed worse than the nonlesioned animals on a nonsocial task involving the discrimination between abstract forms.

The latter observation reminds us that, although research is beginning to pinpoint the systems involved in gaze following and social perception, the specificity of these systems for social versus nonsocial processing has still to be definitively examined. One recent study, though, has addressed a related issue in imaging research on human gaze following. Hooker (2002) used whole-brain fMRI to compare neural activity in response to: (1) horizontal eye movement stimuli that provide directional information about where a visual stimulus would appear, (2) arrow stimuli that provided equivalent directional information, and (3) eye movements that did not provide directional information. Hooker (2002) observed more activity in the STS in the first condition than in either of the other conditions. Alternatively, Hooker (2002) reported more activity in the fusiform gyrus and prefrontal cortex in the eye-motion control condition (condition 3) than in the other conditions. These data were consistent with the notion that the STS may develop a specialization for processing gaze-related, social–spatial orientation information.

One puzzling aspect of the imaging research on gaze following has recently been noted by Calder et al. (2002). Theoretically, gaze-following behavior reflects aspects of social-cognitive processes (Baron-Cohen, 1995). In this regard, recent imaging studies have suggested that, in addition to *ventral* "social brain" activation, social cognition is most consistently associated with activation of the *dorsal* medial frontal cortex (BA 8,9) and the anterior cingulate (AC; Frith & Frith, 1999, 2001; Mundy, 2003). So why haven't studies of gaze following observed a link with frontal dorsal medial activation? Calder et al. (2002) suggested that perhaps task difficulty needs to be considered in this regard. Most studies have examined passive gaze following on tasks that did not require the perception or inference of intentions on the basis of eye gaze. These authors suggested that more complex presentations of sequences of gaze-direction stimuli may elicit this type of processing and provide evidence of more dorsal contributions to the neural substrate of gaze following. To this end Calder et al. (2002) used positron emission tomography (PET) to examine the neural responses of 9 female volunteers to a relatively complex sequence of faces with varying gaze-averted, gaze-direct, and gaze-down orientations. It wasn't completely clear from the methods described in this study how these stimuli might have elicited more inferences of gaze-related intentions than were found in previous studies. Nevertheless, the results provided evidence of activation in the dorsal medial frontal cortex (BA 8,9) and medial frontal cortex proximal to the AC (BA 32), as well as areas of the STS, in response to horizontal gaze aversion.

Two other studies have more clearly indicated that, when the interpretation of intentions is an overt feature of the demands of a gaze-processing task, activation of the dorsal medial frontal cortex appears to be involved. In a functional magnetic resonance imaging (fMRI) study, Baron-Cohen et al. (1999) presented 6 individuals with Asperger syndrome and 12 typical controls with the "eyes test" that requires inferring people's emotional states or gender from pictures of their eyes. The results of this study indicated that, in addition to activity in the orbitofrontal cortex, amygdala, and STS, activation of the left and right dorsal medial frontal cortex was also a specific correlate of performance on this task in the typical sample. Interestingly, the autism group failed to display amygdala activation and may not have shown as much right dorsal medial activation in response to this gaze-interpretation task. Russell et al. (2000) also employed the "eyes test" (Baron-Cohen et al., 1999) in an fMRI study of the neural characteristics of individuals affected by schizophrenia. The control sample displayed relatively more activity in the medial frontal lobe (BA 9, 45) in association with performance on this task relative to the individuals with schizophrenia. In addition, more ventral "social brain" components of the left inferior frontal gyrus (BA 44, 45, 47) and the left middle and superior temporal gyri (BA 21, 22) contributed to clinical group differences on performance on this task.

Thus the emerging literature on gaze following indicates that the most consistent correlates of basic gaze following and RJA skill appear to involve "social brain" neural clusters in the STS and parietal lobes (see Table

11.1 for summary). However, when tasks involve interpretation of the meaning of direction of gaze (e.g., social-cognitive inference of intentions), more dorsal medial cortical systems may be brought to bear in processing gaze-related stimuli. This difference across basic and more complex studies of RJA-related behaviors is interesting because it is consistent with developmental studies that suggest that gaze following may not reflect social-cognitive activity per se initially but, rather, that it comes to do so over time and experience (Brooks & Meltzoff, 2002; Moore, 1996; Woodward, 2003). It is also consistent with the notion that elements of RJA may reflect an early developing, more reflexive posterior attention-control system but that over time it may become influenced by a more intentional anterior attention-control system (Mundy et al., 2000).

In contrast to RJA, there is little evidence of parietal or temporal activation in the few studies of IJA that are available. Alternatively, the data from these studies suggest that IJA may reflect important contributions of the development of the anterior attention system to social development.

THE NEURAL SUBSTRATES OF IJA

The study of processes involved in the initiation of social behavior is as important as, but perhaps more difficult than, the study of processes involved in the perception of social behavior. It is fairly easy to set up a controlled study of the neural correlates of a *responsive* social behavior, such as gaze following, by presenting an analogue (e.g., video of a face with moving eyes) that may be used in electrophysiological or imaging paradigms. Alternatively, to study the initiation of a social behavior, one typically needs a more interactive paradigm that provides ecologically valid contexts that motivate individuals to generate social goals and behaviors. The development of virtual-environment paradigms may be one way to address this methodological difficulty (Eisenberger, Lieberman, & Williams, 2003). Currently, though, this methodological issue has limited the exploration of the neural correlates of self-initiated social behaviors such as IJA.

Nevertheless, important data have been provided in a study of the behavioral outcome of 13 infants who underwent hemispherectomies in an attempt to treat their intractable seizure disorders (Caplan et al., 1993). PET data were gathered prior to surgical intervention with the infants, and the ESCS was used to assess the postsurgical development of IJA and RJA, as well as the tendency for infants to initiate behavior requests (IBR). In addition to comparing IJA and RJA, it may also be important to consider IBR in research on joint attention. Whereas IJA reflects the social use of attention-directing behavior (e.g., directing attention to show or share interest in

TABLE 11.1. Summary of Neurobehavioral Research on Gaze Following, Joint Attention, and Related Behaviors

Study	Participants	Measure/method	Observations
Campbell et al. (1990); Eacott et al. (1993); Heywood & Cowey (1992)	Primates	Gaze following; neurolesion	STS involvement
Hoffman & Haxby (2000); Hooker (2002); Puce et al. (1998); Wicker et al. (2002)	Adults	Gaze following; imaging	STS involvement
Senju et al. (2005)	Children with autism	Gaze following; ERP/EEG	Right-hemisphere STS
George et al. (2001)	Adults	Direct versus averted gaze; imaging	Fusiform involvement
Kingstone et al. (2000)	Split-brain patients	Gaze following; neuropsychology	Temporal-parietal involvement in face and gaze processing
Calder et al. (2002)	Adults	Gaze direction inferences; imaging	Dorsal medial frontal cortex
Caplan et al. (1993)	Infants	IJA, RJA, IBR; imaging	Frontal involvement in IJA development
McEvoy et al. (1993); Griffith et al. (1999)	Children with autism	IJA, RJA; neuropsychology	Association with dorsolateral inhibition processes
Dawson et al. (2002)	Children with autism	RJA, IJA; neuropsychology	Association with ventromedial reward perception and learning
Mundy et al. (2000)	Infants	IJA, RJA, IBR; resting EEG	Dorsal medial frontal involvement with IJA, parietal involvement with RJA
Henderson et al. (2002)	Infants	IJA, IBR pointing; resting EEG	Dorsal medial and ventromedial frontal involvement with IJA

an object), IBR involves the instrumental use of attention-directing behavior (e.g., directing attention to elicit aid in obtaining an object or event). Hence, by comparing IJA behaviors (e.g., showing a jar containing toys) with IBR behaviors (e.g., giving a jar containing toys to request aid in opening the jar), brain systems associated with the spontaneous initiation of "social" joint-attention bids versus "instrumental" joint-attention bids may be examined.

The results of the Caplan et al. (1993) study indicated that metabolic activity in the frontal hemispheres, especially the left frontal hemisphere, predicted the development of IJA skill. However, the postsurgical development of the capacities to respond to joint-attention bids (RJA) or to initiate requesting bids (IBR) was not observed to relate to any of the PET indices of cortical activity. Moreover, metabolic activity recorded from other brain regions, including ventral "social brain" regions of the orbital, temporal, parietal, and occipital cortices, was not significantly associated with IJA or other social-communication skills in this study. Thus dorsal anterior activity appeared to be specifically related to the development of the tendency to spontaneously initiate social joint-attention bids to share experience with others in infants with neurological impairment.

Mundy et al. (2000) followed up on these clinical observations with a study of the links between EEG activity and joint-attention development in typical infants between 14 and 18 months of age. As previously noted, one result of this study was the observation that resting EEG activity at parietal sites at 14 months predicted differences in RJA skill development at 18 months. Alternatively, individual differences in 18-month IJA were predicted by a different and complex pattern of 14-month resting EEG activity at left medial frontal electrode sites, as well as indices of right central deactivation, left occipital activation, and right occipital deactivation. Although the source location of the EEG data could not be definitively determined in this study, the frontal correlates of IJA reflected activity only from electrodes at F3 of the 10/20 placement system. These electrodes were positioned above a point of confluence of BA 8 and 9 of the medial-frontal cortex of the left hemisphere (Martin, 1996). This area includes aspects of the frontal eye fields and supplementary motor cortex commonly observed to be involved in an anterior system of attention control (Posner & Petersen, 1990).

Another important step in the study of the neural correlates of IJA was taken by Henderson et al. (2002). This research group also employed the ESCS to examine the degree to which 14-month resting EEG data predicted 18-month joint-attention development in 27 typically developing infants. However, to improve the spatial resolution of their EEG data, Henderson et al. (2002) used a higher density array of 64 electrodes than did Mundy et al. (2000). Moreover, they reasoned that, because the total ESCS scores for measures of IJA and other domains were composites of several behaviors, the exact nature of the associations with EEG activity observed by Mundy et al. (2000) were unclear. To address this issue, Henderson et al. (2002) compared the EEG correlates of only two types of behaviors—self-initiated pointing to share experience with respect to an active mechanical toy (IJA pointing) and self-initiated pointing to elicit aid in obtaining an out-of-reach object (IBR pointing). In the ESCS, IJA pointing involves pointing to a toy that is within easy reach of a child, and IBR pointing involves pointing to a toy that is out of the reach of a child.

In their study, Henderson et al. (2002) did not observe any significant correlations between any of the 14-month EEG data and IBR pointing at 18 months. With regard to IJA, though, data in the 3- to 6-Hz band of 14-month resting EEG, indicative of greater brain activity over the medial frontal cortex, was strongly associated with more 18-month pointing to share attention and experience with an adult social partner. These correlations involved electrodes that were placed above cortical regions corresponding to BA 8, 9, and 6. Henderson et al. (2002) also analyzed data from the 6- to 9-Hz band that revealed 15 significant correlations between 14-month resting EEG data and 18-month IJA pointing. Again, higher bilateral activity corresponding to the previously identified medial frontal sites were strong predictors of IJA pointing at 18 months. In addition, though, IJA pointing at 18 months was also predicted by activity in this bandwidth from regions of the orbitofrontal, temporal, and dorsolateral frontal cortical regions. Thus this study suggested that IJA development may reflect an integration of dorsal cortical functions (Mundy et al., 2000) with ventral "social brain" and dorsolateral functions identified in other studies (Dawson et al., 2002; Griffith et al., 1999). However, there was no evidence for parietal involvement in IJA in this study.

The contribution of Henderson et al. (2002) also provided information about the social specificity of the link between IJA and dorsal cortical brain activity. As previously noted, the specific medial frontal cortical areas of involvement suggested by data from Mundy et al. (2000) and by some of the data from Henderson et al. (2002) correspond to aspects of both the frontal eye fields and supplementary motor cortex associated with the control of saccadic eye movement and motor planning (Martin, 1996). Therefore, these associations could simply reflect the motor control of the eye movements and/or gestural behaviors that are intrinsic to joint-attention behavior. However, the simple elegance of the Henderson et al. (2002) study controls for this possible interpretation. The gross motor topography of IJA pointing and IBR pointing are virtually identical on the ESCS. Therefore, a neuromotor explanation of the different cortical correlates of IJA and IBR appears unlikely. Instead, because IJA pointing and IBR pointing appear to serve different social-communicative functions, it is reasonable to assume that the difference in EEG correlates of these infant behaviors also reflects differences in the neurodevelopmental substrates of these social-communicative functions.

Several other neuropsychological studies have provided information on the functions and brain systems that may be involved with IJA. Two studies have reported that executive control, and especially the flexible inhibition of learned responses, which may be associated with dorsolateral activity, is also associated with RJA and IJA performance in children with autism and those with typical development (Griffith et al., 1999; McEvoy, Rogers, & Pennington, 1993). However, there was little evidence in these studies that this component played a role in the joint-attention deficits of children with autism. Dawson et al. (2002) have also reported a neuropsychological study that examined the hypothesis that IJA impairment in autism may be related to a disturbance in reward sensitivity and/or the ability to learn to flexibly associate rewards with elements in the environment (Dawson et al., 2002; Mundy, 1995). To examine this hypothesis Dawson et al. (2002) observed the performance of children with autism and controls on a delayed nonmatching-to-sample (DNMS) task that measures the ability of the child to learn to associate novel signs with the location of rewards in a forced-choice task. Previous research indicates that DNMS performance is associated with functions of an orbitofrontal circuit that is involved in reward perception and learning (e.g., Diamond & Goldman-Rakic, 1989; Rolls, Hornak, Wade, & McGrath, 1994). Consistent with the involvement of reward responsiveness in joint attention, DNMS performance was significantly associated with performance on a combined measure of RJA/IJA in children with autism and with typical development. However, although the children with autism displayed joint-attention impairment, they were not impaired on the DNMS measure. So it was not clear from this study whether reward responsiveness played a specific role on autistic joint-attention impairment. Moreover, the joint-attention measure used in this study was a composite of two RJA measures and one IJA measure, and thus it was also unclear whether DNMS performance was related to IJA, RJA, or both skill domains.

Some clarification on the latter issue has been provided by a recent study of typically developing children (Nichols, Fox, & Mundy, 2005). Nichols et al. (2005) worked with 39 typically developing infants and examined the relations of DNMS task performance with measures of IJA and RJA in the 14- to 18-month period. However, because previous research had implicated the dorsomedial cortex with IJA, the researchers also included a behavioral task that theoretically may be related to activity in this brain system. The dorsomedial cortex appears to play a fundamental role in self-monitoring and self-awareness (Buch, Luu, & Posner, 2000; Craik et al., 1999; Frith & Frith, 1999, 2001; Johnson et al., 2002; Stuphorn, Taylor, & Schall, 2000). So, for example, recent research indicates that the dorsal medial frontal cortex plays a role in encoding and recalling words and actions that involve self-reference rather than those that do not involve self-reference (Craik et al., 1999; Johnson et al., 2002). Therefore, Nichols et al. (2005) included a measure of infant self-recognition to examine the possible correlates of early self-awareness and self-monitoring with IJA. They hypothesized that if the data from Henderson et al. (2002) were correct, then it was likely that variance in both an orbital frontal-related behavior (DNMS) and a putative dorsal medial-related behavior (self-recognition) would make a unique contribution to the explanation of variance in IJA development. Consistent with these hypotheses, both a composite of the DNMS and self-recognition tasks (combined 14-, 16-, and 18-month data) made significant contributions to a multiple regression for 18-month IJA. However, these measures did not contribute to the explanation of 18-month RJA data. Hence, consistent with the resting EEG data from Henderson et al. (2002), these behavioral data suggest that psychological functions associated with both orbitofrontal and dorsal medial frontal systems may make a contribution to IJA development. The integrated functioning of these two-brain systems may be critical not only for IJA development but also for later developing aspects of social engagement and social competence (Mundy & Sigman, 2006; Mundy & Acra, 2006; Vaughan & Mundy, in press).

IJA, THEORY OF MIND, AND THE FRONTAL CORTEX

Additional information pertinent to understanding the neural correlates of joint attention is provided by recent research on the brain systems involved in social cognition as measured with theory-of-mind (ToM) task performance. Several lines of theory suggest that, by the second year of development, the infant capacity for joint attention involves an elementary social-cognitive understanding that others possess covert mental intentions that may be directed or shared (Tomasello, 1999; Wellman, 1993). Similarly, several researchers have suggested that deficits in both joint attention and theory of mind observed in children with autism reflect common social-cognitive paths of disturbance (e.g., Baron-Cohen, 1995; Mundy, Sigman, & Kasari, 1993). Surprisingly, little empirical data has been provided on the connections between joint attention and social-cognitive development. One study, though, followed a sample of 13 typically developing infants from 20 to 44 months of age as part of a study on the early identification of autism (Charman et al., 2000). At 20 months, an alternating-gaze measure was employed that involved children spontaneously initiating eye contact with a tester or parent after gazing at an interesting toy spectacle (see Figure 11.2c). Alternating-gaze measures are often used as indexes of IJA (e.g., Mundy et al., 1986; Tomasello, 1995). After controlling for differences in IQ and language development, the 20-month IJA alternating-gaze measure was observed to be a significant predictor of 44-month ToM performance.

If IJA in infants displays longitudinal continuity with ToM performance in preschool children, then imaging studies of ToM-related task performance may provide information about the neural systems involved in IJA. Indeed, recent imaging research indicates that brain activity in the dorsal medial cortex (BA 8,9) and adjacent subcortical areas of the AC is the most consistent correlate of ToM task performance (Frith & Frith, 1999, 2001). This is true for both verbal (Fletcher et al., 1995; Goel, Grafman, Sadato, & Hallett, 1995) and nonverbal measures of social cognition (Brunet, Sarfati, Hardy-Bayle & Decety, 2000; Castelli, Happé, Frith, & Frith, 2000; Gallagher et al., 2000). In addition, areas of the orbitofrontal and temporal cortices may also be involved in solving social-cognitive tasks (see Mundy, 2003, for a review). This pattern of activation has considerable overlap with the cortical areas that research suggests are involved in IJA. Indeed, because IJA and ToM abilities have long been linked theoretically, the imaging data on ToM task performance lends credence to observations of dorsal medial frontal, as well as more orbitofrontal and temporal, contributions to IJA.

IJA AND FUNCTIONS OF THE ANTERIOR ATTENTION SYSTEM

The foregoing research suggests that IJA is associated with a neural system involving the dorsomedial frontal cortex and AC (DMFC/AC), which forms a significant component of what has been referred to as the anterior attention system (Rothbart & Posner, 2001). It is thought that this system becomes functional after the posterior parietal system does and that it makes numerous contributions to the planning, self-initiation, and self-monitoring of goal-directed behaviors such as the intentional control of visual orienting (Mundy, 2003; Rothbart, Posner, & Rosicky, 1994; Vaughan & Mundy, in press). In particular, the anterior attention system is thought to play a significant role in the capacity to share attention across dual tasks or foci of attention (Stuss, Shallice, Alexander, & Picton, 1995), especially with respect to the capacity to maintain and flexibly switch between goal representations in working memory (e.g., Birrell & Brown, 2000; Rushworth, Hadland, Paus, & Siplia, 2002). This anterior capacity likely contributes to the development of infants' ability to maintain representations of self, a social partner, and an interesting object spectacle while flexibly switching attention between these foci in initiating joint-attention behaviors (Mundy et al., 2000). This attention-switching facility of the anterior system makes a critical contribution to the supervisory attention system (SAS; Norman & Shallice, 1986) that functions to guide behavior, especially attention deployment, *depending on the motivational context of the task* (e.g., Amador, Schlag-Rey, & Schlag, 2000; Buch et al., 2000). In this regard this system ultimately comes to participate in monitoring and representing the self and in directing attention to internal and external events (Faw, 2003).

At least two lines of research link the DMFC/AC system with self-representation and self-monitoring. For example, with respect to the former, Craik et al. (1999) and Johnson et al. (2002) have reported studies that reveal that self-referenced memory processes preferentially activate the dorsal medial frontal cortical component of this anterior system. With respect to self-monitoring, research has led to the observation that, when people make erroneous saccadic responses in an attention-deployment task, there is a negative deflection in the stimulus and response locked evoked response potential (ERP) called the error-related negativity, or ERN (Luu, Flaisch, & Tucker, 2000; Buch et al., 2000). Source location suggests that the ERN emanates from an area of the DMFC proximal to the anterior cingulate cortex (Luu et al., 2000). Observations of ERN suggest that there are not only specific cell groups within the DMFC/AC that are active in initiating a behavioral act, such as orienting to a stimulus, but also distinct cell groups involved in the processing of the positive or negative outcome of the response behavior (i.e., accuracy and reward or reinforcement information; e.g., Amador et al., 2000; Holroyd & Coles, 2002).

ERN is thought to reflect a crucial component of the AC's significant role in learning. In this regard Holroyd and Coles (2002) have recently presented a comprehensive and heuristic model. Very briefly, Holroyd and Coles (2002) suggest that distinct cortical areas control different adaptive motor-output functions, such as searching for immediate reinforcement, inhibiting motor action in favor of delayed reinforcement, avoiding pain at all cost, and more complex behavior patterns such as navigating social encounters. The AC is somatotopically connected to these distinct cortical motor-control areas and acts as a selective switch that enables one or more of the cortical motor controllers to take command at a particular time to select and initiate goal-directed behaviors that are most adaptive for a given set of environmental demands. This AC regulator function of motor output appears to be related to the SAS (Norman & Shallice, 1986), which guides behavior, especially attention deployment, depending on the motivational context of the task According to Holroyd and Coles (2002), the activity of the AC in this regard is most prominent in the earliest stages of learning, and the AC itself is "trained" to recognize which cortical control area(s) need to be given command per situation via reinforcement signals conveyed by a mesencephalic dopamine system. These reinforcement signals contribute to error detection (and the ERN), which allows specific types of motor behavior to be shaped to its most effective and adaptive configuration depending on reward or nonreward contingencies during motor activity. The AC also receives projections from limbic structures (e.g., the amygdala), providing a pathway for emotional and motivational factors to influence AC regulations of cortical motor-controller activation and inhibition (see Holroyd & Coles, 2002, for additional details).

The nature of the distinct cortical motor controllers was not discussed in detail by Holroyd and Coles (2002). It may bear noting, though, that developmental theory suggests that, with experience, motor activity becomes internalized as representational thinking (Piaget, 1952). So, ultimately, different cortical motor-control areas also become associated with the mediation of different types of motor representation, or cognition. Faw (2003) has attempted to describe the distinct frontal motor-cognitive units and has suggested that the dorsomedial/AC system functions to represent the self in spatial temporal coordinates and to direct attention to internal and external events. Related to this notion, Frith and Frith (1999, 2001) have argued that the DMFC integrates proprioceptive information from the self (e.g., goal-directed motor behaviors) with exteroceptive perceptions processed by the STS about the goal-directed behaviors and emotions of others. This integrative activity may be facilitated by the abundance of connections between the DMFC, the AC, and the STS (Morecraft, Guela, & Mesulam, 1993). Indeed, cell groups in and around BA 8 and 9 may be especially well connected to the STS (Ban, Shiwa, & Kawamura, 1991). We have described this putative facility for the integration of proprioceptive self-information with exteroceptive social-other perceptions as a social-executive function (SEF) of the dorsal medial frontal cortex (Mundy, 2003). Hypothetically this SEF utilizes the DMFC facility for the maintenance of representation of multiple goals in working memory to compare and integrate the actions of self and others. This integration gives rise to the capacity to infer the intentions of others by matching them with representations of self-initiated actions or intentions (Stich & Nichols, 1992). Indeed, Lau, Rogers, Haggard, and Passingham (2004) and recently reported that activity in the supplementary eye fields of the DMFC, but not in the parietal activity, is associated with the representation of self-intention. As the self–other integration begins to occur in the DMFC, a fully functional, adaptive human social-cognitive system emerges with experience (Frith & Frith, 1999, 2001).

According to the model of Holroyd and Coles (2002), though, this integrative development may not occur if some disturbance in the motor-control system occurs early in development that prevents DMFC/AC "learning" of the adaptive functions of social initiations, such as directing visual attention to social partners or bidding for attention from social partners (e.g., IJA). Without social initiations it is difficult for the DMFC system to gain the information required to develop a relational representation of self and other (Mundy et al., 1993; Vaughan & Mundy, in press). Although many details related to this process are unclear at this time, we have hypothesized that a developmental disturbance in control functions of the DMFC/AC system makes a significant contribution to the etiology of autism (Mundy, 2003). Of course, this hypothesis does not preclude the distinct possibility that a disturbance of temporal and parietal "other" processing systems is also integral to autism (e.g., Castelli, Frith, Happé, & Frith, 2002; Senju et al., 2005; Townsend et al., 2001). Nevertheless, several lines of research support the DMFC/AC hypothesis of autism. Two recent studies have reported that individual differences in the fMRI and PET indicators of activity in the DMFC and AC are specific correlates of the relative intensity of social symptom impairments displayed by children with autism (Haznedar et al., 2000; Ohnishi et al., 2000). In a related finding, Henderson et al. (in press) observed that an ERN index of DMFC/AC activity associated with self-monitoring was related to social impairments among higher functioning children with autism. Happé et al. (1996) and Castelli et al. (2002) have also observed that atypical DMFC/AC activation on social-cognitive tasks is characteristic of some individuals with autism. Consistent with this possibility, Ernst, Zametkin, Matochik, Pascualvaca, and Cohen (1997) have observed a disturbance of dopaminergic activity in the dorsal medial frontal cortices of children with autism. Morphometric studies have also revealed atypical gray matter density in components of the DMFC/AC system (i.e., AC, paracingulate sulcus, left superior frontal gyrus), as well as the amygdala, temporal lobe, left inferior parietal lobe, and cerebellum (Abell et al., 1999; Hardan et al., 2002). Finally, lesions or impairments of components of the DMFC/AC complex have been observed to produce a variety of symptoms that are similar to those displayed by some people with autism, including: akinetic mutism or a lack of will or motivation to generate behavior, excessive preoccupation with motor output and related ideation as in obsessive–compulsive disorder, inattention, dysregulation of autonomic functions, emotional instability, and variability in pain sensitivity (Buch et al., 2000; Holroyd & Coles, 2002).

CLINICAL IMPLICATIONS AND APPLICATIONS

As many of the chapters in this volume make eminently clear, behavioral research on early joint-attention disturbance has had a positive impact on developing more effective diagnostic and intervention methods for children with autism. Therefore, one reasonable question to raise at this juncture is: Does research on the neural correlates of joint attention add anything of significance to clinically relevant knowledge about the nature of autism? A complete answer to this question is not yet available because research on the neural development of joint attention has just begun, and consequently interpretation of this research is highly speculative. Nevertheless, this literature begins to raise meaningful hypotheses about the neuropsychological functions involved in autism. These hypotheses, in turn, hold considerable promise for guiding future intervention-related research and theory development with young children with autism. Examples of some of these hypotheses are presented in the remainder of this chapter.

AUTISM AND LEARNING

First of all, the putative connections between IJA and functions of the DMFC/AC as previously described are consistent with the notion that a disturbance of early neurodevelopmental learning processes may contribute to autism. Dawson, for example, has suggested that rule learning between stimuli and reward is critical to social development, including joint attention, and that an impairment in the capacity to connect stimuli and rewards plays a significant role in the development of social impairments in children with autism (Dawson et al., 2002). Related to this idea is the notion that children with autism may suffer from a specific deficit in their early sensitivity to the reward value of social stimuli (Mundy, 1995; Panksepp, 1979). A disturbance of learning functions of the DMFC/AC may contribute to either the more general stimulus–reward association impairment (Dawson et al., 2002) or the more specific social stimulus–reward association impairment (Mundy, 1995; Panksepp, 1979).

In either case, problems with establishing and maintaining stimulus–reward associations have long been recognized as a significant complication in intervention with children with autism (Dawson, Osterling, Rinaldi, Carver, & McPartland, 2001). It may be that work on the neural correlates of IJA will lead to a better understanding of the neural systems that underlie this general problem. For example, by linking the neural learning model of Holroyd and Coles (2002) to joint-attention development, the possibility is raised that a disturbance in the relations between the mesencephalic dopamine system and the DMFC/AC may play a role in impairments in this domain and related social domains in autism. This possibility is quite consistent with ongoing research on drug treatments for autism that address the role of dopaminergic systems in the pathophysiology of autism (McDougle et al., 2001). Moreover, the types of effects that may be reasonably expected from pharmacological manipulations of dopamine-related systems may be clarified by this model. Because activity of the AC is most prominent in the earliest stages of learning (Holroyd & Coles, 2002), it may be that the most obvious effects of rectifying the dopaminergic system in autism would be revealed in the context of interventions designed to promote new learning. That is, it may be unreasonable to expect pharmacological interventions, by themselves, to have significant effects on the adaptive social behavior of children with autism, especially in short-term trials (e.g., less than several months). Alternatively, it may be that dopaminergic pharmacological interventions may augment the capacity of children with autism to appreciate stimulus–reward associations (and perhaps specifically social stimulus–reward associations) and, therefore, display enhanced speed and maintenance of learning within a behavioral intervention paradigm.

INTERVENTION WITH RJA AND IJA IN AUTISM

Given that pharmacological interventions may augment the ability of the child with autism to respond to behavioral intervention, the question then becomes what types of behavioral interventions may best address joint-attention and related social-developmental impairments in autism. Recall that research suggests that RJA and IJA are two distinct forms of joint-attention skills that dissociate in the development of autism. Research also suggests that the neurodevelopment of joint attention may be described in terms of a dual-process model (Mundy et al., 2003; Vaughan & Mundy, in press). By the second year of life, RJA may be primarily mediated by the posterior parietal attention system (Rothbart & Posner, 2001) that is integrated with temporal circuits specific to social attention and social information processing (Vaughan & Mundy, in press). Theoretically, one characteristic of the posterior attention system is that it is a relatively nonvolitional system that automatically responds with shifts in attention to *external* biologically significant stimuli (Rothbart et al., 1994). Accordingly, posterior attention system behaviors such as RJA should be relatively open to modification through the manipulation of external stimulus conditions and stimulus contingencies. Alternatively, the link between IJA and the anterior attention system suggests that this type of behavior involves self-initiation and self-monitoring of goal-directed behaviors that may be under endogenous rather than exogenous motivational constraint (Mundy, 1995; Mundy & Acra, 2006; Mundy & Sigman, 2006). Hence the contextual constraints that motivate a child with autism to initiate a social behavior such as IJA may be different from those that might be effective in eliciting more responsive behaviors such as RJA. Let us consider these differences, starting with RJA.

Research with normally developing children supports the notion that RJA is a highly responsive social behavior that may be relatively easily affected by external stimulus contingencies. Corkum and Moore (1998) worked with a sample of 8-month-old infants who displayed as many incorrect as correct responses to a gaze-following task. These researchers then established stimulus conditions for the infants such that, whenever an infant displayed a correct gaze-following response, he or she was "rewarded" with an interesting event that occurred in his or her line of sight (i.e., a dark Plexiglas box would be illuminated, revealing an active, cymbal-clapping mechanical toy monkey). The results of this study indicated that infants who had not mastered gaze following quickly acquired this skill under optimized conditions of contingent external reward. The study by Corkum and Moore (1998) is important for a number of reasons, not the least of which is that it suggests that it may be possible to develop intervention paradigms that manipulate stimulus–reward contingencies that lead to the more rapid acquisition of RJA skill among children with autism.

Surprisingly, we know of no published intervention studies on the effects of manipulating external reward contingency as a specific intervention for RJA development in children with autism. Nevertheless, consistent with previous research (Mundy et al., 1994), Leekam and colleagues (2001) have reported that children with autism vary in their gaze-following RJA skill, with better skill displayed by children with higher mental ages and IQs. Perhaps more important, Leekum and colleagues (2001) also reported that the performance of 40% of their sample of children with autism improved in gaze following when illuminated targets such as those used by Corkum and Moore (1998) appeared in response to correct gaze shifts. This observation suggests that a substantial number of children with autism may be sensitive to modifications of nonsocial external contingencies that facilitate RJA development.

This observation of improved performance on a gaze-following task is not well recognized in the intervention literature on autism, but it may be very significant for several reasons. First, children do not only *learn to* control gaze following/RJA, but they also *learn from* engagement in this pattern of motor behavior. That is, young children's own behavior becomes a critical source of information for subsequent executive and conceptual development (e.g., Piaget, 1952). In this regard, consider the heuristic set of observations from comparative research reviewed by Calder et al. (2002). Different sets of cells in the STS of macaque monkeys appear to contribute to the processing of gaze direction versus the processing of the direction and orientation of limb movements (Perrett, Heitenen, Oram, & Benson, 1992). However, a subset of limb movement cells appears to be modulated by activity of the gaze-following system (Jallema, Baker, Wicker, & Perrett,

2000). Jallema et al. (2000) interpret these data to suggest that the *combined* analysis of direction of visual attention and body movements of others provides an important source of information that gives rise to the capacity to detect intentionality in others. Translated to human development, this finding suggests that gaze following does not occur in isolation but rather as an integrated element of processing of additional dimensions of social-behavioral information about others. According to Jallema et al. (2000), this is consistent with the observation that, in addition to its social information processing specialization, the STS may also include polysensory areas involved in attending to and processing information synchronously from multiple modalities. The integrated processing of others' direction of gaze, limb and postural direction, and vocal behavior ultimately may be an important, if not critical, source of information that enables the young child to learn about self, others, and social intentions. For example, with respect to gaze following, Jallema et al. (2000) suggested that one major lesson learned from gaze following is, "Where the eyes go, behavior follows." In this regard we have also suggested that neural connections between the posterior attention system and anterior attention system make it plausible that social and cognitive information that is gleaned as part of RJA development is fed forward to support the development of the self-initiation of critical social behaviors such as IJA (Vaughan & Mundy, in press). So the early facilitation of RJA may be an important goal for intervention that targets social-cognitive disturbance in young children with autism.

RJA may also serve a self-organizing function that is specific to language development by reducing referential mapping errors and maximizing relevant social information processing in language-related incidental-learning opportunities (Baldwin, 1995). Observations consistent with the self-organizing role of RJA in the development of children with autism have been provided by Bono, Daley, and Sigman (2004). These researchers examined the treatment responsiveness of 23 children with autism to varying intensities of intervention over a 1-year period (6–43 hours per week). ESCS data were collected at baseline, and the Reynell Language Development Scales (Reynell & Gruber, 1990) were used to assess outcome. The results revealed that ESCS scores from both the IJA and RJA scales predicted individual differences in language outcome. Surprisingly, differences in intervention intensity were not associated with language outcomes. However, a significant interaction between intervention intensity and RJA was observed. Children with autism who more consistently responded correctly on RJA trials displayed more evidence of benefiting from higher intensities of intervention (i.e., more social learning opportunities) than did children with less consistent RJA skills.

These observations suggest that the adequate development of RJA may contribute to the capacity of the child with autism to profit from additional intervention. Moreover, recall that both behavioral research (Corkum & Moore, 1998; Leekam et al., 2001) and research linking RJA development to the posterior attention system (e.g., Mundy et al., 2000) suggest that RJA skills may be sensitive to external rewards (cf. Leekam et al., 2001). Therefore, RJA appears to be a domain that is pivotal to the development of the child with autism and that can also be targeted relatively easily. In contrast, as previously discussed, neural research on IJA is consistent with the notion that this domain of development may be more sensitive to endogenous motivation and executive constraints. Hence effective intervention strategies for IJA-related aspects of development may be more complicated than those for RJA. However, considering the neurodevelopmental functions that may be associated with IJA development, it may be that effective intervention in this domain is at least as important as intervention for RJA.

NEURODEVELOPMENT, IJA, AND THE SELF-SYSTEM IN AUTISM

In examining the development of behaviors displayed in Figure 11.2, researchers may ask at least two different questions: How are infants able to share attention and experience with others? and Why do infants share attention and experiences with others? The second question leads to reflection on the motivation factors and processes that contribute to the human tendency to share experience with others. For example, consider the following vignette. You are going to be part of the audience at an event that you are sure you will thoroughly enjoy (a play, a concert, a sporting event, etc.). You have a choice: You can go alone, or take a friend along. Many, if not most, people will choose the company of a friend. Moreover, during the event, there is a strong likelihood that you and your friend will exchange eye contact and experience a sense of relatedness at some point in response to your shared experience of an especially interesting or emotionally stimulating incident that occurs during the event. In that moment, the two of you are socially engaged in joint attention, much like the infant in Figure 11.2c. Why do we, as infants, children, and adults, engage in this behavior even when viewing the event by ourselves would be pleasurable? Does the sharing of experience with others hold some positive reward value that motivates people to engage in acts of joint attention throughout the lifespan? Does this motivation system assist in bootstrapping the development of joint attention and its critical early self-organizing functions in human social development? Some would respond with an unequivocal *yes* to these questions and go on to suggest that human beings have an intrinsic motivation for sharing of experience, or intersubjectivity, and that this motivation is important for the early organization of social and cognitive development (e.g., Trevarthen & Aitken, 2001). Extrapolating from this theory, others have suggested that a disturbance of the intrinsic motivation for sharing experience with others makes a very significant contribution to IJA impairments and related components of the social-developmental disorder of autism (Hobson, 1993, 2002; Mundy, 1995; Mundy & Burnette, 2005).

At least one study directly supports this hypothesis. Kasari and her colleagues (1990) integrated ESCS ratings of joint attention with systematic ratings of facial affect and made several important observations. First, in the typical control sample, infants conveyed positive affect significantly more often to social partners in the context of IJA bids compared with IBR or RJA behaviors. Alternatively, children with Down syndrome and autism did not display differences in affect across IJA and IBR measures, but the reasons they did not are different. The children with Down syndrome displayed equally high rates of positive affect across both IJA and IBR bids, but the children with autism displayed equally low rates of positive affect in IJA and IBR. Positive affect was not a major component of RJA for any group. These results suggested that the sharing of positive affective experiences with others is a major component of IJA behavior in typical development and that an attenuation of positive affect sharing may be an important component of IJA deficits in children with autism (Kasari et al., 1990).

Surprisingly few, if any, studies have been implemented to replicate and extend these important observations. Nevertheless, the basic observation that IJA involves affective sharing to a significantly greater degree than RJA or other forms of nonverbal communication in typically developing children has been replicated (Mundy et al., 1993) and appears to become codified in the behavioral repertoire of children between 8 and 10 months of age (Venezia, Messinger, Thorp, & Mundy, 2004). The data from these studies may be interpreted to suggest that IJA assessments provide an operational definition of the development of secondary intersubjectivity, or the tendency of children to initiate episodes of positive affective sharing with a social partner (see Figure 11.2c). Also, evidence consistent with the notion that intrinsic factors affect IJA has been presented by Vaughan et al. (2003), who have observed that individual differences in IJA development are specifically sensitive to temperamental factors associated with emotional reactivity in infants. Just because intrinsic factors may be involved in IJA development, however, does not mean that IJA is not sensitive to environmental factors. Indeed, in this regard research suggests that relative to RJA, IBR, or other social-communication skills, IJA is specifically sensitive to a complex system of factors involved in the degree of nurturing and positive social-emotional caregiving experienced by young children (e.g.,

Claussen, Mundy, Malik, & Willoughby, 2002; Kroupina, Kuefner, Iverson, & Johnson, 2003; Wachs & Chan, 1986).

Trevarthen and Aitken (2001) suggested that the development of intersubjectivity is affected by motivation systems theoretically mediated by orbital frontal and temporal brain systems involved in the perception of social stimuli (e.g., facial affect) and the association of these stimuli with positive reward value. According to this model, sensitivity to the reward value of these stimuli is inherent to human beings and possibly mediated by a neuropeptide-based endogenous social-reward system (Panksepp, 1979). The identification of these brain systems in this regard is consistent with some of the neurodevelopment data and theory on IJA and its disturbance in autism (Dawson et al., 2002; Henderson et al., 2002; Mundy, 1995). However, the social-reward system involved in joint attention likely goes beyond the ventral brain systems to include more dorsal cortical regions, including the AC (Eisenberger et al., 2003; Mundy, 2003). Moreover, the disturbance of IJA development in autism may reflect a disruption of the functions of the self-system. Specifically, IJA and related social impairments may reflect a disturbance in one or more of the DMFC facilities for: self-monitoring and/or the capacity to integrate the monitoring of self-related intentions with STS/parietal processing of information about the behavior of others (Mundy et al., 1993; Mundy, 2003; also see Faw, 2003; Frith & Frith, 2001). Problems in these putative DMFC functions may contribute to what some have described as a core disturbance in the ability of people with autism to perceive and identify with the bodily expressed psychological attitudes of other people (Hobson, 1993, 2002), and to what others describe as a fundamental impairment in the capacity to simulate the behavior of others (Frith & Fith, 2001; Mundy, 2003).

This literature affords a view of the characteristics of successful interventions with autism. For example, it is consistent with the findings of those who have recognized that optimal intervention programs with autism will need to target the motivational substrates of the tendency to initiate social behaviors (Koegel, Koegel, & McNeary, 2001). In addition, the hypothesis that autism may involve impairments in self-monitoring and/or in integrating self-monitoring with processing the behavior of others may also help to explain why mirroring or imitation of the behavior of young children with autism has been observed to be a useful early intervention technique in bootstrapping social awareness and social behavior (Dawson & Adams, 1984; Dawson & Galpert, 1990). That is, in addition to having a disturbance in orienting to others, young children with autism may be less aware of when other people are orienting to them. This problem, though, may be mitigated to some degree when social partners simplify their behavior and emphasize their own attention to a child through mirroring the behavior of the child.

Of course, neurological theory and research that suggest a biological attenuation of the basic social motivation system (Dawson et al., 2002; Hobson, 1993; Mundy, 1995) and/or difficulty in self-monitoring and apprehending the relations between self and other behavior (Hobson, 1993; Mundy, 2003) also hint at the magnitude of the obstacles that need to be overcome in effective intervention with IJA-related social deficits in children with autism. Nevertheless, recent research on the responsiveness of IJA to nurturing and especially to the affective tone of caregiving (Claussen et al., 2002; Kroupina et al., 2003; Wachs & Chan, 1986) also provides some hope and direction for effective intervention development.

In programmatic efforts in this regard, researchers and clinicians will need to identify a developmental sequence of techniques that have a positive impact on critical social behaviors, such as IJA. Several research groups have already begun to make headway in this regard (Kasari, Freeman, & Paparella, 2001; Yoder & Warren, 2002). Indeed, it may be important to test a set of related hypotheses that: (1) available techniques may be modified to provide effective intervention paradigms for RJA development in young children with autism (e.g., Leekam et al., 2001), (2) effective intervention with RJA will have a positive impact on children's social information processing and the capacity to perceive relations between self and others, and (3) improvement in these domains will facilitate subsequent language and social development, including IJA development, in a significant number of young children with autism.

It may also be important to develop methods to saturate the environment of children with autism with developmentally appropriate learning opportunities that magnify the salience of social-emotional responses to the child's behavior and increase the child's awareness of other people. Parent training will be a critical component of any effective intervention. This training will likely involve increasing the salience and frequency of caregiver positive affective responses to the behaviors of the child with autism in an attempt to compensate for biologically based impairments in social-perception and/or social-reward sensitivity (Gutstein & Sheely, 2002; Greenspan & Wieder, 2000; Siller & Sigman, 2002). Programmatic research here will need to provide evidence in support of this hypothesis (i.e., that increasing the salience and frequency of affective responses has a significant impact on development in young children with autism). It is also likely that optimally effective intervention of this kind will involve (1) training parents to understand the nature and role of social motivation in developing the capacity for intersubjectivity in children with autism and (2) providing parents with a developmentally sequenced system of techniques that they can use in relatively natural interactions with their children throughout the day to optimize social-emotional development and self–other awareness. Indeed, as is exemplified by relationship development intervention (RDI; Gutstein & Sheely, 2002), creative and informed strides have already been made in developing such a manualized intervention system. However, like many new and promising intervention methods, RDI awaits thorough empirical examination before its effectiveness can fully be appreciated.

Of course, many would agree that it is unlikely that any single type of intervention will be sufficient to mitigate the complex developmental disturbances of autism. Rather, future effective intervention may need to combine both biological (e.g., pharmacological) and behavioral approaches to most effectively address the needs of children with autism. Understanding the biological substrates of early social-communication skills, such as IJA and RJA, may be critical to guiding the development of effective intervention strategies within both modalities.

NEURODEVELOPMENT AND INDIVIDUAL DIFFERENCES IN AUTISM

It is also important to note that the neurodevelopmental research on joint attention may contribute to an understanding of individual differences in social development and treatment responsiveness among children with autism. The research reviewed in this chapter suggests that the capacity to share experience with others (e.g., IJA skill) is a complex aspect of development that stems from the confluence of multiple neural systems (e.g., orbitofrontal, temporal/parietal, DMFC/AC systems) involved in learning, motivation, and affective processes, as well as intersubjectivity and self–other monitoring. It may be anticipated that individuals, including children with autism, display differences in the integrity and functioning of this array of neural systems. Some criterion level of dysfunction across these systems may give rise to autism. However, the pattern of dysfunction across systems, or the relative intensity of dysfunctions within systems, may vary among individuals with autism.

This variation may be manifested in the different types of social growth patterns that are exhibited by children with autism. Since the late 1970s, before many of the contemporary forms of early intervention were available, it has been recognized that children with autism vary in their social presentation and outcomes, with some children displaying a maximally aloof social style and others displaying an active but odd style that involves a relatively high frequency of attempts to initiate social interactions with others (Wing & Gould, 1979). It seems likely that some aspects of these social individual differences in autism may be linked to variability in the functioning of the neural systems associated with joint attention and intersubjective processes in social development. For example, given what we are beginning to understand about the DMFC/AC, it may well be that variation in the functioning of this system affects the capacity for social learning in autism. In some children this system may be moderately impaired but sufficiently intact to respond to concerted attempts to enrich their social-emotional environmental stimulation. For other children, however, the DMFC/AC system may be so impaired that all facets of learning are disrupted. These children may require a more structured sequence of intervention to establish even basic stimulus–reward mechanisms, as well as self-monitoring and self-regulatory functions.

Support for the notion that children with autism vary in the functioning of these neural systems is provided by previously noted research, which observed that biological activity in the DMFC/AC brain system has been linked to variation in social symptom presentation in children with autism (Haznedar et al., 2000; Henderson et al., in press; Ohnishi et al., 2000). It is important to recognize, though, that the DMFC/AC system is not only associated with social development but is also strongly linked to basic learning and cognitive processes (Holroyd & Coles, 2002). Indeed, this may be emphasized by developmental observations that link individual differences in infant joint attention to childhood intellectual outcomes in at-risk children (Neal et al., 2005; Ulvund & Smith, 1996). The point here is that it would be a mistake to leave the reader with the impression that the neural systems that we believe to be involved in joint-attention, intersubjectivity, and experience-sharing disturbances in autism are only social-emotional systems. Rather, we believe that one value of the neurodevelopmental literature on joint attention is that it strongly suggests that the brain systems involved in this critical act of development, such as the DMFC/AC systems, are as integral to learning and cognition as they are to social development (Frith & Frith, 2001; Holroyd & Coles, 2002). Specifically, we believe that the putative links between behavioral markers of autism such as IJA disturbance and neural systems involving the functions of AC (Holroyd & Coles, 2002) raise an important hypothesis. That is, disturbances in the functions of the AC and related cortical systems may contribute not only to the social deficits of autism but also to the frequent association between autism and mental retardation. If so, one can well imagine why differences in intensity of DMFC/AC dysfunction may have a significant impact on the treatment responsiveness of children with autism.

Finally, we also believe that investigating the functional relations between anterior brain systems and social development may be important to understanding the wide range of phenotypic presentation in autism and related differences in the treatment responsiveness of these children. A recent study in our laboratory suggests that higher-functioning children with autism display individual differences in anterior cortical brain activity and that these are related to significant differences in their social symptoms, self-awareness, and cognitive style (Sutton et al., 2005). The Sutton et al. (2005) study was based on an integration of research and theory that suggested that measures of resting anterior EEG asymmetry reflect complex brain processes associated with approach or avoidance motivation (e.g., Sutton & Davidson, 1997) and that approach–avoidance motivation may be related to the development of the tendency to initiate and engage in social behaviors in children with autism (Mundy, 1995). Basically, the literature on EEG asymmetry suggests that individuals with more left anterior than right anterior resting cortical activity tend to show motivational tendencies associated with more behavioral activation and the initiation of more social interactions, whereas a bias to right anterior activation is associated with behavioral inhibition and lower social interactive tendencies (Sutton & Davidson, 1997). Early versions of this theory lead us to suggest that relative left frontal activation may be associated with social-emotional motivation in children with autism that is related to their tendency to initiate social interactions with others (Mundy, 1995).

This integration of research and theory led to a study of the relations among resting anterior asymmetry, social impairment, and social anxiety in 23 high-functioning children with autism (HFA) and 20 verbal IQ- and age-matched controls (age range 9–14 years). Sutton et al. (2005) observed that these groups were significantly different on the measures of anterior asymmetry, social symptoms, and anxiety-related measures. Moreover, children with HFA who displayed right frontal asymmetry (RFA group) displayed more symptoms of social impairments and better visual analytical skills than did children who displayed left frontal asymmetry (LFA group). Alternatively, although the LFA group displayed fewer symptoms of social impairment, they also reported greater levels of social anxiety and social stress and lower satisfaction with interpersonal relations than did the RFA group (Sutton et al., 2005). A second study with larger samples has replicated the observations that children with autism and LFA display greater levels of social anxiety and social stress and lower satisfaction with their social relations (Burnette et al., 2005). These children also reported a greater sense of internal locus of control, and parents reported that their first concerns occurred at a much later point in development for children with LFA and RFA. However, this study did not replicate the observations of associations between asymmetry and cognition or executive functions reported in Sutton et al. (2005).

These observations suggest that anterior EEG asymmetry may be a marker of motivation and emotion processes that refract the autism taxon into important individual differences in social ability and presentation in children with autism. Specifically, it raises the hypothesis that variation in left and right anterior brain systems, possibly including the DMFC/AC complex, is related to variation in the tendency of children to be motivated to interact with others and to be self-aware of their interactions with others. If this is correct, those children with autism who show greater biologically based social motivation and self-awareness may be expected to be responsive to different types of social interventions than those with lower social motivation and self-awareness.

SUMMARY

Over the past few years several research groups, including our own, have been attempting to better understand the neural substrates of autism. For our own part we have started with observations on the nature of the critical early social-behavioral difficulties of children affected by autism, and then we have begun to try to identify the neural systems that may contribute to the developments in these critical behavior domains. From time to time, though, we ask ourselves what the immediate value of this line of inquiry is. As part of this chapter, we have tried to address this question. The answer appears to be that integrating brain–behavior research with developmental studies of joint attention can assist in revealing new perspectives and raising new hypotheses about the nature and treatment of autism. The research in this regard has just begun; hence the hypotheses that have been raised are clearly in their formative stage. Nevertheless, this approach is clearly heuristic, and its immediate value lies in its potential to stimulate, as well as corroborate, new approaches to understanding treatment and individual differences in autism.

ACKNOWLEDGMENTS

The preparation of this chapter was supported, in part, by Grant No. HD38052 from the National Institutes of Health (Peter Mundy, Principal Investigator) and by State of Florida funding for the University of Miami Center for Autism and Related Disabilities (UM-CARD).

REFERENCES

Abell, F., Krams, M., Ashburner, J., Passingham, R., Friston, K., Frackowiak, R., et al. (1999). The neuroanatomy of autism: A voxel-based whole-brain analysis of structure scans. *Neuroreport, 10*, 1647–1651.

Adamson, L. (1995). *Communication development in infancy.* Madison, WI: Brown & Benchmark.

Adolphs, R. (2001). The neurobiology of social cognition. *Current Opinion in Neurobiology, 11*, 231–239.

Amador, N., Schlag-Rey, M., & Schlag, J. (2000). Reward predicting and reward detecting neuronal activity in the primate supplementary eye field. *Journal of Neurophyisology, 84,* 2166–2170.

American Psychiatric Association. (2000). *Diagnostic and statistical manual of mental disorders* (4th ed., text rev.). Washington, DC: Author.

Bakeman, R., & Adamson, L. (1984). Coordinating attention to people and objects in mother–infant and peer–infant interaction. *Child Development, 55,* 1278–1289.

Baldwin, D. A. (1995). Understanding the link between joint attention and language. In C. Moore & P. J. Dunham (Eds.), *Joint attention: Its origins and role in development* (pp. 131–158). Hillsdale, NJ: Erlbaum.

Ban, T., Shiwa, T., & Kawamura, K. (1991). Cortico-cortical projections from the prefrontal cortex to the superior temporal sulcal area (STS) in the monkey studied by means of HRP method. *Archives of Italian Biology, 129,* 259–272.

Baron-Cohen, S. (1995). *Mindblindness.* Cambridge, MA: MIT Press.

Baron-Cohen, S., Ring, H., Wheelwright, S., Bullmore, E., Brammer, M., Simmons, A., et al. (1999). Social intelligence in the normal and autistic brain: An fMRI study. *European Journal of Neuroscience, 11,* 1891–1898.

Bates, E. (1976). *Language and context: The acquisition of performatives.* New York: Academic Press.

Birrell, J., & Brown, V. (2000). Medial-frontal cortex mediates perceptual attention set shifting in the rat. *Journal of Neuroscience, 20,* 4320–4324.

Bono, M., Daley, T., & Sigman, M. (2004). Relations among joint attention, amount of intervention, and language gain in early autism. *Journal of Autism and Developmental Disorders, 34,* 495–505.

Brooks, R., & Meltzoff, A. (2002). The importance of eyes: How infants interpret adult looking behavior. *Developmental Psychology, 38,* 958–966.

Brothers, L. (1990). The social brain: A project for integrating primate behavior and neurophysiology in a new domain. *Concepts in Neuroscience, 1,* 27–51.

Brunet, E., Sarfati, Y., Hardy-Bayle, M.C., & Decety, J. (2000). A PET investigation of the attribution of intentions with a nonverbal task. *Neuroimage, 11,* 157–166.

Buch, G., Luu, P., & Posner, M. (2000). Cognitive and emotional influences in the anterior cingulate cortex. *Trends in Cognitive Science, 4,* 214–222.

Burnette, C., Sutton, S., Meyer, J., Henderson, H., Schwartz, C., Zahka, N., et al. (2005, April). *Frontal asymmetry groups and cognitive processes in autism.* Paper presented at the meeting of the Society for Research in Child Development, Atlanta, GA.

Calder, A., Lawrence, A., Keane, J., Scott, S., Owen, A., Christoffels, I., et al. (2002). Reading the mind from eye gaze. *Neuropsychologia, 40,* 1129–1138.

Campbell, R., Heywood, C., Cowey, A., Regard, M., & Landis, T. (1990). Sensitivity to eye gaze in prosopagnosic patients and monkeys with superior temporal sulcus ablation. *Neuropsychologia, 28,* 1123–1142.

Caplan, R., Chugani, H., Messa, C., Guthrie, D., Sigman, M., Traversay, J., et al. (1993). Hemispherectomy for early onset intractable seizures: Presurgical cerebral glucose metabolism and postsurgical nonverbal communication patterns. *Developmental Medicine and Child Neurology, 35,* 582–592.

Carper, R., & Courchesne, E. (2000). Inverse correlation between frontal lobe and cerebellum sizes in children with autism. *Brain, 123,* 836–844.

Castelli, F., Frith, C., Happé, F., & Frith, U. (2002). Autism, Asperger syndrome, and brain mechanisms for the attribution of mental states to animated shapes. *Brain, 125,* 1839–1849.

Castelli, F., Happé, F., Frith, U., & Frith, C. (2000). Movement and mind: A functional imaging study of perception and interpretation of complex intentional movement patterns. *Neuroimage, 12,* 314–325.

Charman, T., Baron-Cohen, S., Swettenham, J., Baird, G., Cox, A., & Drew, A. (2000). Testing joint attention, imitation, and play infancy precursors to language and theory of mind. *Cognitive Development, 15,* 481–498.

Charwarska, K., Klin, A., & Volkmar, F. (2003). Automatic attention cuing through eye movement in 2–year-old children with autism. *Child Development, 74,* 1108–1123.

Claussen, A. H., Mundy, P. C., Malik, S. A., & Willoughby, J. C. (2002). Joint attention and disorganized attachment status in infants at risk. *Development and Psychopathology, 14,* 279–291.

Corkum, V., & Moore, C. (1998). The origins of joint visual attention in infants. *Developmental Psychology, 34,* 28–38.

Courchesne, E., Townsend, J., Akshoomoff, N., Yeung-Courchesne, G., Murakami, J., Lincoln, A., et al. (1994). A new finding: Impairment in shifting attention in autistic and cerebellar patients. In E. Broman & E. Grafman (Eds.), *Atypical cognitive deficits in developmental disorder: Implications for brain function* (pp. 101–137). Hillsdale, NJ: Erlbaum.

Craik, F., Moroz, T., Moscovich, M., Stuss, D., Winocur, G., Tulving, E., et al. (1999). In search of the self: A positron emission tomography study. *Psychological Science, 10,* 26–34.

Critchley, H., Daly, E., Bullmore, E., Williams, S., Van Amelsvoort, T., Robertson, D., et al. (2000). The functional neuroanatomy of social behavior: Changes in the cerebral blood flow when people with autistic disorder process facial expressions. *Brain, 123,* 2203–2212.

Dawson, G., & Adams, A. (1984). Imitation and social responsiveness in autistic children. *Journal of Abnormal Child Psychology, 12,* 209–226.

Dawson, G., & Galpert, L. (1990). Mother's use of imitative play for the facilitation of social responsiveness and toy play in young autistic children. *Development and Psychopathology, 2,* 151–162.

Dawson, G., Munson, J., Estes, A., Osterling, J., McPartland, J., Toth, K., et al. (2002). Neurocognitive function and joint attention ability in young children with autism spectrum disorder versus developmental delay. *Child Development, 73,* 345–358.

Dawson, G., Osterling, J., Rinalidi, J., Carver, L., & McPartland, J. (2001). Brief report: Recognition memory and stimulus–reward associations: Indirect support for the role of the ventromedial prefrontal dysfunction in autism. *Journal of Autism and Developmental Disorders, 31,* 337–341.

Diamond, A., & Goldman-Rakic, P. (1989). Comparison of human infants and rhesus monkeys on Piaget's AB task: Evidence for the dependence on dorsolateral prefrontal cortex. *Experimental Brain Research, 74,* 24–40.

Eacott, M., Heywood, C., Gross, C., & Cowey, A. (1993). Visual discrimination impairments following lesions of the superior temporal sulcas are not specific for facial stimuli. *Neuropsychologia, 31,* 609–619.

Eisenberger, N., Lieberman, M., & Williams, K. (2003). Does rejection hurt?: An fMRI study of social exclusion. *Science, 302,* 290–292.

Elgar, K., & Campbell, R. (2001). The cognitive neuroscience of face recognition: Implications for developmental disorders [Annotation]. *Journal of Child Psychology and Psychiatry, 6,* 705–717.

Emery, N. (2000). The eyes have it: The neuroethology, function and evolution of social gaze. *Neuroscience and Biobehavioral Reviews, 24,* 581–604.

Ernst, M., Zametkin, J., Matochik, J., Pascualvaca, D., & Cohen, R. (1997). Low medial prefrontal dopaminergic activity in autistic children. *Lancet, 350,* 638.

Faw, B. (2003). Prefrontal executive committee for perception, working memory, attention, long-term memory, motor control and thinking: A tutorial review. *Consciousness and Cognition, 12,* 83–139.

Fletcher, P., Happé, F., Frith, U., Baker, S., Dolan, R., Frackowiak, R., et al. (1995). Other minds in the brain: A functional imaging study of "theory of mind" in story comprehension. *Cognition, 57,* 109–128.

Frith, C., & Frith, U. (1999). Interacting minds: A biological basis. *Science, 286,* 1692–1695.

Frith, U., & Frith, C. (2001). The biological basis of social interaction. *Current Directions in Psychological Science, 10,* 151–155.

Gallagher, H., Happé, F., Brunswick, P., Fletcher, P., Frith, U., & Frith, C. (2000). Reading the mind in cartoons and stories: An fMRI study of "theory of mind" in verbal and nonverbal tasks. *Neuropsychologia, 38,* 11–21.

George, N., Driver, J., & Dolan, R. (2001). Seen gaze direction modulates fusiform activity and its coupling with other brain areas during face processing. *Neuroimage, 13,* 1102–1112.

Goel, V., Grafman, J., Sadato, N., & Hallett, M. (1995). Modeling other minds. *Neuroreport, 6,* 1741–1746.

Greenspan, S., & Wieder, S. (2000). A developmental approach to difficulties in relating and communication in autism spectrum disorders and related syndromes. In A. Wetherby & B. Prizant (Eds.), *Autism spectrum disorders: Vol. 9. A transactional developmental perspective* (pp. 279–306). Baltimore: Brookes.

Griffith, E., Pennington, B., Wehner, E., & Rogers, S. (1999). Executive functions in young children with autism. *Child Development, 70,* 817–832.

Gutstein, S., & Sheely, R. (2002). *Relationship development intervention with young children: Social and emotional development activities for Asperger syndrome, autism, PDD, and NLD.* London: Kingsley.

Happé, F., Ehlers, S., Fletcher, P., Frith, U., Johansson, M., Gillberg, C., et al. (1996). "Theory of mind" in the brain: Evidence from a PET scan study of Asperger syndrome. *Neuroreport, 8,* 197–201.

Hardan, A., Minshew, N., Diwadkar, V., Yorbik, O., Sahni, S., & Keshavan, M. (2002, November). *A voxel based morphometry study of grey matter in autism.* Paper presented at the International Meeting for Autism Research (IMFAR), Orlando, FL.

Haznedar, M., Buchsbaum, M., Wei, T., Hof, P., Cartwright, C., Bienstock, C., et al.

(2000). Limbic circuitry in patients with autism spectrum disorders studied with positron emission tomography and magnetic resonance imaging. *American Journal of Psychiatry, 157*, 1994–2001.

Henderson, H., Schwartz, C., Mundy, P., Burnette, C., Sutton, S., Zahka, N., et al. (in press). Error monitoring, the anterior cingulate cortex, and differences in social behavior in autism. *Brain and Cognition.*

Henderson, L., Yoder, P., Yale, M., & McDuffie, A. (2002). Getting the point: Electrophysiological correlates of protodeclarative pointing. *International Journal of Developmental Neuroscience, 20*, 449–458.

Heywood, C., & Cowey, A. (1992). The role of the "face cell" area in the discrimination and recognition of faces by monkeys. *Philosophical Transactions of the Royal Society of London, 335*, 31–38.

Hobson, P. (2002). *The cradle of thought: Exploring the origins of thinking.* London: Pan Macmillan.

Hobson, R. P. (1993). *Autism and the development of mind.* Hillsdale, NJ: Erlbaum.

Hoffman, E., & Haxby, J. (2000). Distinct representation of eye gaze and identity in the distributed human neural system for face perception. *Nature Neuroscience, 3*, 80–84.

Holroyd, C., & Coles, M. (2002). The neural basis of human error processing: Reinforcement learning, dopamine and the error related negativity. *Psychological Review, 109*, 679–709.

Hooker, C. (2002). The neurocognitive basis of gaze perception: A model of social signal processing. *Dissertation Abstracts International, 63*, 2058B.

Jellema, T., Baker, C., Wicker, B., & Perrett, D. (2000). Neural representation for the perception of intentionality of actions. *Brain and Cognition, 44*, 280–302.

Johnson, S., Baxter, L., Wilder, L., Pipe, J., Heiserman, J., & Prigatano, G. (2002). Neural correlates of self reflection. *Brain, 125*, 1808–1814.

Kasari, C., Freeman, S., & Paparella, T. (2001). Early intervention in autism: Joint attention and symbolic play. In L. M. Glidden (Ed.), *International review of research in mental retardation: Vol. 23. Autism* (pp. 207–237). San Diego, CA: Academic Press.

Kasari, C., Sigman, M., Mundy, P., & Yirmiya, N. (1990). Affective sharing in the context of joint attention interactions of normal, autistic, and mentally retarded children. *Journal of Autism and Developmental Disorders, 20*, 87–100.

Kawashima, R., Sugiura, M., Kato, T., Nakamura, A., Hatano, K., Ito, K., et al. (1999). The human amygdala plays an important role in gaze monitoring: A PET study. *Brain, 122*, 779–783.

Kingstone, A., Friesen, C.-K., & Gazzaniga, M. (2000). Reflexive joint attention depends on lateralized cortical functions. *Psychological Science, 11*, 159–166.

Klin, A., Jones, W., Schultz, R., & Volkmar, F. (2003). The enactive mind, or from actions to cognition: Lessons from autism. *Philosophical Transactions of the Royal Society of London, 10*, 1–16.

Koegel, R., Koegel, L., & McNeary, E. (2001). Pivotal areas of intervention for autism. *Journal of Community Psychology, 30*, 19–32.

Kroupina, M., Kuefner, D., Iverson, S., & Johnson, D. (2003, April). *Joint attention skills of post-institutionalized children.* Poster presented at the meeting of the Society for Research in Child Development, Tampa, FL.

Lau, H., Rogers, R., Haggard, P., & Passingham, R. (2004). Attention to intention. *Science, 303,* 1208–1210.

LeDoux, J. (1989). Cognitive-emotional interactions in the brain. *Cognition and Emotion, 3,* 267–289.

Leekam, S., Lopez, B., & Moore, C. (2001). Attention and joint attention in preschool children with autism. *Developmental Psychology, 36,* 261–273.

Lord, C., Floody, H., Anderson, D., & Pickles, A. (2003, April). *Social engagement in very young children with autism: Differences across contexts.* Paper presented at the meeting of the Society for Research in Child Development, Tampa, FL.

Lord, C., Risi, S., Lambrecht, L., Cook, E., Leventhal, B., DiLavore, P., et al. (1999). The Autism Diagnostic Observations Schedule—Generic: A standard measure of social and communication deficits associated with autism spectrum disorder. *Journal of Autism and Developmental Disorders, 30,* 205–223.

Luu, P., Flaisch, T., & Tucker, D. (2000). Medial-frontal cortex in action monitoring. *Journal of Neuroscience, 20,* 464–469.

Martin, J. (1996). *Neuroanatomy: Text and atlas* (2nd ed.). New York: McGraw-Hill.

McDougle, C., Scahill, L., McCraken, J., Aman, M., Tierney, E., Arnold, E., et al. (2001). Research Units on Pediatric Psychopharmacology (RUPP) autism network: Background and rationale for an initial controlled study of risperidone. *Child and Adolescent Psychiatric Clinics of North America, 9,* 201–224.

McEvoy, R., Rogers, S., & Pennington, R. (1993). Executive function and social communication deficits in young autistic children. *Journal of Child Psychology and Psychiatry, 34,* 563–578.

Minshew, N., Meyer, J., & Goldstein, G. (2002). Abstract reasoning in autism: A dissociation between concept formation and concept identification. *Neuropsychology, 16,* 327–334.

Moore, C. (1996). Theories of mind in infancy. *British Journal of Developmental Psychology, 14,* 19–40.

Morecraft, R., Guela, C., & Mesulam, M. (1993). Architecture of connectivity within the cingulo-frontal-parietal neurocognitive network for directed attention. *Archives of Neurology, 50,* 279–283.

Mundy, P. (1995). Joint attention and social-emotional approach behavior in children with autism. *Development and Psychopathology, 7,* 63–82.

Mundy, P. (2003). The neural basis of social impairments in autism: The role of the dorsal medial-frontal cortex and anterior cingulate system. *Journal of Child Psychology and Psychiatry, 44,* 793–809.

Mundy, P., & Acra, F. (2006). Joint attention, social engagement and the development of social competence. In P. Marshall & N. Fox (Eds.), *The development of social engagement: Neurobiological perspectives* (pp. 81–117). New York: Oxford University Press.

Mundy, P., & Burnette, C. (2005). Joint attention and neurodevelopmental models of autism. In F. Volkmar, R. Paul, A. Klin, & D. J. Cohen (Eds.), *Handbook of autism and pervasive developmental disorders: Vol. 1. Diagnosis, development, neurobiology, and behavior* (pp. 650–681). Hoboken, NJ: Wiley.

Mundy, P., Card, J., & Fox, N. (2000). EEG correlates of the development of infant joint attention skills. *Developmental Psychobiology, 36*, 325–338.

Mundy, P., & Crowson, M. (1997). Joint attention and early communication: Implications for intervention with autism. *Journal of Autism and Developmental Disorders, 6*, 653–676.

Mundy, P., Delgado, C., Block, J., Venezia, M., Hogan, A., & Seibert, J. (2003). *A manual for the abridged Early Social Communication Scales (ESCS).* (Available from pmundy@miami.edu)

Mundy, P., Hogan, A., & Doehring, P. (1996). *A preliminary manual for the abridged Early Social-Communication Scales.* Coral Gables, FL: University of Miami.

Mundy, P., Kasari, C., & Sigman, M. (1992). Joint attention, affective sharing, and intersubjectivity. *Infant Behavior and Development, 15*, 377–381.

Mundy, P., & Sigman, M. (1989). Specifying the nature of the social impairment in autism. In G. Dawson (Ed.), *Autism: Nature, diagnosis, and treatment* (pp. 3–21). New York: Guilford Press.

Mundy, P., & Sigman, M. (2006). Joint attention, social competence and developmental Psychopathology. In D. Cicchetti & D. Cohen (Eds.), *Developmental psychopathology: Vol. 1. Theory and methods* (2nd ed., pp. 293–332). Hoboken, NJ: Wiley.

Mundy, P., Sigman, M., & Kasari, C. (1993). The theory of mind and joint attention deficits in autism. In S. Baron-Cohen, H. Tager-Flusberg, & D. Cohen (Eds.), *Understanding other minds: Perspectives from autism* (pp. 181–203). Oxford, UK: Oxford University Press.

Mundy, P., Sigman, M., & Kasari, C. (1994). Joint attention, developmental level, and symptom presentation in young children with autism. *Development and Psychopathology, 6*, 389–401.

Mundy, P., Sigman, M., Ungerer, J., & Sherman, T. (1986). Defining the social deficits of autism: The contribution of nonverbal communication measures. *Journal of Child Psychology and Psychiatry, 27*, 657–669.

Neal, R., Mundy, P., Claussen, A., Mallik, S., Scott, K., & Acra, F. (2005). *The relations between infant joint attention skill and cognitive and language outcome in at-risk children.* Manuscript submitted for publication.

Nichols, K., Fox, N., & Mundy, P. (2005). Joint attention, self-recognition and neurocognitive functioning. *Infancy, 7*, 35–51.

Norman, D., & Shallice, T. (1986). Attention to action: Willed and automatic control of behavior. In R. Davidson, G. Schwartz, & D. Shapiro (Eds.), *Consciousness and self-regulation* (pp. 1–18). New York: Plenum.

Ohnishi, T., Matsuda, H., Hashimoto, T., Kunihiro, T., Nishikawa, M., Uema, T., et al. (2000). Abnormal regional cerebral blood flow in childhood autism. *Brain, 123*, 1838–1844.

Osterling, J., Dawson, G., & Munson, J. (2002). Early recognition of 1–year-old infants with autism spectrum disorder versus mental retardation. *Development and Psychopathology, 14*, 239–251.

Panksepp, J. (1979). A neurochemical theory of autism. *Trends in Neurosciences, 2*, 174–177.

Perrett, D., Heitenen, J., Oram, M., & Benson, P. (1992). Organization and functions of cells responsive to faces in the temporal cortex. *Philosophical Transactions of the Royal Society of London, 335,* 23–30.

Piaget, J. (1952). *The origins of intelligence in children.* New York: Norton.

Posner, M., & Petersen, S. (1990). The attention system of the human brain. *Annual Review of Neuroscience, 13,* 25–42.

Puce, A., Allison, T., Bentin, S., Gore, J., & McCarthy, G. (1998) Temporal cortex activation in humans viewing eye and mouth movements. *Journal of Neuroscience, 18,* 2188–2199.

Reynell, J., & Gruber, C. (1990). *Reynell Developmental Language Scales: U.S. edition.* Los Angeles: Western Psychological Services.

Rolls, E., Hornak, J., Wade, D., & McGrath, J. (1994). Emotion related learning in patients with social and emotional changes associated with frontal lobe damage. *Journal of Neurology, Neurosurgery and Psychiatry, 57,* 1518–1524.

Rothbart, M., & Posner, M. (2001). Mechanism and variation in the development of attention networks. In C. Nelson & M. Luciana (Eds.), *The handbook of developmental cognitive neuroscience* (pp. 353–363). Cambridge, MA: MIT Press.

Rothbart, M., Posner, M., & Rosicky, J. (1994). Orienting in normal and pathological development. *Development and Psychopathology, 6,* 635–652.

Rushworth, M., Hadland, K., Paus, T., & Siplia, P. (2002). Role of the human medial frontal cortex in task switching: A combined fMRI and TMS study. *Journal of Neurophysiology, 87,* 2577–2592.

Russell, T., Rubia, K., Bullmore, E., Soni, W., Suckling, J., Brammer, M., et al. (2000). Exploring the social brain in schizophrenia: Left prefrontal underactivation during mental state attribution. *American Journal of Psychiatry, 157,* 2040–2042.

Scaife, M., & Bruner, J. (1975). The capacity for joint visual attention in the infant. *Nature, 253,* 265–266.

Seibert, J. M., Hogan, A. E., & Mundy, P. C. (1982). Assessing interactional competencies: The Early Social Communication Scales. *Infant Mental Health Journal, 3,* 244–245.

Senju, A., Tojo, Y., Yaguchi, K., & Hasegawa, T. (2005). Deviant gaze processing in children with autism: An ERP study. *Neuropsychologia, 43,* 1297–1306.

Sigman, M., Kasari, C., Kwon, J., & Yirmiya, N. (1992). Responses to the negative emotions of others by autistic, mentally retarded and normal children. *Child Development, 63,* 796–807.

Sigman, M., & Ruskin, E. (1999). Continuity and change in the social competence of children with autism, Down syndrome, and developmental delay. *Monographs of the Society for Research in Child Development, 64*(Serial No. 256).

Siller, M., & Sigman, M. (2002). The behaviors of parents of children with autism predict the subsequent development of their children's communication. *Journal of Autism and Developmental Disorders, 22,* 77–89.

Stich, S., & Nichols, S. (1992). Folk psychology: Simulation versus tacit theory. *Mind and Language, 7,* 29–65.

Stuphorn, V., Taylor, T., & Schall, J. (2000). Performance monitoring by the supplementary eye field. *Nature, 408,* 857–860.

Stuss, D., Shallice, T., Alexander, M., & Picton, T. (1995). A multidimensional approach to anterior attention functions. In J. Grafman, K. Holyoak, & F. Boller

(Eds.), *Annals of the New York Academy of Sciences, Vol. 769. Structure and function of the human prefrontal cortex* (pp. 191–211). New York: New York Academy of Sciences.

Sutton, S., Burnette, C., Mundy, P., Meyer, J., Vaughan, A., Sanders, C., et al. (2005). Resting cortical brain activity and social behavior in higher functioning children with autism. *Journal of Child Psychology and Psychiatry, 46,* 211–222.

Sutton, S., & Davidson, R. (1997). Prefrontal brain asymmetry: A biological substrate of the behavioral approach and inhibition systems. *Psychological Science, 8,* 204–210.

Swettenham, J., Baron-Cohen, S., Charman, T., Cox, A., Baird, G., Drew, A., et al. (1998). The frequency and distribution of spontaneous attention shifts between social and nonsocial stimuli in autistic, typically developing, and nonautistic developmentally delayed infants. *Journal of Child Psychology and Psychiatry, 39,* 747–753.

Tomasello, M. (1995). Joint attention as social cognition. In C. Moore & P. Dunham (Eds.), *Joint attention: Its origins and role in development* (pp. 103–130). Hillsdale, NJ: Erlbaum.

Tomasello, M. (1999). *The cultural origins of human cognition.* Boston: Harvard University Press.

Townsend, J., Westerfield, M., Leaver, E., Makeig, S., Tzyy-Ping, J., Pierce, K., et al. (2001). Event-related brain response abnormalities in autism: Evidence for impaired cerebello-frontal spatial attention networks. *Cognitive Brain Research, 11,* 127–145.

Trevarthen, C., & Aitken, K. (2001). Infant intersubjectivity: Research, theory and clinical applications. *Journal of Child Psychology and Psychiatry, 42,* 3–48.

Ulvund, S., & Smith, L. (1996). The predictive validity of nonverbal communication skills in infants with perinatal hazards. *Infant Behavior and Development, 19,* 441–449.

Vaughan, A., & Mundy, P. (in press). Neural systems and the development of gaze following and related joint attention skills. In R. Flom, K. Lee, & D. Muir (Eds.), *The ontogeny of gaze processing in infants and children.* Mahwah, NJ: Erlbaum.

Vaughan, A., Mundy, P., Block, J., Burnette, C., Delgado, C., & Gomez, Y. (2003). Child, caregiver and temperament contributions to infant joint attention. *Infancy, 4,* 603–616.

Venezia, M., Messinger, D., Thorp, D., & Mundy, P. (2004). Timing changes: The development of anticipatory smiling. *Infancy, 6,* 397–406.

Wachs, T., & Chan, A. (1986). Specificity of environmental action, as seen in environmental correlates of infants' communication performance. *Child Development, 57,* 1464–1474.

Watanabe, M. (1999). Neurobiology: Attraction is relative, not absolute. *Nature, 398,* 661–663.

Wellman, H. (1993). Early understanding of mind: The normal case. In S. Baron-Cohen, H. Tager-Flusberg, & D. Cohen (Eds.), *Understanding other minds: Perspectives from autism* (pp. 40–58). Oxford, UK: Oxford University Press.

Wicker, B., Michel, F., Henaff, M., & Decety, J. (2002). Brain regions involved in the perception of gaze. *Neuroimage, 8,* 221–227.

Wing, L., & Gould, J. (1979). Severe impairments of social interaction and associated abnormalities in children: Epidemiology and classification. *Journal of Autism and Developmental Disorders, 9,* 11–29.

Woodward, A. (2003). Infants' developing understanding of the link between looker and object. *Developmental Science, 6,* 297–311.

Yoder, P., & Warren, S. (2002). The effects of prelinguistic milieu teaching and parent responsivity education on dyads involving children with intellectual disabilities. *Journal of Speech, Language and Hearing, 45,* 1158–1174.

Index